Women's Health Rehabilitation Medicine

Editors

SARA JEAN CUCCURULLO
KRISTEN A. HARRIS
HAYK PETROSYAN

PHYSICAL MEDICINE AND REHABILITATION CLINICS OF NORTH AMERICA

www.pmr.theclinics.com

Consulting Editor
BLESSEN C. EAPEN

May 2025 • Volume 36 • Number 2

ELSEVIER

1600 John F. Kennedy Boulevard ● Suite 1800 ● Philadelphia, Pennsylvania, 19103-2899

http://www.theclinics.com

PHYSICAL MEDICINE AND REHABILITATION CLINICS OF NORTH AMERICA Volume 36, Number 2
May 2025 ISSN 1047-9651, 978-0-443-31668-5

Editor: Megan Ashdown
Developmental Editor: Nitesh Barthwal

Publication information: *Physical Medicine and Rehabilitation Clinics of North America* (ISSN 1047-9651) is published quarterly by Elsevier, 230 Park Avenue, Suite 800, New York, NY 10169. Periodicals postage paid at New York, NY and additional mailing offices. USA POSTMASTER: Send address changes to *Physical Medicine and Rehabilitation Clinics of North America*, Elsevier Customer Service Department, 3251 Riverport Lane, Maryland Heights, MO 63043, USA. Months of issue are February, May, August, and November. Subscription price per year is $359.00 (US individuals), $100.00 (US students), $408.00 (Canadian individuals), $100.00 (Canadian students), $516.00 (foreign individuals), and $210.00 (foreign students). For institutional access pricing please contact Customer Service via the contact information below. Foreign air speed delivery is included in all *Clinics* subscription prices. All prices are subject to change without notice. Orders, claims, and journal inquiries: Please visit our Support Hub page https://service.elsevier.com for assistance.

Physical Medicine and Rehabilitation Clinics of North America is indexed in *Excerpta Medica, MEDLINE/PubMed (Index Medicus), Cinahl, and Cumulative Index to Nursing and Allied Health Literature.*

Contributors

CONSULTING EDITOR

BLESSEN C. EAPEN, MD
Chief, VA Greater Los Angeles Health Care System, Associate Clinical Professor, Division of Physical Medicine and Rehabilitation, Department of Medicine, David Geffen School of Medicine at UCLA, Los Angeles, California

EDITORS

SARA JEAN CUCCURULLO, MD
Professor and Chair, Residency Program Director, Department of Physical Medicine and Rehabilitation, Hackensack Meridian School of Medicine, Rutgers Robert Wood Johnson Medical School, New Brunswick, New Jersey; Medical Director, VP, JFK Johnson Rehabilitation Institute at Hackensack Meridian Health, Physician in Chief, HMH Rehabilitation Care Transformation Services, Edison, New Jersey

KRISTEN A. HARRIS, MD
Assistant Professor, Department of Physical Medicine and Rehabilitation, JFK Johnson Rehabilitation Institute, Hackensack Meridian School of Medicine, Rutgers-Robert Wood Johnson Medical School, Edison, New Jersey

HAYK PETROSYAN, PhD
Associate Professor, Department of Physical Medicine and Rehabilitation, JFK Johnson Rehabilitation Institute, Hackensack Meridian School of Medicine, Rutgers-Robert Wood Johnson Medical School, Edison, New Jersey

AUTHORS

AMANDA APPEL, MD, MPH
Physician, Departments of Pediatric Rehabilitation Medicine, and Pediatrics, Children's Hospital Colorado, Department of Physical Medicine and Rehabilitation, University of Colorado Anschutz School of Medicine, Aurora, Colorado

ALBA M. AZOLA, MD
Assistant Professor, Pediatrics Division of Adolescent Medicine, Department of Physical Medicine and Rehabilitation, Director of the Long COVID Chronic Fatigue Syndrome Clinic, Johns Hopkins University School of Medicine, Baltimore, Maryland

RAISA BAKSHIYEV, MD
Physical Medicine and Rehabilitation Physician, Department of Physical Medicine and Rehabilitation, Hackensack Meridian Johnson Rehabilitation Institute at Ocean University Medical Center, Brick, New Jersey

STACEY BENNIS, MD, CAQ-SM
Assistant Professor of Physical Medicine and Rehabilitation, Departments of Orthopedic Surgery and Rehabilitation, and Obstetrics and Gynecology, Loyola University Chicago, Maywood, Illinois

ARIELLE BERKOWITZ, DO
Brain Injury Medicine Fellow, Department of Physical Medicine and Rehabilitation, JFK Johnson Rehabilitation Institute, Hackensack Meridian Health, Edison, New Jersey

MICHAEL BOVA, MD
Pain Medicine Fellow, Department of Physical Medicine and Rehabilitation, JFK Johnson Rehabilitation Institute, Edison, New Jersey

JESSIE P. CHAN, MD
PM&R Resident Physician, Department of Physical Medicine and Rehabilitation, JFK Johnson Rehabilitation Institute, Hackensack Meridian Health, Edison, New Jersey

SUANN CHEN, MD
Medical Director, Chair, Department of Physical Medicine and Rehabilitation, Hackensack Meridian Johnson Rehabilitation Institute at Ocean University Medical Center, Brick, New Jersey

JENNIFER CHUI, MD
Spinal Cord Injury Medical Director, Department of Physical Medicine and Rehabilitation, JFK Johnson Rehabilitation Institute, Hackensack Meridian Health, Edison, New Jersey

SARA JEAN CUCCURULLO, MD
Professor and Chair, Residency Program Director, Department of Physical Medicine and Rehabilitation, Hackensack Meridian School of Medicine, Rutgers Robert Wood Johnson Medical School, New Brunswick, New Jersey; Medical Director, VP, JFK Johnson Rehabilitation Institute at Hackensack Meridian Health, Physician in Chief, HMH Rehabilitation Care Transformation Services, Edison, New Jersey

LAURENT V. DELAVAUX, MD
Program Director, Pain Medicine Fellowship, Assistant Professor, Department of Physical Medicine and Rehabilitation, JFK Johnson Rehabilitation Institute, Hackensack Meridian School of Medicine, Clinical Assistant Professor, Rutgers Robert Wood Johnson Medical School, New Brunswick, New Jersey

ALLY FERBER, MD
PM&R Resident Physician, Department of Physical Medicine and Rehabilitation, JFK Johnson Rehabilitation Institute, Hackensack Meridian Health, Edison, New Jersey

COLLEEN FITZGERALD, MD
Professor of Physical Medicine and Rehabilitation, Department of Obstetrics and Gynecology, Loyola University Chicago, Maywood, Illinois

TALYA K. FLEMING, MD
Associate Professor, Department of Physical Medicine and Rehabilitation, JFK Johnson Rehabilitation Institute at Hackensack Meridian Health, Edison, New Jersey

MICHAEL GALIBOV, DO
Resident Physician, Department of Physical Medicine and Rehabilitation, JFK Johnson Rehabilitation Institute, Edison, New Jersey

MATTHEW C. GLENN, MD, MS
Resident Physician, Department of Physical Medicine and Rehabilitation, Rusk NYU Langne Health, New York, New York

PHILLIP GORDON, MD
SCI Fellow Physician, Department of Physical Medicine and Rehabilitation, Mount Sinai Hospital, New York, New York

CRYSTAL GRAFF, MD
Fellow Physician, Department of Orthopedics and Rehabilitation, University of Iowa Sports Medicine, Iowa City, Iowa

CHRISTINE GREISS, DO
Clinical Associate Professor, Department of Physical Medicine and Rehabilitation, JFK Johnson Rehabilitation Institute, Hackensack Meridian Health, Edison, New Jersey

MAURA GUYLER, BA
Medical Student, Case Western University School of Medicine, Cleveland, Ohio

REBECCA HINE, PT, DPT
Oncology Clinical Specialist, Department of Inpatient Therapy, Carolinas Rehabilitation Atrium Health, Charlotte, North Carolina

VIVIEN HSU, MD
Professor, Acting Chief, Division of Rheumatology, Department of Medicine, Director, Rutgers Robert Wood Johnson Scleroderma Program, Rutgers Robert Wood Johnson Medical School, New Brunswick, New Jersey

JACLYN JOKI, MD
Assistant Professor, Department of Physical Medicine and Rehabilitation, Hackensack Meridian School of Medicine, Nutley, New Jersey; Clinical Assistant Professor, Department of Physical Medicine and Rehabilitation, Rutgers Robert Wood Johnson Medical School, New Brunswick, New Jersey; Director, PM&R Consult Service at RWJUH, HMH JFK Johnson Rehabilitation Institute, Edison, New Jersey

LISA LAURENZANA, MD
Resident Physician, Department of Physical Medicine and Rehabilitation, McGaw Medical Center of Northwestern University, Chicago, Illinois

PAGE P. MACK, PT, MPT, CLT
Clinical Coordinator of Rehabilitation Services, Department of Supportive Care, Section of Cancer Rehabilitation, Atrium Health Levine Cancer, Charlotte, North Carolina

SEEMA MALKANA, DO
Assistant Professor, Division of Rheumatology, Rutgers Robert Wood Johnson Medical School, New Brunswick, New Jersey

STEVEN MARKOS, MD
Attending Physician, Department of Physical Medicine and Rehabilitation, JFK Johnson Rehabilitation Institute, Edison, New Jersey; Assistant Professor, Rutgers Robert Wood Johnson Medical School, New Brunswick, New Jersey; Assistant Professor, Hackensack Meridian School of Medicine, Nutley, New Jersey

SARAH MULLAN, MS, OTR/L
Manager of Cancer Rehabilitation and PsychoOncology, Department of Supportive Care Section of Cancer Rehabilitation, Atrium Health Levine Cancer, Charlotte, North Carolina

BHAVESH D. PATEL, DO
Clinical Assistant Professor, Department of Orthopaedics and Rehabilitation Medicine, Wake Forest University School of Medicine, Winston-Salem, North Carolina; Department of Supportive Care, Section of Cancer Rehabilitation, Atrium Health Levine Cancer, Carolinas Rehabilitation Atrium Health, Charlotte, North Carolina

HAYK PETROSYAN, PhD
Associate Professor, Department of Physical Medicine and Rehabilitation, JFK Johnson Rehabilitation Institute, Hackensack Meridian School of Medicine, Rutgers-Robert Wood Johnson Medical School, Edison, New Jersey

SOFIYA PRILIK, MD
Clinical Assistant Professor, Department of Rehabilitation Medicine, NYU Grossman School of Medicine, Director, Transplant Rehabilitation, Clinical Director of Cardiac and Pulmonary Rehabilitation, Department of Physical Medicine and Rehabilitation, Rusk NYU Langne Health, New York, New York

TERRENCE PUGH, MD
Clinical Associate Professor, Department of Orthopaedic Surgery and Rehabilitation, Winston-Salem, North Carolina; Vice-Chief of Cancer Rehabilitation, Department of Supportive Care, Section of Cancer Rehabilitation, Atrium Health Levine Cancer Director of Oncology Rehabilitation, Carolinas Rehabilitation Atrium Health, Charlotte, North Carolina

VISHWA S. RAJ, MD
Clinical Professor, Department of Orthopaedics and Rehabilitation Medicine, Wake Forest University School of Medicine, Winston-Salem, North Carolina; Chief, Section of Cancer Rehabilitation, Department of Supportive Care, Atrium Health Levine Cancer, Medical Director, Carolinas Rehabilitation Atrium Health, Charlotte, North Carolina

CARLY ROTHMAN, DO
Assistant Professor, Department of Pediatric Physical Medicine and Rehabilitation, Joseph M. Sanzari Children's Hospital, Hackensack Meridian Health, Hackensack, New Jersey

CASEY SCHOENLANK, MD
Attending Physiatrist, Director, Rehab Consult Services, Department of Physical Medicine and Rehabilitation, Hackensack Meridian Johnson Rehabilitation Institute at Ocean University Medical Center, Brick, New Jersey

ALLISON N. SCHROEDER, MD
Assistant Professor, Department of Physical Medicine and Rehabilitation, MetroHealth Rehabilitation Institute and Case Western Reserve University, Case Western University School of Medicine, Cleveland, Ohio

ALEXANDER SHUSTOROVICH, DO
Associate Program Director, Pain Medicine Fellowship, Assistant Professor, Department of Physical Medicine and Rehabilitation, JFK Johnson Rehabilitation Institute, Hackensack Meridian School of Medicine, Clinical Assistant Professor, Rutgers Robert Wood Johnson Medical School, New Brunswick, New Jersey

ALPHONSA THOMAS, DO
Director, Outpatient Clinical Services, Department of Physical Medicine and Rehabilitation, Hackensack Meridian Johnson Rehabilitation Institute at Ocean University Medical Center, Brick, New Jersey

MONICA VERDUZCO-GUTIERREZ, MD
Professor and Distinguished Chair, Department of Rehabilitation Medicine, University of Texas Health Science Center at San Antonio, San Antonio, Texas

JONATHAN H. WHITESON, BSc, MD
Professor, Department of Physical Medicine and Rehabilitation, Rusk, NYU Grossman School of Medicine, Medical Director, Cardiac and Pulmonary Rehabilitation, Rusk Rehabilitation, NYU Langone Health, New York, New York

Contents

> Stroke is the third leading cause of death of women in the United States, and women have a higher lifetime risk of stroke than men. Studies show that women live longer but with poorer functional outcomes and higher rates of disability compared with men. Sex-specific disparities exist between clinical symptoms, medical evaluation, and management after stroke. Stroke rehabilitation strategies specific to women should take into consideration both physiologic and psychosocial demands more common in women to improve functional outcomes. Additional resources for education, clinical research, and implementation of best practices are needed to eliminate gender-related disparities in poststroke care.

> Cardiovascular disease is the leading cause of morbidity and mortality in women globally. Cardiac rehabilitation (CR)—a comprehensive program including supervised progressive exercise, education, support, behavior modification, and nutritional guidance over 36 individual sessions—positively impacts morbidity, mortality, function, and quality of life. Overall, less than 30% of those who qualify are referred and participate in CR—referral and completion rates are significantly less in women compared with men despite evidence supporting equal benefit. Barriers contributing to these disparities have been identified, and CR programs can be modified to enhance the participation of women.

> This review highlights the physiological, hormonal, and hematological changes following traumatic brain injury (TBI) in women. Younger women may experience worse outcomes due to higher cerebral pressures, while hormonal changes during menstruation, pregnancy, and menopause further influence TBI recovery. Postmenopausal women face higher risks of osteoporosis and fall-related TBIs. Psychological impacts include higher rates of depression, anxiety, and posttraumatic stress disorder. Social challenges and sexual dysfunction are prevalent, impacting community

and vocational reintegration. Tailored rehabilitation addressing these gender-specific factors is crucial for improving outcomes for female patients with TBI across their lifespan.

As the prevalence of female cancer survivors increases, their quality of life (QOL) and function have become key areas of focus in the context of survivorship and rehabilitation needs. Although behavioral modifications may help to decrease the development of malignancy, women are still at increased risk of developing a cancer diagnosis in their lifetime. Cancer and its treatment can lead to significant functional impairments and symptomatic challenges. However, rehabilitation interventions and medical management provide options to address these issues throughout the oncological continuum of care. With appropriate treatment, women are enabled to experience improved QOL and performance status.

Although men are more commonly affected than women with spinal cord injuries (SCIs), women comprise a growing portion of the population of individuals with SCIs. Guidelines for primary care and SCI issues are generally non-sex specific, and there are differences in the medical and rehabilitation needs of women compared with men. Consideration of these differences can optimize function and health for women with SCI and improve quality of life.

This article discussed the anatomic, physiologic, hormonal, and psychosocial factors unique to the female athelte that can affect a female athlete's injury risk and rehabilitation trajectory. A review of considerations unique to different stages of life in the female athlete and a discussion of the prevalence of certain injuries in female athletes are discussed. The purpose of this narrative review is to highlight how understanding the unique characteristics of the female athlete can allow for optimization of rehabilitation protocols.

There is well-established epidemiologic evidence demonstrating variance in the pain disorders affecting women compared with men, although limited conclusive evidence exists regarding the pathophysiologic mechanisms to account for this difference. Six of the most common pain disorders affecting women include migraine headache, fibromyalgia, endometriosis, interstitial cystitis, temporomandibular disorders, and osteoarthritis. The sex-specific prevalence, risk factors, triggers, presentations, and treatments of these disorders are critical for physicians to appreciate and understand to provide the highest standard of care when treating these common pain conditions.

Chronic pelvic pain is a complex diagnosis that has a significant impact on quality of life and function in women of all ages. Symptoms often span across numerous organ systems and involve several types of pain including visceral, neuropathic, musculoskeletal, and psychological, making management and treatment difficult. To adequately assess and recognize etiologies of pelvic pain, it is critical to first understand the specialized skills required for history taking and physical examination. This article aims to serve as a guide to understanding the physiatrist's approach to history taking and examination of pelvic pain.

Pelvic pain is a complex diagnosis that can be related to numerous etiologies across several specialties. This chapter aims to explore diagnosis and management of common neuromusculoskeletal causes of pelvic pain including pelvic floor myofascial pain, vulvodynia, nerve injuries, pelvic girdle pain, and coccydynia. Pelvic floor physical therapy is often the first-line treatment of many musculoskeletal causes of pelvic pain. Depending on examination findings, diagnosis, and response to physical therapy, additional medical management may include neuromodulation in oral or topical form, vaginal muscle relaxants, or pelvic floor botulinum toxin or trigger point injections.

This article discusses rheumatologic conditions in women including rheumatoid arthritis, lupus, Sjogren's syndrome, inflammatory myopathies, systemic sclerosis, and polymyalgia rheumatica. These conditions, often affecting muscles, joints, and other organ systems, require early diagnosis and multidisciplinary management. Treatment includes medications, braces, therapy services, education, and lifestyle modifications including energy conservation techniques. These conditions can also impact pregnancy and require close monitoring and careful disease control. It also highlights the benefits of pulmonary rehabilitation that can be helpful for patients with chronic respiratory disease secondary to their rheumatologic conditions.

PHYSICAL MEDICINE AND REHABILITATION CLINICS OF NORTH AMERICA

FORTHCOMING ISSUES

August 2025
Pediatric Rehabilitation
David Cancel, *Editor*

November 2025
Headache Management
Udai Nanda and Miriam Segal, *Editors*

February 2026
Adaptive and Para Sports
Melissa J. Tinney and Alexander M. Senk, *Editors*

RECENT ISSUES

February 2025
Enhancing Care After Spinal Cord Injury
Camilo M. Castillo Diaz, *Editor*

November 2024
Amputation Rehabilitation
Alex Donaghy and Alberto Miranda, *Editors*

August 2024
Traumatic Brain Injury Rehabilitation
Amy Hao and Blessen C. Eapen, *Editors*

SERIES OF RELATED INTEREST

Orthopedic Clinics
https://www.orthopedic.theclinics.com/
Neurologic Clinics
https://www.neurologic.theclinics.com/
Clinics in Sports Medicine
https://www.sportsmed.theclinics.com/

VISIT THE CLINICS ONLINE!
Access your subscription at:
www.theclinics.com

Foreword

A Comprehensive Review of Women's Health Rehabilitation

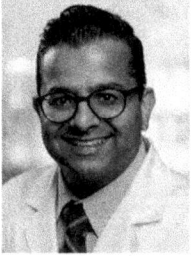

Blessen C. Eapen, MD
Consulting Editor

Women's Health Rehabilitation is a dynamic and growing subspeciality within the field of Physical Medicine and Rehabilitation that focuses on addressing the unique rehabilitation needs of women. This issue aims to provide comprehensive insights into the many facets of women's rehabilitation and emphasizes the crucial role in managing conditions that disproportionately affect women, such as osteoporosis, pelvic floor dysfunction, and musculoskeletal conditions of the female athlete. In addition, the authors review special rehabilitation considerations for women after stroke, traumatic brain injury, spinal cord injury, neurodegenerative disorders, and cancer. Furthermore, the authors outline reproductive and sexual health considerations for adolescent women with disabilities.

As women are facing an increasing incidence of pelvic floor disorders, rheumatologic conditions, long COVID, pain disorders, and cardiac conditions thus highlighting the critical role of the *physiatrist* in managing these complex disorders. These conditions not only affect mobility and quality of life but also present unique rehabilitation considerations demanding a carefully crafted rehabilitation plan and underscore the importance of the multidisciplinary team approach to rehabilitation and the need for specialized interventions.

This special issue aims to shine a light on these critical issues, providing both a scientific foundation and clinical expertise for addressing the rehabilitation needs of women across a wide spectrum of conditions. We want to thank Drs Cuccurullo, Harris, and Petrosyan and esteemed authors for leading this special issue and for

Phys Med Rehabil Clin N Am 36 (2025) xv–xvi
https://doi.org/10.1016/j.pmr.2025.02.002
1047-9651/25/© 2025 Published by Elsevier Inc.

pmr.theclinics.com

sharing their valuable experience and expertise with the physical medicine and rehabilitation community!

Blessen C. Eapen, MD
Division of Physical Medicine
and Rehabilitation
David Geffen School of Medicine at UCLA
VA Greater Los Angeles Health Care System
11301 Wilshire Boulevard
Los Angeles, CA 90073, USA

E-mail addresses:
beapen@ucla.mednet.edu; blessen.eapen2@va.gov

Preface

Rehabilitation Management Considerations for Women

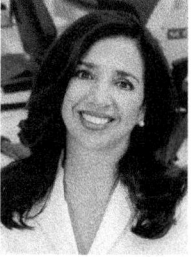

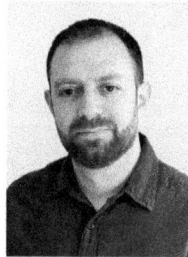

Sara Jean Cuccurullo, MD   Kristen A. Harris, MD   Hayk Petrosyan, PhD
Editors

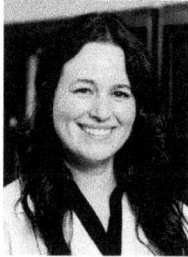

We are pleased to present this issue of *Physical Medicine and Rehabilitation Clinics of North America* on "Women's Health—Rehabilitation Medicine." Sex differences impacting epidemiology, patient care, and outcomes have been demonstrated across many diagnoses in medicine. Women's experiences in rehabilitation medicine differ significantly from men's due to variations in symptom presentation, patient experience, and treatment needs. Recognizing and addressing these unique needs is crucial for providing optimal care and improving women's rehabilitation outcomes. Rehabilitation medicine considerations specific to women include stroke, musculoskeletal disorders, cardiovascular issues, neurologic issues, pain management, and pregnancy/postpartum issues to name a few. Educational initiatives, research efforts, and advocacy initiatives should prioritize understanding the biological, social, and psychological factors influencing women's experiences in rehabilitation, leading to the development of evidence-based interventions and improved health care delivery. Addressing these disparities requires a multifaceted approach encompassing education for health care providers, further research, and patient advocacy.

This issue presents further background on specific issues related to women's health within the field of rehabilitation medicine, and current treatment paradigms for both musculoskeletal and neurologic conditions. Readers will find that a broad range of topics are included, from both established and emerging fields within rehabilitation. It is our hope that the content contained in this issue will help contribute to an improved understanding of unique considerations for the rehabilitation management of women. Ultimately, it is the editors' goal that increased attention and knowledge to these issues will lead to decreased disparities in patient care.

The authors are all extremely knowledgeable and established in their respective fields. They have shared excellent content in a clear manner for our readers. We

Phys Med Rehabil Clin N Am 36 (2025) xvii–xviii
https://doi.org/10.1016/j.pmr.2025.02.001
1047-9651/25/© 2025 Published by Elsevier Inc.

appreciate the time and effort they have spent sharing their expertise. Special thanks to Dr Blessen Eapen, who invited us to edit this issue, and to Megan Ashdown and Nitesh Barthwal from Elsevier, who guided us through every step of the process. We are grateful for the opportunity to compile such an important and necessary issue dedicated to the rehabilitation of women.

DISCLOSURES

The authors have no financial conflicts of interest to disclose.

Sara Jean Cuccurullo, MD
Department of Physical Medicine
and Rehabilitation
Hackensack Meridian School of Medicine
Rutgers- Robert Wood Johnson
Medical School
JFK Johnson Rehabilitation Institute
HMH Rehabilitation Services
65 James Street
Edison, NJ 08820, USA

Kristen A. Harris, MD
Department of Physical Medicine
and Rehabilitation
Hackensack Meridian School of Medicine
Rutgers–Robert Wood Johnson
Medical School
JFK Johnson Rehabilitation Institute
65 James Street
Edison, NJ 08820, USA

Hayk Petrosyan, PhD
Department of Physical Medicine
and Rehabilitation
Hackensack Meridian School of Medicine
Rutgers–Robert Wood Johnson
Medical School
JFK Johnson Rehabilitation Institute
65 James Street
Edison, NJ 08820, USA

E-mail addresses:
sara.cuccurullo@hmhn.org (S. Jean Cuccurullo)
kristen.harris@hmhn.org (K.A. Harris)
hayk.petrosyan@hmhn.org (H. Petrosyan)

Unique Characteristics of Stroke in Women and Rehabilitation Considerations

Talya K. Fleming, MD*, Sara Jean Cuccurullo, MD,
Hayk Petrosyan, PhD

KEYWORDS

- Stroke • Cerebrovascular accident • Women • Stroke rehabilitation
- Stroke recovery • Sex • Gender

KEY POINTS

- Gender disparities after stroke have been well-documented and reveal distinct risk factors specific to women.
- Health care must address the various gaps in care for women, with initiatives to eliminate gender disparities.
- Continued education for patients, care partners, and health care providers is imperative to improve clinical awareness of stroke in women and their unique challenges.

INTRODUCTION

Each year, an average of 795,000 people are diagnosed with a new or recurrent stroke in the United States.[1] Stroke is the third leading cause of death in women in the United States and is a leading cause of disability.[2] Although the prevalence of stroke increases with advancing age for both men and women,[1] it is estimated that 55,000 more women than men have a stroke, largely because of an average longer life expectancy in women.[2] Overall, women have a higher lifetime risk of stroke than men. In the Framingham Heart Study, the lifetime risk of stroke among those 55 to 75 years of age was 1 in 5 for women (95% confidence interval [CI], 20%–21%) and approximately 1 in 6 for men (95% CI, 14%–17%).[3] As the population ages between 2012 and 2030, nearly 4% of the US population is projected to have had a stroke; estimated total direct medical stroke-related costs are projected to triple, from $71.55 billion to $184.13 billion.[4] While we recognize that there are differences in the rates of stroke

JFK Johnson Rehabilitation Institute at Hackensack Meridian Health, Department of Physical Medicine and Rehabilitation, 65 James Street, Edison, NJ, USA
* Corresponding author.
E-mail address: Talya.Fleming@hmhn.org

Phys Med Rehabil Clin N Am 36 (2025) 209–221
https://doi.org/10.1016/j.pmr.2024.11.001
pmr.theclinics.com

between men and women, the etiologies of those differences are being studied by the clinical and research communities.

RISK FACTORS FOR STROKE IN WOMEN

Gender differences in stroke have been studied extensively, demonstrating gender disparities in clinical presentation and modifiable and nonmodifiable risk factors, revealing distinct unique risk factors specific to women (**Fig. 1**).

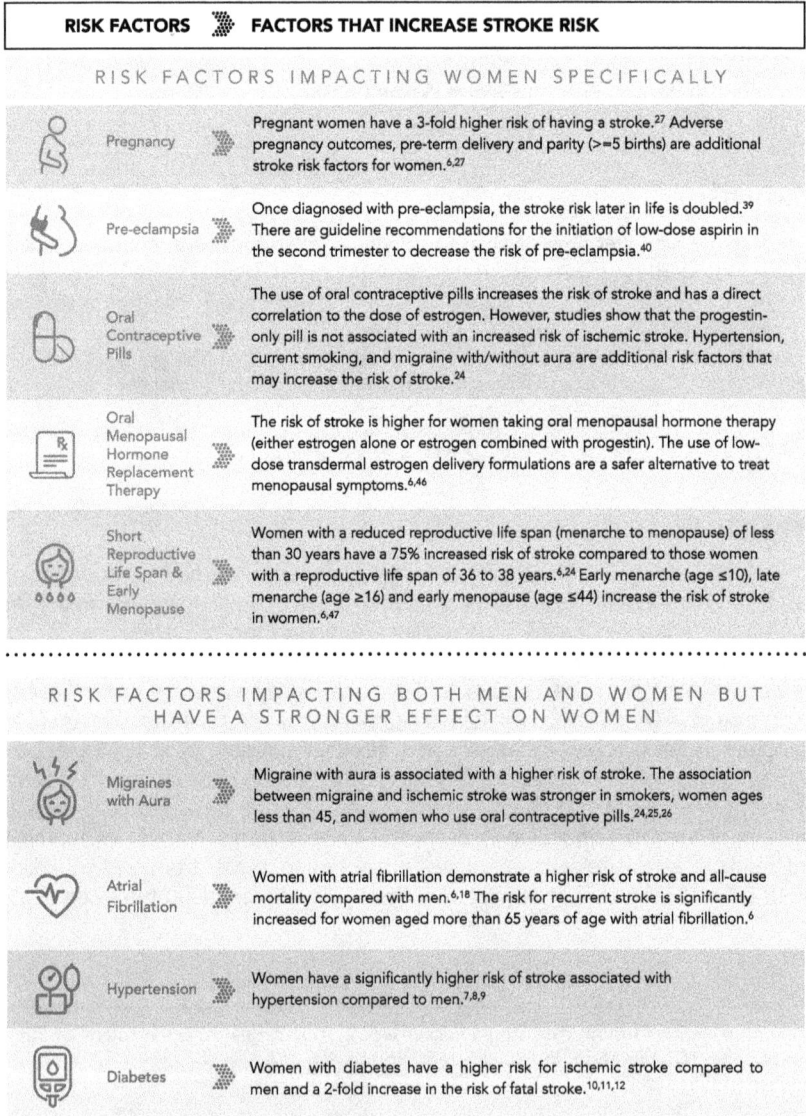

RISK FACTORS	🐾 FACTORS THAT INCREASE STROKE RISK

RISK FACTORS IMPACTING WOMEN SPECIFICALLY

Pregnancy	🐾	Pregnant women have a 3-fold higher risk of having a stroke.[27] Adverse pregnancy outcomes, pre-term delivery and parity (>=5 births) are additional stroke risk factors for women.[6,27]
Pre-eclampsia	🐾	Once diagnosed with pre-eclampsia, the stroke risk later in life is doubled.[39] There are guideline recommendations for the initiation of low-dose aspirin in the second trimester to decrease the risk of pre-eclampsia.[40]
Oral Contraceptive Pills	🐾	The use of oral contraceptive pills increases the risk of stroke and has a direct correlation to the dose of estrogen. However, studies show that the progestin-only pill is not associated with an increased risk of ischemic stroke. Hypertension, current smoking, and migraine with/without aura are additional risk factors that may increase the risk of stroke.[24]
Oral Menopausal Hormone Replacement Therapy	🐾	The risk of stroke is higher for women taking oral menopausal hormone therapy (either estrogen alone or estrogen combined with progestin). The use of low-dose transdermal estrogen delivery formulations are a safer alternative to treat menopausal symptoms.[6,46]
Short Reproductive Life Span & Early Menopause	🐾	Women with a reduced reproductive life span (menarche to menopause) of less than 30 years have a 75% increased risk of stroke compared to those women with a reproductive life span of 36 to 38 years.[6,24] Early menarche (age ≤10), late menarche (age ≥16) and early menopause (age ≤44) increase the risk of stroke in women.[6,47]

RISK FACTORS IMPACTING BOTH MEN AND WOMEN BUT HAVE A STRONGER EFFECT ON WOMEN

Migraines with Aura	🐾	Migraine with aura is associated with a higher risk of stroke. The association between migraine and ischemic stroke was stronger in smokers, women ages less than 45, and women who use oral contraceptive pills.[24,25,26]
Atrial Fibrillation	🐾	Women with atrial fibrillation demonstrate a higher risk of stroke and all-cause mortality compared with men.[6,18] The risk for recurrent stroke is significantly increased for women aged more than 65 years of age with atrial fibrillation.[6]
Hypertension	🐾	Women have a significantly higher risk of stroke associated with hypertension compared to men.[7,8,9]
Diabetes	🐾	Women with diabetes have a higher risk for ischemic stroke compared to men and a 2-fold increase in the risk of fatal stroke.[10,11,12]

Fig. 1. Risk factors that increase stroke risk. Several stroke risk factors impact women specifically. There are additional stroke risk factors that affect men and women but have a stronger effect on women.

Although women share major nonmodifiable risk factors with men such as age, race, and family history of stroke, their impact differs by gender. For example, the influence of age as a stroke risk factor varies throughout the patient's lifetime and impacts women more substantially in a bimodal distribution, with women experiencing a higher incidence of stroke than men both at ages under 30 years and when over 70 years old.[5,6]

Among modifiable risk factors, there are substantial gender disparities, with several factors presenting a more significant risk of stroke in women than in men. The most prevalent modifiable risk factor for stroke, hypertension, has significant gender disparity in prevalence and the risk associated with stroke. Several large cohort studies report a significantly higher risk of stroke associated with hypertension in women compared with men.[7–9] These results are influenced by factors such as age, race, and ethnicity; nevertheless, it underscores the need for a tailored approach to management and early screening for women. Similarly, the association of diabetes mellitus with ischemic stroke is stronger in women than in men, with large systematic reviews and meta-analyses reporting a 27% higher risk of stroke in women than men, and a twofold increased risk of fatal stroke in women with diabetes mellitus compared with men.[10–12]

Another dominant modifiable risk factor for stroke is atrial fibrillation (AF), which is an established factor associated with increased risk of stroke, cardiovascular disease, and mortality for men and women.[13–15] A substantial body of evidence shows that AF has a significantly greater impact on women than men.[16–18] A large meta-analysis study revealed that AF is associated with twice the relative risk of stroke in women compared with men.[19] In addition, the female gender is identified as an independent risk factor associated with thromboembolism, stroke, cardiovascular diseases, and mortality attributable to AF.[12,20] As a result, it is considered an independent variable in the stratification of risks such as in the CHA2DS2-VASc score.[20,21]

Traditional risk factors such as elevated body mass index (BMI) and obesity also have a stronger association in women compared with men. Studies report that obesity increases the risk of ischemic stroke in women by approximately 30% compared with men.[22,23] Migraines, especially those with aura, increase the risk of stroke for men and women. However, women are more vulnerable to these risks. Among people who experience migraines with aura, the risk of stroke is higher for women, especially those who are under 45 years of age and those who use oral contraceptive pills or smoke.[23–26]

Importantly, in addition to traditional modifiable and nonmodifiable risk factors that affect both genders, women face unique female-specific risk factors that substantially elevate the risk of stroke (**Fig. 1**). During pregnancy, the risk of stroke is 3 times higher than the rate for age-matched adults,[27] with studies demonstrating that 30 out of every 100,000 pregnancies are affected by stroke.[28–30] Furthermore, women with adverse pregnancy outcomes, preterm delivery, gestational hypertension, placental abruption, and stillbirth are at increased risk for cerebrovascular and cardiovascular morbidity and mortality.[31–34] Additionally, a large population cohort study suggests that a history of 5 or more births is associated with an increased risk of stroke, coronary heart disease, and myocardial infarction.[6,31,35] Another pregnancy-related risk factor is pre-eclampsia, which significantly increases the risk of stroke in women. Systematic review and meta-analysis studies demonstrated that pre-eclampsia was associated with an approximately twofold higher risk of stroke and future cardiovascular and cerebrovascular disease-related mortality compared to women with no history of pre-eclampsia.[36–39] Clinical recommendations advise the use of low-dose aspirin to decrease the risk of pre-eclampsia during pregnancy.[40]

The use of oral contraceptive pills (OCPs) poses a significant risk of stroke, with data showing an increased risk for ischemic and hemorrhagic stroke.[41,42] The risk of stroke is directly associated with the dose of estrogen, with OCPs that contain a lower dose of estrogen potentially contributing to a lower stroke risk compared to those with a higher dose of estrogen.[43] Progestin-only pills, on the other hand, have not shown any correlation with an increased risk of ischemic stroke.[41,43] Crucially, the risk of stroke further increases by additional factors such as smoking, hypertension, history of migraines, or age older than 35 for women taking OCPs.[24,41]

Additionally, the administration of oral hormone therapy for menopause increases the risk of ischemic stroke in women, regardless of whether it is estrogen alone or in combination with progestin.[44,45] As an alternative, studies have demonstrated that low-dose transdermal estrogen delivery formulations may offer a safer alternative for managing menopausal symptoms without increasing the risk of stroke.[46]

Furthermore, according to a recent meta-analysis, women who have a reduced reproductive life span of less than 30 years are at a 75% higher risk of stroke, compared to those with a reproductive life span of 36 to 38 years.[47] Women with a reproductive life span of 32 to 35 years are also at a higher risk of stroke although to a lesser extent.[47,48] Additionally, age at menarche presents a U-shaped association with increased risk of stroke in women who experience early menarche (age ≤ 10) or late menarche (age ≥ 16) at higher risk of stroke, Moreover, early menopause (age ≤ 44) is also associated with at an increased risk of stroke.[47]

CLINICAL PRESENTATIONS AND SYMPTOMS OF STROKE IN WOMEN

Regrettably, the diagnosis of stroke within the emergency department continues to be a persistent challenge, with studies reporting stroke being the fourth most common misdiagnosis.[49,50] The early recognition of stroke symptoms is critical to confirm diagnosis and to initiate treatments promptly to maximize recovery and prevent long-term disability. Recent studies estimated that approximately 9% to 12% of all strokes are not recognized in the emergency department at initial presentation.[51,52] Misdiagnosis of stroke leads to significantly worse outcomes, including severe disability and death.[53,54]

Women encounter distinct challenges compared with men. A recent large cross-sectional study demonstrated that women have 25% higher odds of misdiagnosis than men.[51] Additionally, numerous studies have reported considerable gender disparities in clinical presentation, received in-hospital services, and poor functional outcomes for women compared with men.[55–57] One of the major factors influencing the misdiagnosis of stroke in women is the manifestation of nontraditional symptoms in addition to conventional stroke symptoms[58–60] (**Fig. 2**). Women often present with atypical symptoms such as dizziness, headaches, nausea, confusion, fatigue, disorientation, and generalized weakness, posing challenges in differentiating actual strokes from stroke-like mimics.[6,58,59,61] Additionally, several studies reported that women often present with non-neurological symptoms such as chest pain and palpitations.[61]

Women face an increased risk of not identifying strokes at initial presentation because of often exhibiting nontraditional symptoms and signs. A large multiregional population-based study analyzing emergency department misdiagnosis revealed that headaches and dizziness were the 2 most common symptoms leading to stroke hospital readmissions.[52] Other studies demonstrated that patients presenting with motor symptoms have the lowest rates for misdiagnosis, at about 4%, whereas 35% of patients presenting with dizziness and 50% of those presenting with isolated dizziness with no other neurologic symptoms are misdiagnosed.[52,62,63] An international multicenter cohort study demonstrated that early MRI within 1 week of presentation led

SYMPTOMS OF STROKE

SYMPTOMS COMMON
FOR MEN/WOMEN

NON-TRADITIONAL
SYMPTOMS IN
WOMEN

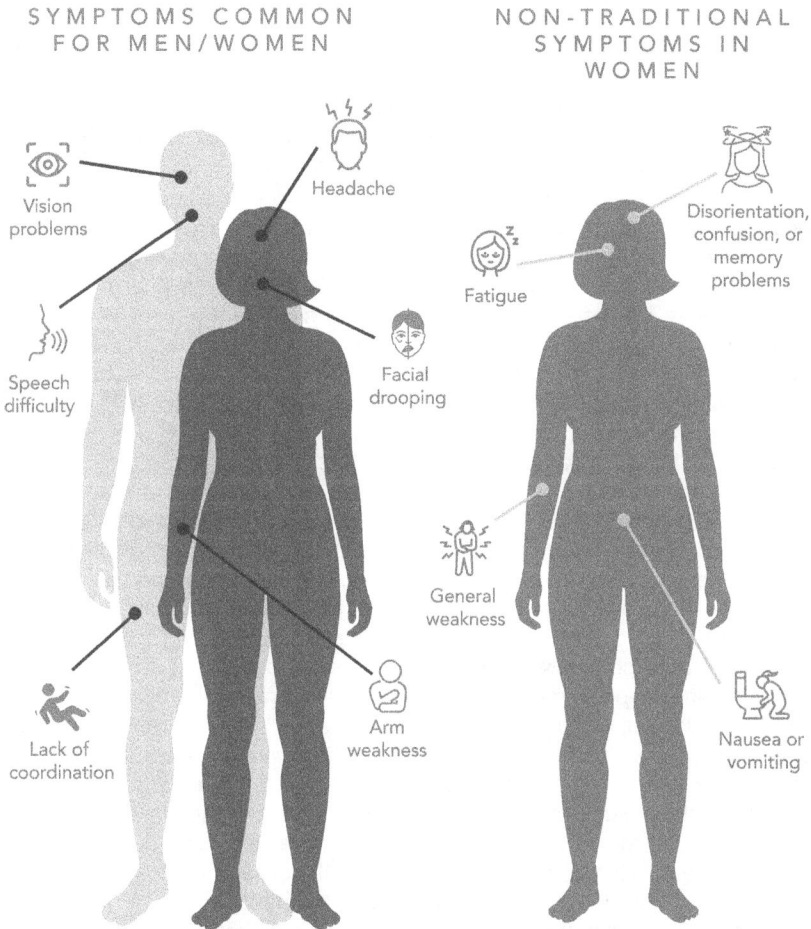

Vision problems

Headache

Disorientation, confusion, or memory problems

Fatigue

Speech difficulty

Facial drooping

Lack of coordination

General weakness

Arm weakness

Nausea or vomiting

Fig. 2. Symptoms of stroke. Although the most recognized signs of stroke are common for men and women (gray), there are nontraditional clinical signs of stroke that should be recognized in women (pink).

to a change in the diagnosis for 30% of cases such as transient ischemic attack and stroke mimic, based on the results of MRI.

It is crucial to raise awareness among health care professionals of the nontraditional symptoms of stroke in women to enable early diagnosis and timely intervention. This highlights the critical need and importance of developing and implementing standardized diagnostic approaches for identifying stroke symptoms, especially understanding gender-specific manifestations of stroke symptoms.

DIFFERENCES IN STROKE REHABILITATION AND OUTCOMES FOR WOMEN

Sex disparities exist for women starting in the early stages of the medical evaluation and carry through their course of recovery, negatively influencing their overall clinical outcomes. Women are more likely to present nontraditional stroke symptoms and may have a delayed clinical presentation to the acute care hospital.[64] Women have higher intracerebral hemorrhage scores than men at initial emergency department presentation[65] and have a significantly shorter acute care hospital length of stay (median 3 days) even when controlled for age compared with men (median 4 days).[66] While hospitalized, they are less likely to receive a comprehensive medical evaluation and diagnostic studies (eg, carotid imaging and echocardiography) required to adequately diagnose and treat acute stroke.[67] Studies have shown that women may be as much as 30% less likely to be treated with thrombolytics when presenting with acute stroke compared with men, despite considering patient eligibility, geographic/regional location, and after controlling for age, stroke severity, and comorbidities.[25] Female patients undergoing endovascular therapy are more likely to have prestroke disability, and to live alone, which results in delays between symptom onset and activation of the emergency response system compared with men.[68] Even after controlling for age, women with intracerebral hemorrhage were significantly more likely to die or enter hospice.[66] Upon hospital discharge, a study reviewing Medicare Advantage poststroke discharge patterns revealed that women were more likely to be discharged to a skilled nursing facility rather than an inpatient rehabilitation facility,[68,69] while men were more likely to be discharged to home.[66]

Concerning clinical outcomes, women have lesser functional recovery and inferior quality of life compared with men after stroke.[24,70–73] Studies show that women live longer but with poorer functional outcomes and higher rates of disability compared with men.[64,74] Older women are generally more prone to physical disability than men and tend to survive longer with disability.[64] This may be partially explained, because older female patients may experience greater socioeconomic disadvantage than men and be more affected by changes in social networks and support.[64] In addition to functional outcomes, women are more likely to experience poststroke depression (78%)[24] and other mental health symptoms like anxiety, compared with men.[64] After multivariable adjustment for stroke severity, age at stroke onset, and functional activity limitations, women were still more likely to have a significantly higher prevalence, incidence, or symptoms of depression than men.[24] Furthermore, preliminary data from a cohort study of community-dwelling adults in the United States found that women endure more cognitive deficits after stroke, even after controlling for prestroke cognitive measures, predominantly during the early poststroke period.[24]

Factors that may contribute to sex-specific differences with a less favorable outcome for women after stroke include more severe strokes at symptom onset, disparities in acute stroke treatment, advanced age, poorer prestroke function, more serious medical comorbidities, less social support, and higher likelihood of being a widow without a care partner to help during the recovery process.[24,67,70] Despite psychosocial factors, preclinical and clinical evidence demonstrates that the combination of factors including exposure to sex hormones and the microenvironment of the brain and vasculature may contribute to sex differences in cellular mechanisms of stroke injury.[64]

STROKE REHABILITATION STRATEGIES FOR WOMEN

Stroke rehabilitation strategies should be tailored for the individual and be an integral part of a comprehensive treatment plan. Several subgroups of women have additional needs that should factor into developing a comprehensive approach to rehabilitation. Women who are pregnant and/or breastfeeding should consult with their health care provider regarding the risks and benefits when considering certain treatment options used for the treatment of stroke-related disability including neurostimulants for cognitive and attention deficits,[75] medication for neuropathic pain,[76] and medication for the treatment of mood disorders[77] after stroke. Causes of self-reported increasing spasticity include the menstrual cycle, mental stress, and bowel/bladder dysfunction.[78] Pelvic floor muscle training has proven beneficial for the management of urinary incontinence in female stroke survivors.[79] The use of physical activity is foundational to neurorehabilitation, but also for a reduced risk of cardiovascular/cerebrovascular disease.[71,80,81] Lifestyle modifications that encourage a healthy diet, physical activity, smoking cessation, and maintenance of a healthy BMI have been shown to decrease stroke incidence in women and improve outcomes after stroke in men and women.[70,82] Invariably, clinicians should evaluate how the individual's functional, cognitive, and psychological deficits after stroke may negatively affect quality of life, especially if if the patient is a caregiver for another person.

DISCUSSION

Women bear a disproportionate burden of stroke, with a higher lifetime risk of stroke and poorer outcomes after stroke.[83] It is imperative to educate stroke survivors, care partners, and health care providers to acknowledge sex-specific differences after stroke and implement clinical best practices to address these disparities. Building clinical awareness of stroke symptoms, poststroke care, and stroke rehabilitation strategies for women may lead to improved outcomes and possibly a reduced incidence of stroke in women. Beyond secondary prevention, women-specific risk factors should be considered when developing preventive approaches targeted to women.[24,84]

Several subpopulations of women warrant special attention. The intersection of gender with race,[85] ethnicity, age, and socioeconomic status creates an additional barrier to health care services and outcomes. In the United States, stroke is a leading cause of death for women, but may vary by race/ethnicity: Non-Hispanic Black women (third, 6.5%), Hispanic women (third, 6,5%), Non-Hispanic Asian women (third, 7.6%), Non-Hispanic Native Hawaiian or Pacific Islander women (third, 7.2%), Non-Hispanic white women (fifth, 6.0%), and Non-Hispanic American Indian or Alaska Native women (seventh, 4.5%)[86]

Studies demonstrate that the index stroke rate may vary between genders by age:[86]

- Ages 15 to 24, no difference
- Ages 25 to 34, more women had strokes than men (incidence rate ratio: men:-women, 0.70 [95% confidence interval (CI)], 0.57–0.86)
- Ages 35 to 44, more women had strokes than men (incidence rate ratio: men:-women, 0.87 [95% CI, 0.78–0.98])
- Ages 45 to 54, more men had strokes (incidence rate ratio, 1.25 [95% CI, 1.16–1.33]
- Ages 55 to 64, more men had strokes (incidence rate ratio, 1.41 [95% CI, 1.18–1.34])
- Ages 65 to 74; more men had strokes (incidence rate ratio, 11.18 [95% CI, 1.12–125])
- Ages 75 years old and up – no difference.

In a UK study, women of lower socioeconomic status were approximately 20% more likely to experience any stroke, mainly ischemic stroke.[23] In a systematic review and meta-analysis, the lowest educational level, income, occupation, and composite socioeconomic status were associated with an increased risk of stroke mortality.[87,88] As these societal conditions are more likely to affect women, the numerous health care disparities compound to have an even greater negative impact on overall outcomes for women.[89] Recognizing that sex refers to biological factors, while gender refers to social roles, behaviors, and expressions,[68] future work within the medical community should clarify the factors that contribute to physiologic and societal differences between genders.

Unfortunately, women are under-represented in clinical research trials,[90] and more well-designed clinical trials powered to detect sex-based differences are required to evaluate the underlying mechanisms responsible for these differences.[24] As with many areas of health care, increased support is needed to increase the number of researchers who examine the health care needs specific to women. The study of nontraditional along with traditional risk factors may give additional insight into sex-specific comorbidities that lead to differences in outcomes.[91,92] Furthermore, additional resources specifically targeted toward increasing the number of women who lead stroke clinical trials[93] may help to advance the clinical research trial design and enrollment of women after stroke.

SUMMARY

Acute and postacute stroke care is complex, multifaceted, and should be highly personalized. Clinicians should be cognizant of gender-specific differences between risk factor management, clinical symptoms, and rehabilitation strategies to provide competent poststroke care and diminish health care disparities.

CLINICS CARE POINTS

Several risk factors for stroke are specific to women (eg, pregnancy, pre-eclampsia, OCPs, menopausal hormonal replacement therapy, and reproductive life span), while other risk factors impact both men and women, but have a stronger effect on women (eg, migraines with aura, AF, hypertension, and diabetes).

- Beyond the common symptoms of stroke, clinicians should be aware of alternate clinical symptoms in women (eg, fatigue, disorientation, confusion, memory problems, nausea, vomiting, and general weakness).
- Stroke rehabilitation strategies should be tailored for the individual; women have additional physiologic and psychosocial considerations that factor into developing a comprehensive approach to rehabilitation.

DISCLOSURE

None.

REFERENCES

1. Tsao CW, Aday AW, Almarzooq ZI, et al. Heart disease and stroke statistics-2023 update: a report from the American Heart Association. Circulation 2023;147(8): e93–621.
2. Demel SL, Kittner S, Ley SH, et al. Stroke risk factors unique to women. Stroke 2018;49(3):518–23.
3. Seshadri S, Beiser A, Kelly-Hayes M, et al. The lifetime risk of stroke: estimates from the Framingham Study. Stroke 2006;37(2):345–50.
4. Ovbiagele B, Goldstein LB, Higashida RT, et al. Forecasting the future of stroke in the United States: a policy statement from the American Heart Association and American Stroke Association. Stroke 2013;44(8):2361–75.

5. Vyas MV, Silver FL, Austin PC, et al. Stroke incidence by sex across the lifespan. Stroke 2021;52(2):447–51.

6. Rexrode KM, Madsen TE, Yu AYX, et al. The impact of sex and gender on stroke. Circ Res 2022;130(4):512–28.

7. Madsen TE, Howard G, Kleindorfer DO, et al. Sex differences in hypertension and stroke risk in the regards study: a longitudinal cohort study. Hypertension 1979; 74(4):749–55.

8. Howard VJ, Madsen TE, Kleindorfer DO, et al. Sex and race differences in the association of incident ischemic stroke with risk factors. JAMA Neurol 2019;76(2): 179–86.

9. Foy CG, Lovato LC, Vitolins MZ, et al. Gender, blood pressure, and cardiovascular and renal outcomes in adults with hypertension from the Systolic Blood Pressure Intervention Trial. J Hypertens 2018;36(4):904–15.

10. Peters SAE, Huxley RR, Woodward M. Diabetes as a risk factor for stroke in women compared with men: a systematic review and meta-analysis of 64 cohorts, including 775,385 individuals and 12,539 strokes. Lancet Lond Engl 2014;383(9933):1973–80.

11. Stevens RJ, Coleman RL, Adler AI, et al. Risk factors for myocardial infarction case fatality and stroke case fatality in type 2 diabetes: UKPDS 66. Diabetes Care 2004;27(1):201–7.

12. Madsen TE, Howard VJ, Jiménez M, et al. Impact of conventional stroke risk factors on stroke in women: an update. Stroke 2018;49(3):536–42.

13. Wolf PA, Abbott RD, Kannel WB. Atrial fibrillation as an independent risk factor for stroke: the Framingham Study. Stroke 1991;22(8):983–8.

14. Benjamin EJ, Wolf PA, D'Agostino RB, et al. Impact of atrial fibrillation on the risk of death: the Framingham Heart Study. Circulation 1998;98(10):946–52.

15. Chugh SS, Havmoeller R, Narayanan K, et al. Worldwide epidemiology of atrial fibrillation: a global burden of disease 2010 study. Circulation 2014;129(8): 837–47.

16. Wang TJ, Larson MG, Levy D, et al. Temporal relations of atrial fibrillation and congestive heart failure and their joint influence on mortality: the Framingham Heart Study. Circulation 2003;107(23):2920–5.

17. Mikkelsen AP, Lindhardsen J, Lip GYH, et al. Female sex as a risk factor for stroke in atrial fibrillation: a nationwide cohort study. J Thromb Haemost JTH 2012;10(9): 1745–51.

18. Sulzgruber P, Wassmann S, Semb AG, et al. Oral anticoagulation in patients with non-valvular atrial fibrillation and a CHA2DS2-VASc score of 1: a current opinion of the European society of cardiology working group on cardiovascular pharmacotherapy and European society of cardiology council on stroke. Eur Heart J Cardiovasc Pharmacother 2019;5(3):171–80.

19. Emdin CA, Wong CX, Hsiao AJ, et al. Atrial fibrillation as risk factor for cardiovascular disease and death in women compared with men: systematic review and meta-analysis of cohort studies. BMJ 2016;532:h7013.

20. Ko D, Rahman F, Schnabel RB, et al. Atrial fibrillation in women: epidemiology, pathophysiology, presentation, and prognosis. Nat Rev Cardiol 2016;13(6): 321–32.

21. January CT, Wann LS, Alpert JS, et al. 2014 AHA/ACC/HRS guideline for the management of patients with atrial fibrillation: a report of the American College of Cardiology/American Heart Association Task Force on Practice Guidelines and the Heart Rhythm Society. Circulation 2014;130(23):e199–267.

22. Rodríguez-Campello A, Jiménez-Conde J, Ois Á, et al. Sex-related differences in abdominal obesity impact on ischemic stroke risk. Eur J Neurol 2017;24(2): 397–403.

23. Peters SAE, Carcel C, Millett ERC, et al. Sex differences in the association between major risk factors and the risk of stroke in the UK Biobank cohort study. Neurology 2020;95(20):e2715–26.

24. Yoon CW, Bushnell CD. Stroke in women: a review focused on epidemiology, risk factors, and outcomes. J Stroke 2023;25(1):2–15.

25. Cherian L. Women and ischemic stroke: disparities and outcomes. Neurol Clin 2023;41(2):265–81.

26. Schürks M, Rist PM, Bigal ME, et al. Migraine and cardiovascular disease: systematic review and meta-analysis. BMJ 2009;339:b3914.

27. Camargo EC, Singhal AB. Stroke in pregnancy: a multidisciplinary approach. Obstet Gynecol Clin North Am 2021;48(1):75–96.

28. Swartz RH, Cayley ML, Foley N, et al. The incidence of pregnancy-related stroke: a systematic review and meta-analysis. Int J Stroke 2017;12(7):687–97.

29. Leffert LR, Clancy CR, Bateman BT, et al. Hypertensive disorders and pregnancy-related stroke: frequency, trends, risk factors, and outcomes. Obstet Gynecol 2015;125(1):124–31.

30. Yoshida K, Takahashi JC, Takenobu Y, et al. Strokes associated with pregnancy and puerperium: a nationwide study by the Japan Stroke Society. Stroke 2017; 48(2):276–82.

31. Grandi SM, Filion KB, Yoon S, et al. Cardiovascular disease-related morbidity and mortality in women with a history of pregnancy complications. Circulation 2019; 139(8):1069–79.

32. Heida KY, Bots ML, de Groot CJ, et al. Cardiovascular risk management after reproductive and pregnancy-related disorders: a Dutch multidisciplinary evidence-based guideline. Eur J Prev Cardiol 2016;23(17):1863–79.

33. Robbins CL, Hutchings Y, Dietz PM, et al. History of preterm birth and subsequent cardiovascular disease: a systematic review. Am J Obstet Gynecol 2014; 210(4):285–97.

34. Ranthe MF, Andersen EAW, Wohlfahrt J, et al. Pregnancy loss and later risk of atherosclerotic disease. Circulation 2013;127(17):1775–82.

35. Parikh NI, Gonzalez JM, Anderson CAM, et al. Adverse pregnancy outcomes and cardiovascular disease risk: unique opportunities for cardiovascular disease prevention in women: a scientific statement from the American Heart Association. Circulation 2021;143(18):e902–16.

36. Wu P, Haththotuwa R, Kwok CS, et al. Pre-eclampsia and future cardiovascular health: a systematic review and meta-analysis. Circ Cardiovasc Qual Outcomes 2017;10(2):e003497.

37. Bellamy L, Casas JP, Hingorani AD, et al. Pre-eclampsia and risk of cardiovascular disease and cancer in later life: systematic review and meta-analysis. BMJ 2007;335(7627):974.

38. Søndergaard MM, Hlatky MA, Stefanick ML, et al. Association of adverse pregnancy outcomes with risk of atherosclerotic cardiovascular disease in postmenopausal women. JAMA Cardiol 2020;5(12):1390–8.

39. Leslie MS, Briggs LA. Pre-eclampsia and the risk of future vascular disease and mortality: a review. J Midwifery Wom Health 2016;61(3):315–24.

40. ACOG Committee Opinion No. 743: low-dose aspirin use during pregnancy. Obstet Gynecol 2018;132(1):e44–52. https://doi.org/10.1097/AOG. 0000000000002708.

41. Xu Z, Li Y, Tang S, et al. Current use of oral contraceptives and the risk of first-ever ischemic stroke: a meta-analysis of observational studies. Thromb Res 2015;136(1):52–60.
42. Xu Z, Yue Y, Bai J, et al. Association between oral contraceptives and risk of hemorrhagic stroke: a meta-analysis of observational studies. Arch Gynecol Obstet 2018;297(5):1181–91.
43. Li F, Zhu L, Zhang J, et al. Oral contraceptive use and increased risk of stroke: a dose-response meta-analysis of observational studies. Front Neurol 2019;10:993.
44. Wassertheil-Smoller S, Hendrix SL, Limacher M, et al. Effect of estrogen plus progestin on stroke in postmenopausal women: the Women's Health Initiative: a randomized trial. JAMA 2003;289(20):2673–84.
45. Manson JE, Chlebowski RT, Stefanick ML, et al. Menopausal hormone therapy and health outcomes during the intervention and extended poststopping phases of the Women's Health Initiative randomized trials. JAMA 2013;310(13):1353–68.
46. Renoux C, Dell'aniello S, Garbe E, et al. Transdermal and oral hormone replacement therapy and the risk of stroke: a nested case-control study. BMJ 2010;340: c2519.
47. Mishra SR, Chung HF, Waller M, et al. Association between reproductive life span and incident nonfatal cardiovascular disease: a pooled analysis of individual patient data from 12 studies. JAMA Cardiol 2020;5(12):1410–8.
48. Ley SH, Li Y, Tobias DK, et al. Duration of reproductive life span, age at menarche, and age at menopause are associated with risk of cardiovascular disease in women. J Am Heart Assoc 2017;6(11):e006713.
49. Tarnutzer AA, Lee SH, Robinson KA, et al. ED misdiagnosis of cerebrovascular events in the era of modern neuroimaging: a meta-analysis. Neurology 2017; 88(15):1468–77.
50. Schiff GD, Hasan O, Kim S, et al. Diagnostic error in medicine: analysis of 583 physician-reported errors. Arch Intern Med 2009;169(20):1881–7.
51. Newman-Toker DE, Dy FJ, Stanton VA, et al. How often is dizziness from primary cardiovascular disease true vertigo? A systematic review. J Gen Intern Med 2008; 23(12):2087–94.
52. Newman-Toker DE, Moy E, Valente E, et al. Missed diagnosis of stroke in the emergency department: a cross-sectional analysis of a large population-based sample. Diagn Berl Ger 2014;1(2):155–66.
53. Tarnutzer AA, Berkowitz AL, Robinson KA, et al. Does my dizzy patient have a stroke? A systematic review of bedside diagnosis in acute vestibular syndrome. CMAJ Can Med Assoc J 2011;183(9):E571–92.
54. Kowalski RG, Claassen J, Kreiter KT, et al. Initial misdiagnosis and outcome after subarachnoid hemorrhage. JAMA 2004;291(7):866–9.
55. Reeves MJ, Bushnell CD, Howard G, et al. Sex differences in stroke: epidemiology, clinical presentation, medical care, and outcomes. Lancet Neurol 2008; 7(10):915–26.
56. Niewada M, Kobayashi A, Sandercock PAG, et al, International Stroke Trial Collaborative Group. Influence of gender on baseline features and clinical outcomes among 17,370 patients with confirmed ischaemic stroke in the international stroke trial. Neuroepidemiology 2005;24(3):123–8.
57. Gall SL, Donnan G, Dewey HM, et al. Sex differences in presentation, severity, and management of stroke in a population-based study. Neurology 2010; 74(12):975–81.
58. Lisabeth LD, Brown DL, Hughes R, et al. Acute stroke symptoms: comparing women and men. Stroke 2009;40(6):2031–6.

59. Jerath NU, Reddy C, Freeman WD, et al. Gender differences in presenting signs and symptoms of acute ischemic stroke: a population-based study. Gend Med 2011;8(5):312–9.

60. Bushnell CD, Chaturvedi S, Gage KR, et al. Sex differences in stroke: challenges and opportunities. J Cereb Blood Flow Metab 2018;38(12):2179–91.

61. Ali M, van Os HJA, van der Weerd N, et al. Sex differences in presentation of stroke: a systematic review and meta-analysis. Stroke 2022;53(2):345–54.

62. Morgenstern LB, Lisabeth LD, Mecozzi AC, et al. A population-based study of acute stroke and TIA diagnosis. Neurology 2004;62(6):895–900.

63. Lever NM, Nyström KV, Schindler JL, et al. Missed opportunities for recognition of ischemic stroke in the emergency department. J Emerg Nurs 2013;39(5):434–9.

64. Xu M, Amarilla Vallejo A, Cantalapiedra Calvete C, et al. Stroke outcomes in women: a population-based cohort study. Stroke 2022;53(10):3072–81.

65. Ganti L, Shameem M, Houck J, et al. Gender disparity in stoke: women have higher ICH scores than men at initial ED presentation for intracerebral hemorrhage. J Natl Med Assoc 2023;115(2):186–90.

66. Craen A, Mangal R, Stead TG, et al. Gender differences in outcomes after non-traumatic intracerebral hemorrhage. Cureus 2019;11(10):e5818.

67. Chavez AA, Simmonds KP, Venkatachalam AM, et al. Health care disparities in stroke rehabilitation. Phys Med Rehabil Clin N Am 2024;35(2):293–303.

68. Ospel JM, Schaafsma JD, Leslie-Mazwi TM, et al. Toward a better understanding of sex- and gender-related differences in endovascular stroke treatment: a scientific statement from the American heart association/American stroke association. Stroke 2022;53(8):e396–406.

69. Hayes HA, Mor V, Wei G, et al. Medicare advantage patterns of poststroke discharge to an inpatient rehabilitation or skilled nursing facility: a consideration of demographic, functional, and payer factors. Phys Ther 2023;103(4):pzad009.

70. Bushnell C, McCullough LD, Awad IA, et al. Guidelines for the prevention of stroke in women: a statement for healthcare professionals from the American Heart Association/American Stroke Association. Stroke 2014;45(5):1545–88.

71. Madsen TE, Samaei M, Pikula A, et al. Sex differences in physical activity and incident stroke: a systematic review. Clin Ther 2022;44(4):586–611.

72. Thomas Q, Crespy V, Duloquin G, et al. Stroke in women: when gender matters. Rev Neurol (Paris) 2021;177(8):881–9.

73. White BM, Magwood GS, Burns SP, et al. Sex differences in patient-reported poststroke disability. J Womens Health (Larchmt) 2018;27(4):518–24.

74. Hubbard IJ, Vo K, Forder PM, et al. Stroke, physical function, and death over a 15-year period in older Australian women. Stroke 2016;47(4):1060–7.

75. Zhang Y, Gong F, Liu P, et al. Effects of prenatal methamphetamine exposure on birth outcomes, brain structure, and neurodevelopmental outcomes. Dev Neurosci 2021;43(5):271–80.

76. Zerfas I, McGinn R, Smith MA. Pharmacologic management of cancer-related pain in pregnant patients. Drugs 2023;83(12):1067–76.

77. Fischer Fumeaux CJ, Morisod Harari M, Weisskopf E, et al. Risk-benefit balance assessment of SSRI antidepressant use during pregnancy and lactation based on best available evidence - an update. Expert Opin Drug Saf 2019;18(10):949–63.

78. Phadke CP, Balasubramanian CK, Ismail F, et al. Revisiting physiologic and psychologic triggers that increase spasticity. Am J Phys Med Rehabil 2013;92(4):357–69.

79. Shin DC, Shin SH, Lee MM, et al. Pelvic floor muscle training for urinary incontinence in female stroke patients: a randomized, controlled and blinded trial. Clin Rehabil 2016;30(3):259–67.
80. Oguma Y, Shinoda-Tagawa T. Physical activity decreases cardiovascular disease risk in women: review and meta-analysis. Am J Prev Med 2004;26(5):407–18.
81. Cuccurullo SJ, Fleming TK, Petrosyan H. Integrating cardiac rehabilitation in stroke recovery. Phys Med Rehabil Clin N Am 2024;35(2):353–68.
82. Cuccurullo SJ, Fleming TK, Zinonos S, et al. Stroke recovery program with modified cardiac rehabilitation improves mortality, functional & cardiovascular performance. J Stroke Cerebrovasc Dis 2022;31(5):106322.
83. Lundberg GP, Volgman AS. Burden of stroke in women. Trends Cardiovasc Med 2016;26(1):81–8.
84. Christensen H, Bushnell C. Stroke in women. Contin Minneap Minn 2020;26(2): 363–85.
85. Jiménez MC, Manson JE, Cook NR, et al. Racial variation in stroke risk among women by stroke risk factors. Stroke 2019;50(4):797–804.
86. CDC, Health Equity, Women's Health. Leading cause of death. 2018. Available at: https://www.cdc.gov/women/lcod/2018/all-races-origins/index.htm. Accessed April 22, 2024.
87. Wang S, Zhai H, Wei L, et al. Socioeconomic status predicts the risk of stroke death: a systematic review and meta-analysis. Prev Med Rep 2020;19:101124.
88. Kim YD, Jung YH, Caso V, et al, Women's Disparities Working Group. Countries with women inequalities have higher stroke mortality. Int J Stroke 2017;12(8): 869–74.
89. Ospel J, Singh N, Ganesh A, et al. Sex and gender differences in stroke and their practical implications in acute care. J Stroke 2023;25(1):16–25.
90. Strong B, Pudar J, Thrift AG, et al. Sex disparities in enrollment in recent randomized clinical trials of acute stroke: a meta-analysis. JAMA Neurol 2021;78(6): 666–77.
91. Jacobs MM, Ellis C. Stroke in women between 2006 and 2018: demographic, socioeconomic, and age disparities. Womens Health Lond Engl 2023;19: 17455057231199061. https://doi.org/10.1177/17455057231199061.
92. Leppert MH, Ho PM, Burke J, et al. Young women had more strokes than young men in a large, United States claims sample. Stroke 2020;51(11):3352–5.
93. Carcel C, Reeves M. Under-enrollment of women in stroke clinical trials: what are the causes and what should be done about it? Stroke 2021;52(2):452–7.

Cardiac Rehabilitation for Women with Heart Disease

Jonathan H. Whiteson, BSc, MD[a,b,*], Sofiya Prilik, MD[c,d,e],
Matthew C. Glenn, MD, MS[e]

KEYWORDS

- Heart disease • Women • Cardiac rehabilitation • Aerobic exercise • Barriers
- Disparities

KEY POINTS

- Heart disease is the most common cause of morbidity and mortality in women.
- Women have worse outcomes from cardiovascular disease due to disparities in: research; understanding of prevalence and presentation of cardiovascular conditions in women; appropriate therapeutic interventions; poor referral for cardiac rehabilitation.
- Despite being under-referred, women completing CR have equivalent benefit to men from participation including improved aerobic fitness, enhanced cardiovascular risk factor profile, reduced risk for secondary cardiovascular events and use of health services, and improved morbidity.
- CR programs configured to meet the specific needs of women support the referral, enrollment, participation, and outcomes from the CR intervention.

INTRODUCTION

Cardiac rehabilitation (CR) reduces the risk of cardiovascular disease mortality and improves cardiovascular function by limiting the physiologic and psychological stresses associated with cardiovascular disease. CR helps patients optimize their health, function, and quality of life. While significant research has been conducted on the etiology of cardiovascular disease and the benefit of CR, there has been a paucity of research focused on women. To optimize outcomes from CR for women with heart disease (HD), it is essential for the physician practicing CR to understand the unique differences between HD in women and men. Similarly, CR programs have to be tailored

[a] Department of Medicine and Rehabilitation Medicine, NYU Grossman School of Medicine;
[b] Cardiac and Pulmonary Rehabilitation, Rusk Rehabilitation, NYU Langone Health, New York, NY 10016, USA; [c] Department of Rehabilitation Medicine, NYU Grossman School of Medicine; [d] Transplant Rehabilitation; [e] Department of Physical Medicine and Rehabilitation, Rusk NYU Langne Health, 240 East 38th Street, 15th Floor, New York, NY 10016, USA
* Cor‑ponding author. Department of Physical Medicine and Rehabilitation, Rusk NYU Langne Health, 240 East 38th Street, 15th Floor, New York, NY 10016.
E-mail address: jonathan.whiteson@nyulangone.org

Phys Med Rehabil Clin N Am 36 (2025) 223–238
https://doi.org/10.1016/j.pmr.2024.11.005
1047-9651/25/© 2024 Elsevier Inc. All rights reserved, including those for text and data mining, AI training, and similar technologies.

to the specific needs of women to achieve the goals of secondary prevention, optimal function, and quality of life.

CR should be prescribed for all individuals diagnosed with qualifying HD or following specified cardiac procedures (**Box 1**).[1]

Some private insurances will cover additional diagnoses including arrhythmias, heart failure with preserved ejection fraction (HFpEF), myomectomy, or surgery to the major cardiac vessels.

Heart Disease in Women—Etiology, Incidence, and Diagnosis

HD is the leading cause of morbidity and mortality in women globally.[2] Over 60 million women (44%) have some form of HD in the United States.[2] In 2017, 21.8% of deaths in females in the United States were due to HD and a further 6.2% were due to cerebro-vascular disease.[2] HD in women includes coronary artery disease (CAD), valvular heart disease (VHD), arrhythmias, and cardiomyopathies (CMs)/heart failure (HF). Athero-sclerotic vascular disease of the brain and PAD should also be considered if CAD has been diagnosed but are beyond the focus of this article.

While the heart in structure and function is the same in both genders, difference in female anatomy, physiology, and the hormonal milieu result in significant differences in risk factors, presentation, course, and outcomes. The general lack of understanding of these differences stems in part from an under-representation of women in clinical research trials and biases underestimating the incidence and impact of HD in women. This has resulted in disparities in diagnosis, referral, and management of HD in women as evidenced by the higher mortality from CAD and other HDs in women than in men.[3] In 2021, 1 in 5 deaths in women was related to HD yet just over half of US women know that HD is the leading cause of death in women.[4]

Coronary Artery Disease in Women

In all women over age 20 years, 5.8% have CAD. Prevalence of CAD increases with age with over 40% having CAD by age 80 years old and 80% of women ages 40 to 60 have one or more risk factors for CAD.[5] CAD and its risk factors demonstrate gender specificity.[5] While there are standard CAD risk factors common in both genders, these risk factors may contribute more significantly to the development of CAD in women than in men.

Hypertension

Globally there are an estimated 600 million women with hypertension (HTN). One-third of all US women between the ages of 30 to 79 years old have HTN.[6] HTN is often

---

Box 1
Medicare covered diagnoses for outpatient cardiac rehabilitation

Myocardial infarction (MI)

Coronary artery bypass surgery (CABG)

Current stable angina

Heart valve repair or replacement

Coronary angioplasty or coronary stent

Heart or heart-lung transplant

Stable chronic heart failure with reduced ejection fraction (HFrEF) $\leq$ 35%

Peripheral arterial disease (PAD)

underdiagnosed and undertreated in women with control rates under 25%. HTN is often undertreated in women compared with men resulting in a greater risk of developing HF.[6]

Diabetes

In 2021, over 14% (>18 million) of US female adults had diabetes with more—3.9% (5 million)—undiagnosed compared to men with 2.8% (3.7 million) undiagnosed.[7] Women with diabetes demonstrate a 44% greater risk for the development of CAD compared to men with diabetes.[7] Gestational diabetes is also an independent risk factor for CAD.

Dyslipidemia

Over 50 million US women (40.4%) had dyslipidemia in 2018[8]—a diagnosis often recognized later in women compared with men and often more poorly controlled compared with men.

Overweight/obesity

In 2018, 27.5% of US women were overweight and 41.9% were obese. More women (11.5%) have severe obesity than men (9.2%).[9]

Physical inactivity

In 2020, only 20.4% of women met the physical activity guidelines for aerobic and strength exercise compared with 28.3% of men.[10] The compliance with exercise guidelines in women decreases significantly with age—28.7% of women aged 18 to 34 years old met the guidelines whereas only 10.8% aged 65 years and older met the guidelines.[10]

Metabolic syndrome

Metabolic syndrome[11] is diagnosed when any 3 of the following conditions are present: obesity; hypertriglyceridemia; low high-density lipoprotein; HTN; elevated blood glucose. It has been reported in over 40% of all US women in 2018 and the prevalence continues to increase.

Tobacco use

In 2021, fewer women (10.1%) than men (13.1%) reported regular tobacco use.[12] However, women who smoke tobacco have a 25% increased risk of CAD compared to men who smoke, the risk increasing by a factor of 10 in women who smoke combined with oral contraceptive use.[13]

There are also "nontraditional" risk factors seen more commonly in, or uniquely in, women (**Fig. 1**).[14]

Unique risk factors for CAD in women are often overlooked and include gender-specific hormonal fluctuations, polycystic ovary syndrome (PCOS), gestational diabetes, pre-eclampsia, preterm delivery, breast cancer therapies, and autoimmune disorders.[15]

Premenopausal women are noted to have lower rates of CAD than men of similar age cohorts and when compared to postmenopausal women, believed to be due to a cardio-protective effect of estrogen.[16] Hormonal irregularities including early menopause, hysterectomy, and PCOS are associated with higher incidence of CAD. Estrogen's cardio-protective benefits are related to antioxidant and antiplatelet effects which improve vasodilation via endothelial pathways. Estrogen has also been shown to increase nitric oxide, regulate prostaglandin production, and inhibit smooth muscle proliferation all of which reduced CAD risk.[17] Pre-eclampsia results in an increased risk of HF, CAD, and cardiovascular mortality, and this is more significant if the pre-eclampsia occurs before 34 weeks of pregnancy.[18]

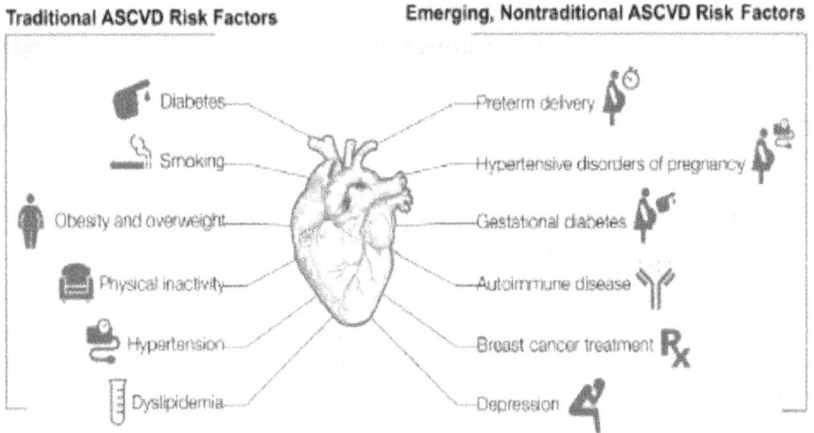

Fig. 1. Traditional and nontraditional risk factors for CAD in women.[14] Mariana Garcia et al., Cardiovascular Disease in Women. Circulation Research 2016-04-15 118(8): 1273-1293. https://doi.org/10.1161/CIRCRESAHA.116.307547.

While there is overlap in symptoms and signs, HD in women can present differently to men in part, related to differences in pathophysiology. Women are more likely to develop microvascular CAD with endothelial dysfunction and preserved myocardial ejection fraction (EF) resulting in atypical cardiac symptoms, whereas men are more likely to develop macrovascular CAD, have myocardial infarction (MI), and reduced EF resulting in more typically recognized cardiac symptoms.[19] Women are more likely to develop unique coronary syndromes. Spontaneous coronary artery dissection (SCAD) has a 90% female preponderance[20] and is not uncommonly associated with pregnancy.[21] The pathogenesis of SCAD is not well understood but is likely associated with fibromuscular hyperplasia—a condition seen more commonly in women. SCAD has been poorly managed due to a lack of established, evidence-based treatment pathways. Women are at a 5 times greater risk than men having a myocardial infarction with nonobstructive coronary arteries (MINOCA). Women with MINOCA are generally younger, less likely to demonstrate traditional risk factors and more likely to have hypercoagulable states.[22] Of note is that current management strategies for MINOCA are based on research studies conducted on men and older patients.

Presenting symptoms of HD may differ between women than in men. One study indicated 37% of women with an acute coronary syndrome (ACS) report no chest pain compared with 27% of men.[23] A recent meta-analysis reported that compared with men, women with ACS had higher odds of presenting with pain between the shoulder blades (OR, 2.15; 95% CI, 1.95–2.37), nausea or vomiting (OR, 1.64; 95% CI, 1.48–1.82), and shortness of breath (OR, 1.34; 95% CI, 1.21–1.48).[18] Women had lower odds of presenting with chest pain (OR, 0.70; 95% CI, 0.63–0.78) and diaphoresis (OR, 0.84; 95% CI, 0.76–0.94).[24]

Successful and timely diagnosis of CAD and ACS in women requires an understanding of the unique risk factors and presentations discussed earlier, as well as overcoming conscious and subconscious biases.[25] It is vital to consider the risk for HD in women despite atypical symptoms and with recognition that risk factor identification and mitigation, as well as CAD preventive measures are underutilized in women compared with men.[26] This has resulted in a plateau in the rate of decrease in cardiovascular deaths in women and an increase in younger women with one-third of cardiovascular events noted in women younger than 65 years old.[27] A recent review addresses this topic in more detail.[28]

Standard diagnostic testing and management protocols for HD have been described elsewhere and should be adhered to similarly in both genders.[29–31] Of note, the interpretation of diagnostic tests has been reported to be less reliable in women compared to men.[32] As well, disparities are noted in medication prescriptions for the management of HD and CAD with women less likely to be prescribed aspirin, statins, and angiotensin-converting enzyme inhibitors and more likely to be prescribed diuretics.[33]

Valvular Heart Disease in Women

With the decline in rheumatic valve disease noted in high income countries, the prevalence of age-related degenerative causes of cardiac VHD is rising as the population ages. As women are living longer than men, the proportion of women with VHD is increasing. VHD is most often diagnosed in individuals over 65 years old.[34] Women are more likely to develop mitral valve diseases and less likely to develop aortic valve diseases compared to men. Of note, the majority of patients with aortic stenosis over 80 years old are women due to their greater longevity. Epidemiology, diagnosis, and treatment of VHD in women compared to men are summarized in **Fig. 2**.[34] Of note, women are often under-represented in VHD research studies, have smaller hearts than men resulting in inaccurate quantification of VHD, often have greater symptom burden but are referred for surgical intervention later than men.[34] Further multifactorial gender disparities that have resulted in poorer outcomes from the management of VHD in women are reviewed in detail elsewhere.[34] Recent developments resulting in an increased use of transcatheter valve repair and replacement approaches are resulting in decreased gender-based differences in VHD management outcomes.

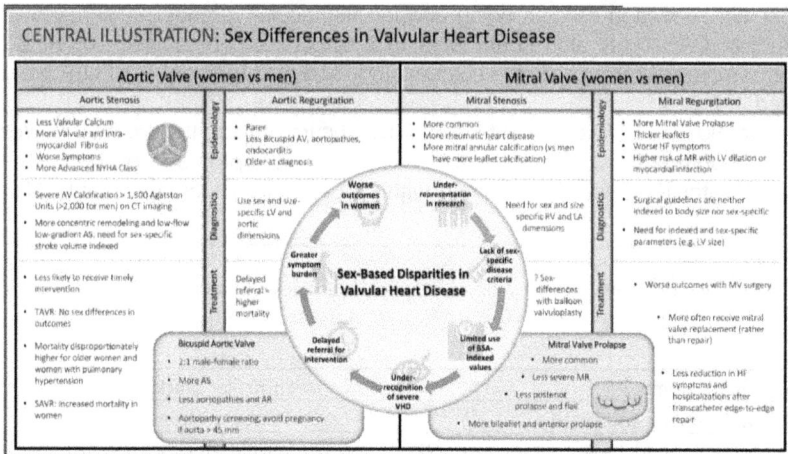

Fig. 2. Sex differences in VHD. AR, aortic regurgitation; AS, aortic stenosis; AV, aortic valve; BSA, body surface area; CT, computed tomography; HF, heart failure; LA, left atrium; LV, left ventricle; MR, mitral regurgitation; MV, mitral valve; NYHA, New York Heart Association; RV, right ventricle; SAVR, surgical aortic valve replacement; TAVR, transcatheter aortic valve replacement; VHD, valvular heart disease.[34] Jacqueline T. DesJardin et al., Sex Differences and Similarities in Valvular Heart Disease. Circulation Research, 130 (4), 2022; 455-473. https://doi.org/10.1161/CIRCRESAHA.121.319914.

Arrhythmias in Women

For over 100 years, differences in cardiac electrophysiology between women and men have been appreciated. Fluctuations in gender-specific sex-hormones, differences in autonomic function and differences in body size and cardiac mass contribute, resulting in a variable prevalence of specific arrhythmias between women and men (**Table 1**).

A detailed review of incidence, presentation, and management of arrhythmias in women is provided elsewhere.[35] Of note, atrial fibrillation (AF) is the most common arrhythmia globally, and females consistently report greater symptoms and worse quality of life due to AF than males. Outcomes associated with AF, including HF and cognitive decline (but not stroke risk), are more common in women. Risk of an arrhythmogenic (ventricular fibrillation) sudden cardiac death resulting from an acute coronary event is less in women (1.9x increased risk) compared with men (3.3x increased risk).[35]

Cardiomyopathies and Heart Failure in Women

HF affects over 2.6 million women (and 3.4 million men) in the United States.[36] Gender-related differences in the prevalence, response to treatment, and outcomes of management are noted. Peripartum cardiomyopathy (PPCM) is only seen in women, whereas other CMs with significant gender differences include stress-induced (Takotsubo's) cardiomyopathy, hypertrophic cardiomyopathy (HCM), and CMs related to sarcoidosis and amyloidosis. Despite women having a lower lifetime risk (5.8%) for heart failure with reduced ejection fraction (HFrEF) compared with men (10.6), women are more likely to have a worse quality of life, similar risk for hospitalization and lower mortality when compared with men. Gender differences in the epidemiology and management of HFrEF are summarized in **Fig. 3**.[36]

HFpEF is more prevalent in women (2.42%) compared with men (0.88%) most likely related to age-related factors and a greater impact of HTN and obesity in women.[36] Gender differences in cardiac aging and left ventricular remodeling in response to obstructive CAD likely also contributes to the increased prevalence of HFpEF in women. Gender differences in the epidemiology and management of HFpEF are summarized in **Fig. 4**.[36]

Of note, 80% to 90% of patients with amyloid cardiomyopathy are men.[37] Women with HCM compared with men are older with more symptoms at presentation and have a greater mortality risk. Women with cardiac sarcoidosis have lower risk for

---

Table 1
Gender-related differences in prevalence of specific cardiac arrhythmias—women compared with men

Higher	Lower
Sick sinus syndrome	Atrioventricular block
Inappropriate sinus tachycardia	Carotid sinus syndrome
Atrioventricular nodal reentry tachycardia (2x)	Atrial fibrillation (1.5–2x)
Supraventricular tachycardia due to *right*-sided accessory pathways (2.8x)	Supraventricular tachycardia due to *left*-sided accessory pathways
Idiopathic right ventricular tachycardia (1.5x)	Wolff-Parkinson-White syndrome
Arrhythmic events in the long-QT syndrome	Reentrant ventricular tachycardia
	Ventricular fibrillation and sudden death
	Brugada syndrome

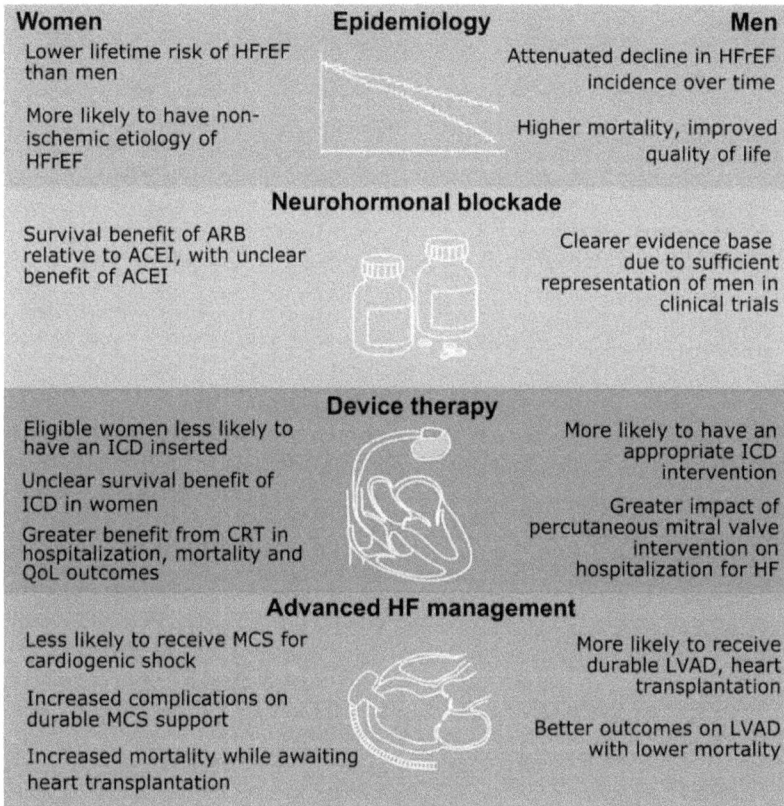

Women	Epidemiology	Men
Lower lifetime risk of HFrEF than men		Attenuated decline in HFrEF incidence over time
More likely to have non-ischemic etiology of HFrEF		Higher mortality, improved quality of life

Neurohormonal blockade

Survival benefit of ARB relative to ACEI, with unclear benefit of ACEI	Clearer evidence base due to sufficient representation of men in clinical trials

Device therapy

Eligible women less likely to have an ICD inserted	More likely to have an appropriate ICD intervention
Unclear survival benefit of ICD in women	Greater impact of percutaneous mitral valve intervention on hospitalization for HF
Greater benefit from CRT in hospitalization, mortality and QoL outcomes	

Advanced HF management

Less likely to receive MCS for cardiogenic shock	More likely to receive durable LVAD, heart transplantation
Increased complications on durable MCS support	Better outcomes on LVAD with lower mortality
Increased mortality while awaiting heart transplantation	

Fig. 3. Sex differences in the pathophysiology and treatment of HFrEF.[36] https://elsevier. proofcentral.com/en-us/landing-page.html?token=91f01646h0cfe00085d7826448ca93.

ventricular arrhythmias but have higher in-hospital mortality rates than men. Takotsubo's cardiomyopathy is more often related to emotional stress in women compared with physical stress in men, and women have better outcomes—lower risk for HF, ventricular arrhythmias, and death—compared with men.

Heart Disease Considerations in Pregnancy

Annually in the United States, there are 50,000 life threatening complications and approximately 700 women die related to pregnancy.[38] The incidence of death increased from 7.2 to 17.2 per 100,000 live births from 1987 to 2015. HTN, CAD–myocardial infarction, cardiomyopathy, and stroke are the leading causes of these complications and death. Arrhythmias and VHD, specifically aortic valve disease, also present or can worsen during pregnancy. Prepregnancy risk factors include age over 40, African American, American Indian, or Alaska Native, overweight/obesity, pre-existing cardiac disease (including congenital HD) and CAD risk factors—diabetes, HTN, sedentary lifestyle, substance use/abuse—drugs, alcohol, tobacco.[38]

PPCM typically presents soon after delivery with HFrEF and is a significant cause of maternal mortality with an incidence of 1:3000 live births in the United States.[38] Risk is increased with greater maternal age, hypertensive complications of pregnancy, twins, Black race, and diabetes. Compared with other CMs, there is an increased risk of intracardiac thrombi and thromboembolic events and so cardiac imaging is essential

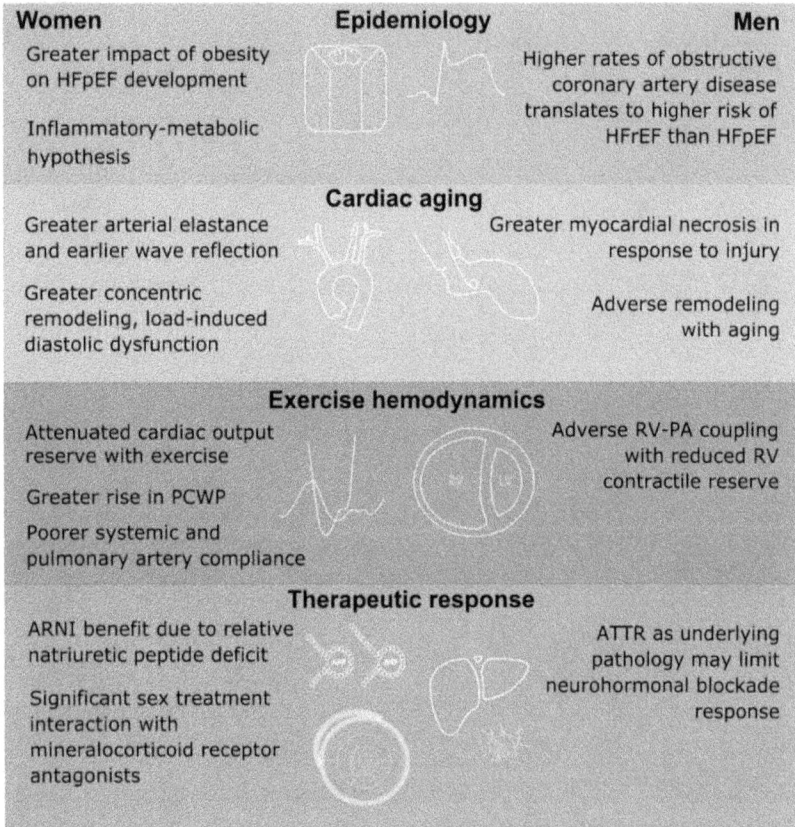

Women	Epidemiology	Men
Greater impact of obesity on HFpEF development		Higher rates of obstructive coronary artery disease translates to higher risk of HFrEF than HFpEF
Inflammatory-metabolic hypothesis		
	Cardiac aging	
Greater arterial elastance and earlier wave reflection		Greater myocardial necrosis in response to injury
Greater concentric remodeling, load-induced diastolic dysfunction		Adverse remodeling with aging
	Exercise hemodynamics	
Attenuated cardiac output reserve with exercise		Adverse RV-PA coupling with reduced RV contractile reserve
Greater rise in PCWP		
Poorer systemic and pulmonary artery compliance		
	Therapeutic response	
ARNI benefit due to relative natriuretic peptide deficit		ATTR as underlying pathology may limit neurohormonal blockade response
Significant sex treatment interaction with mineralocorticoid receptor antagonists		

Fig. 4. Sex differences in the pathophysiology and treatment of HFpEF.[36] https://elsevier.proofcentral.com/en-us/landing-page.html?token=91f01646h0cfe00085d7826448ca93.

to guide management. In the United States, over 50% recover with 2 to 6 months, with greater recovery odds associated with better preserved EF, earlier diagnosis, and non-Black race.[38] Management includes guideline-directed medical therapy for HFrEF and arrhythmias, a wearable or implanted defibrillator, and counseling against further pregnancy. Need for circulatory support with a ventricular assist device or heart transplantation is rare although nearly 50% who progress to transplant are of African American descent.

A detailed review of cardiovascular considerations and complications during pregnancy is provided by the American Heart Association.[38]

Heart Disease in Women—Cardiac Rehabilitation

There are 3 phases of CR in the continuum of care.

Phase 1

Inpatient CR is initiated immediately following a cardiac event or procedure including MI, percutaneous coronary intervention, CABG, left ventricular assist device implantation, or heart transplantation surgery.[39] Early mobilization in the intensive care unit[40] and focus on activities of daily living training is safe and encouraged as it results in better overall patient outcomes.[41] CR therapies include range of motion exercises, light strengthening/resistance training, bed mobility, transfer, balance and posture, gait training and can progress to light aerobic training in preparation for discharge home. The duration of Phase 1 ranges from days to weeks depending on the underlying cardiac diagnosis and procedure, medical complexities and functional deficits and can transition from the acute care hospital to the inpatient rehabilitation facility (IRF) for those meeting recognized IRF admission criteria. The goal of Phase 1 CR is to optimize medical status, improve functional independence and prepare patients and their caregivers for discharge to the community. Education on lifestyle and risk factor modifications is initiated. A referral for outpatient CR should be written at the time of hospital discharge to improve attendance with this next phase of CR.

Phase 2

Outpatient CR is a multidisciplinary comprehensive program including progressive aerobic exercise, education, nutrition guidance, risk factor modification, and psychosocial support. The CR team includes a supervising physician (cardiologist or physiatrist), CR-trained exercise physiologists and physical therapists, nutritionist, nurse, psychologist, and a social worker.

The pre-Phase 2 CR evaluation should include a detailed history and physical examination focusing on cardiovascular risk factors, family history, prior cardiovascular disease, and other conditions resulting from similar risk factors (COPD, stroke, PAD). A detailed psychosocial history can help identify barriers to CR participation in women with caregiver or work responsibilities and financial constraints resulting from co-payments and travel costs.

A review of relevant tests and investigations including the electrocardiogram, cardiac echo, cardiac catheterization, surgical report, blood laboratory tests including blood glucose, lipid studies, electrolytes, and complete blood count is completed. A pre-CR participation exercise stress test (EST) (treadmill or stationary bike) or 6-minute walk test (6MWT) helps determine exercise capacity, level of fitness, and facilitates risk stratification. Cardio-pulmonary (metabolic) exercise stress testing (CPET) when available provides additional diagnostic, physiologic, functional, and prognostic data regarding recurrent cardiac events and mortality.[42]

Intensity of exercise reflected by the training heart rate (THR) and/or rate of perceived exertion from the pre-CR participation EST is based on risk stratification models[43] establishing safety for exercise. The Karvonen formula is commonly used to determine the CR exercise THR based on risk stratification:

$$THR = RHR + [(PHR-RHR) \times Q]$$

THR—Training heart rate.
RHR—Resting heart rate from pre-CR EST.
PHR—Peak heart rate from pre-CR EST.
Q is a coefficient expressed as a percentage based on risk stratification for arrhythmia, ischemia and HF—low, moderate, high.

For patients considered low risk, a Q of 75% to 85% is acceptable. For patients considered moderate risk, a Q of 65% to 75% is selected. For patients considered high risk, a Q of 55% to 65% is selected. For patients on heart-rate limiting beta blockers, those post-heart transplant or ventricular assist device placement, heart rate response and the Karvonen formula are inaccurate. Other methods of setting exercise intensity can be used including the Rate of Perceived Exertion/Borg Scale at 13 to 14—somewhat hard, Dyspnea scales, and percentage of maximal aerobic capacity from CPET.

Aerobic exercise training sessions are physician-supervised and progressive in duration and intensity. The program consists of 36, 1-hour sessions, 2 to 3 times weekly for a total of 36 sessions. Each session is individualized for patients to achieve their THR and includes a warm up, 31 to 60 minutes of monitored exercise and a cool down.

Aerobic exercise can be prescribed as moderate intensity continuous exercise (MICE) or high-intensity interval training (HIIT). Typically, patients interested in and cleared for HIIT will start with MICE for 10 to 18 sessions and then slowly introduce HIIT. HIIT is safe for low and moderate risk patients, helps with long-term exercise adherence,[44] and is acceptable to women participating in CR programs.[45,46] HIIT can be less time-consuming and so a good option for those with caregiver and work commitments.[47]

Other essential elements of Phase 2 CR include education focusing on cardiovascular risk factors, secondary prevention, disease process, management of comorbidities and medications as well as strategies to implement lifestyle changes.[48] Education regarding exercise training and a focus on patient self-efficacy for self-monitored exercise facilitates the transition to independent exercise which is central in Phase 3 CR. Patients undergo nutritional counseling to assist with management of diabetes, weight, hypertension, and lipids.

Psychosocial support guides behavioral change, stress management, and the resolution of barriers to compliance with a heart-healthy lifestyle and CR completion. It increases overall benefits from CR, especially in women. Women are at higher risk for poor outcomes due to stress, anxiety, and depression after a cardiac event. Both individual and group sessions with a psychologist can help develop coping strategies, address stress reduction, and other mental health concerns.[49] A separate referral to a psychologist or a psychiatrist may be necessary based on individual symptoms.

Tobacco cessation when needed requires a multidisciplinary approach and is part of the CR program.[50] Tobacco use impairs endothelial function, increases in oxidative stress, inflammation, coronary vasoconstriction, and reduces oxygen delivery. Tobacco cessation lowers the risk of all-cause mortality, risk of death, recurrent MI and HF. It is imperative to address tobacco use as part of cardiovascular risk reduction[51] through individual and group counseling as well prescribing pharmacologic interventions.[52]

After completing the CR program an exit EST or CPET is recommended to provide objective measure to the gains made during the CR program and to facilitate prescription of an ongoing exercise program and heart-healthy lifestyle.

Phase 3

Maintenance CR is the lifelong continuance of all the elements of a heart healthy lifestyle initiated and progressed in Phase 2 outpatient CR. The lifelong phase is an ongoing partnership between the patient and the CR physician and includes progression of the self-monitored aerobic exercise to meet the physical activity guidelines of at least 150 minutes of moderate intense aerobic exercise and a goal of 300 minutes weekly.[53] Exercise is completed "in the community"—at home, in outdoor recreational areas and parks, and/or in a local gym. On-going monitoring and management of cardiac risk factors, dietary optimization, education, and psychosocial support is essential for long-term success.

Addressing Barriers to Cardiac Rehabilitation in Women

Despite the evidence base supporting Phase 2 outpatient CR, only 11% to 20% of eligible women have engaged in CR over the last 3 decades.[54] Women see similar improvements to men following CR, however, fewer women are referred to CR and fewer women enroll.[55] Referring physician bias that women do not benefit from CR results in low referral rates[56] despite the evidence supporting the benefit of CR for women. Women report that CR was not highly recommended by their physician, and this disparity is even greater for non-white women[57]; African American women are referred to CR at less than half the rate of white women.[58] Overall, men are 1.5x more likely to be referred to CR than women despite similar eligibility.[59] Attrition is high likely due to the pressures of conflicting life-responsibilities, the presence of exercise-limiting comorbidities, insurance issues including co-pays, and a lack of diversity in CR programs. Specificity of CR programs is also an issue as women have unique and differing health profiles compared with men at presentation of their HD and when they need CR. Women tend to be more physically deconditioned, older, widowed, or have an older spouse requiring care at the point of enrolling in CR. Older women lack ingrained exercise behaviors. Younger women entering CR have more tobacco use than older women, as well as worse perceived health, quality of life, hope and optimism, anxiety, depression, and perceived stress.[60] Women experience greater psychosocial impairments following a cardiac event such as impaired adjustment, increased anxiety and depression, sexual dysfunction, and nonreturn to work.[61]

Strategies to address disparities in CR overall also improve access for women. These include automatic referrals to CR at discharge, employing community health workers, lowering cost barriers (eg, "free" transportation, waiving copays, financial incentives for completing), alternative delivery methods (home, virtual, community, equitable access to technology), community partnerships, culturally tailored content, employing health equity metrics, and improving workforce diversity.[55] More women were found to enroll in CR if programs were targeted to older individuals. Programs that provide more social engagement such as support groups, and flexible scheduling may be particularly attractive to women.[58] Home-based CR has been shown to result in improved adherence and completion rates for women compared to in-person programs, with similar functional outcomes. Offering single gender women-only CR may reduce or eliminate the anxiety and depression that can accompany mixed-gender exercise programs. Programs looking to attract more women should also consider offering a wider range of exercise options such as yoga and dance. Women may also prefer not being rushed, crowded, or weighed.[54] Providing symbolic safety with inspirational décor and teaching patients how to check their own pulse may also attract more women to CR.[54]

CR tailored to level of ability is likely beneficial to younger women. Women with SCAD report that the pace of CR is too slow for their preference. HIIT provides faster-paced exercise and is associated with lower dropout rates. HIIT is equal or superior to MICE in improving cardiorespiratory fitness, glycemic control, vascular function, BP, and functional outcomes.[62,63] Additionally, HIIT improves the severity of anxiety, which likely contributes to the cardiovascular burden in women.[64] CR, by improving functional capacity and quality of life is of particular benefit to these psychosocial factors. CR is essential in secondary prevention following a cardiac event. CR improves exercise capacity and results in improvements in cardiovascular mortality and morbidity.[65] Other strategies described that can enable use of CR by women include patient choice of session time, invitations for informal care providers and/or partners to attend exercise sessions, CR staff that have expertise in women and HSs, separate change rooms for women and discussion of CR referral with patients.[66]

SUMMARY

The leading cause of morbidity and mortality in women is cardio-vascular disease. There are significant gender-related differences in risk factors, presenting symptoms and cardiac diagnoses which are often under-appreciated. CR is standard of care in the recovery from acute cardiac events as well as secondary prevention of future events. Fewer women compared with men are referred to and complete CR due to multifactorial reasons. As a result, outcomes in women following a cardiac event are worse compared with men. Outcomes in women completing CR equate to those seen in men. Individualizing the system of patient referral to CR and the CR program itself to meet the specific needs of women results in improved adherence to and optimization of outcomes from CR. Further effort is required to address and resolve these health care disparities in delivering CR to women with HD.

CLINICS CARE POINTS

- Over 60 million (44%) women in the United States have heart disease (HD) contributing to nearly 22% of all deaths in females in 2017.

- Coronary artery disease (CAD) is the most common type of HD in women present in 40% or older women and of note, risk factors for CAD (hypertension, diabetes, dyslipidemia, metabolic syndrome, overweight/obesity, physical inactivity, tobacco use) demonstrate significant gender specificity in terms of impact of development of CAD.

- Often underappreciated, underdiagnosed, and undertreated are the nontraditional risk factors for HD in women including gender-specific hormonal fluctuations, polycystic ovary syndrome, gestational diabetes, pre-eclampsia, preterm delivery, breast cancer therapies, and autoimmune disorders.

- Cardiac rehabilitation (CR) is a continuum of care from the time of the cardiac event if an inpatient—Phase 1, to the outpatient program when stabilized—Phase 2, and continuing in the community lifelong maintenance program—Phase 3.

- Phase 2 is an evidence-based comprehensive program including: exercise—36 sessions of physician supervised aerobic exercise; education—HDs and risk factors and heart-healthy lifestyle; nutrition—heart healthy diet and impact on risk factors; and support—behavioral change and emotional guidance.

- Intensity of the Phase 2 CR exercise is critical to achieve an aerobic stimulus, impact cardiovascular risk factors and is most often based on risk stratification models and reflected in a target training heart rate derived from the Karvonen formula.

- Women are less likely to be referred for, enroll in and complete CR than men, and African American women are referred for CR at half the rate as White women. Referral bias—potential referring physicians believing that women do not benefit from CR—significantly contributes.

- General strategies that improve access to CR for women include automated referrals for CR, lowering of cost barriers, home-based remotely monitored Phase 2 programs, culturally tailored programming, and improved workforce diversity.

- Specific "women-focused" strategies that improve access to CR for women include targeting the program to older individuals, provision of social support and interaction as part of the program, flexible exercise session schedules, home-based programs, single gender women-only sessions, and diverse exercise options including yoga and dance.

- CR in women has equal benefits (improved aerobic capacity; risk factor mitigation; reduction in cardiac events; reduced health care utilization; prolonged survival) to men.

DISCLOSURE

J.H. Whiteson, S. Prilik, and M.C. Glenn have no disclosures or conflicts of interest.

REFERENCES

1. Available at: https://www.medicare.gov/coverage/cardiac-rehabilitation.
2. Tsao CW, Aday AW, Almarzooq ZI, et al. Heart disease and stroke statistics-2023 update: a report from the American heart association [published online ahead of print, 2023 Jan 25]. Circulation 2023. https://doi.org/10.1161/CIR.0000000000001123.
3. Crea F, Battipaglia I, Andreotti F. Sex differences in mechanisms, presentation and management of ischaemic heart disease. Atherosclerosis 2015;241:157–68.
4. Mosca L, Hammond G, Mochari-Greenberger H, et al. American heart association cardiovascular disease and stroke in women and special populations committee of the council on clinical cardiology, council on epidemiology and prevention, council on cardiovascular nursing, council on high blood pressure research, and council on nutrition, physical activity and metabolism. Fifteen-Year trends in awareness of heart disease in women: results of a 2012 American heart association national survey. Circulation 2013;127(11):1254–63, e1–293.
5. Maas AH, Appelman YE. Gender differences in coronary heart disease. Neth Heart J 2010;18(12):598–602.
6. Benjamin EJ, Virani Salim S, Callaway Clifton W, et al. Heart disease and stroke statistics — 2018 update: a report from the American Heart Association. Circulation 2018;137(12):e67–492.
7. Peters SAE, Huxley RR, Woodward M. Diabetes as risk factor for incident coronary heart disease in women compared with men: a systematic review and meta-analysis of 64 cohorts including 858,507 individuals and 28,203 coronary events. Diabetologia 2014;57:1542–51.
8. Patel N, Mittal N, Wilkinson MJ, et al. Unique features of dyslipidemia in women across a lifetime and a tailored approach to management. Am J Prev Cardiol 2024;18:100666.
9. Fryar CD, Carroll MD, Afful J. Prevalence of overweight, obesity, and severe obesity among adults aged 20 and over: United States, 1960–1962 through 2017–2018. NCHS Health E-Stats, Centers for Disease Control and Prevention; 2020. Updated February 8, 2021. . Accessed January 29, 2021.
10. Elgaddal N, Kramarow EA, Reuben C. Physical activity among adults aged 18 and over: United States, 2020. NCHS Data Brief, no 443. Hyattsville, MD: National Center for Health Statistics; 2022.
11. Liang X, Or B, Tsoi MF, et al. Prevalence of metabolic syndrome in the United States national health and nutrition examination survey 2011–18. Postgrad Med 2023;99(1175):985–92.
12. Cornelius ME, Loretan CG, Jamal A, et al. Tobacco product use among adults - United States, 2021. MMWR Morb Mortal Wkly Rep 2023;72(18):475–83.
13. Kaminski P, Szpotanska-Sikorska M, Wielgos M, et al. Cardiovascular risk and the use of oral contraceptives. Neuroendocrinol Lett 2013;34(7):587–9.
14. Garcia M, Mulvagh SL, Merz CNB. Cardiovascular disease in women: clinical perspective. Circ Res 2016;118(8):1273–93.
15. Geraghty L, Figtree GA, Schutte AE, et al. Cardiovascular disease in women: from pathophysiology to novel and emerging risk factors. Heart Lung Circ 2021;30:9–17, 1443-9506/20/$36.00.
16. Lerner DJ, Kannel WB. Patterns of coronary heart disease morbidity and mortality in the sexes: a 26-year follow-up of the Framingham population. Am Heart J 1986; 111(2):383–90.
17. Daniels KM, Arena R, Lavie CJ, et al. Cardiac rehabilitation for women across the lifespan. Am J Med 2012;125(9):937.e1–7.

18. Wu P, Haththotuwa R, Kwok CS, et al. Preeclampsia and future cardiovascular health: a systematic review and meta-analysis. Circ Cardiovasc Qual Outcomes 2017;10(2):e003497.

19. Sara JD, Widmer RJ, Matsuzawa Y, et al. Prevalence of coronary microvascular dysfunction among patients with chest pain and nonobstructive coronary artery disease. JACC Cardiovasc Interv 2015;8(11):1445–53.

20. McAlister C, Alfadhel M, Samuel R, et al. Differences in demographics and outcomes between men and women with spontaneous coronary artery dissection. JACC Cardiovasc Interv 2022;15:2052–61.

21. Ofer Havakuk MD, Sorel Goland MD, Anil Mehra MD, et al. Pregnancy and the risk of spontaneous coronary artery dissection. An analysis of 120 contemporary cases. Circulation: Cardiovascular Interventions 2017;10(3). https://doi.org/10. 1161/CIRCINTERVENTIONS.117.004941.

22. Safdar B, Spatz ES, Dreyer RP, et al. Presentation, clinical profile, and prognosis of young patients with myocardial infarction with nonobstructive coronary arteries (MINOCA): results from the VIRGO study. J Am Heart Assoc 2018;7(13).

23. Canto JG, Goldberg RJ, Hand MM, et al. Symptom presentation of women with acute coronary syndromes: myth vs reality. Arch Intern Med 2007;167(22): 2405–13.

24. van Oosterhout REM, de Boer AR, Maas AHEM, et al. Sex differences in symptom presentation in acute coronary syndromes: a systematic review and meta-analysis. J Am Heart Assoc 2020;9(9). https://doi.org/10.1161/JAHA.119.014733.

25. Johnson HM, Gorre CE, Friedrich-Karnik A, et al. Addressing the bias in cardiovascular care: missed & delayed diagnosis of cardiovascular disease in women. Am J Prev Cardiol 2021;8:100299.

26. Peters SAE, Muntner P, Woodward M. Sex differences in the prevalence of, and trends in, cardiovascular risk factors, treatment, and control in the United States, 2001 to 2016. Circulation 2019;139:1025–35.

27. Ritcheya MD, Wall HK, Georgea MG, et al. US trends in premature heart disease mortality over the past 50 years: where do we go from here? Trends Cardiovasc Med 2020;30:364–74.

28. Johnson HM, Gorre CE, Friedrich-Karnik A, et al. Addressing the bias in cardiovascular care: missed & delayed diagnosis of cardiovascular disease in women. Am J Prev Cardiol 2021;8:100299.

29. Gulati M, Levy PD, Mukherjee D, et al. 2021 AHA/ACC/ASE/CHEST/SAEM/SCCT/ SCMR guideline for the evaluation and diagnosis of chest pain: a report of the American college of cardiology/American heart association joint committee on clinical practice guidelines. Circulation 2021;144(22):e368–454. Epub 2021 Oct 28. Erratum in: Circulation. 2021 Nov 30;144(22):e455. Erratum in: Circulation. 2023 Dec 12;148(24):e281. PMID: 34709879.

30. Virani SS, Newby LK, Arnold SV, et al, Peer Review Committee Members. 2023 AHA/ACC/ACCP/ASPC/NLA/PCNA guideline for the management of patients with chronic coronary disease: a report of the American heart association/American college of cardiology joint committee on clinical practice guidelines. Circulation 2023;148(9):e9–119. Epub 2023 Jul 20. Erratum in: Circulation. 2023 Sep 26;148(13):e148. Erratum in: Circulation. 2023 Dec 5;148(23):e186. PMID: 37471501.

31. Heidenreich PA, Bozkurt B, Aguilar D, et al. 2022 AHA/ACC/HFSA guideline for the management of heart failure: a report of the American college of cardiology/American heart association joint committee on clinical practice guidelines. Circulation 2022;145(18):e895–1032. Epub 2022 Apr 1. Erratum in: Circulation.

2022 May 3;145(18):e1033. Erratum in: Circulation. 2022 Sep 27;146(13):e185. Erratum in: Circulation. 2023 Apr 4;147(14):e674. PMID: 35363499.

32. Mieres JH, Shaw LJ, Arai A, et al. Role of non-invasive testing in the clinical evaluation of women with suspected coronary artery disease. Circulation 2005;111: 682–96.

33. Zhao M, Woodward M, Vaartjes I, et al. Sex differences in cardiovascular medication prescription in primary care: a systematic review and meta-analysis. J Am Heart Assoc 2020;9(11):e014742. Epub 2020 May 20. PMID: 32431190; PMCID: PMC7429003.

34. DesJardin JT, Chikwe J, Hahn RT, et al. Sex differences and similarities in valvular heart disease. Circ Res 2022;130(4):455–73.

35. Zeitler EP, Poole JE, Albert CM, et al. Arrhythmias in female patients: incidence, presentation and management. Circ Res 2022;130:474–95.

36. DeFilippis EM, Beale A, Martyn T, et al. Heart failure subtypes and cardiomyopathies in women. Circ Res 2022;130(4):436–54.

37. Aimo A, Panichella G, Garofalo M, et al. Sex differences in transthyretin cardiac amyloidosis. Heart Fail Rev 2024;29:321–30.

38. Mehta LS, Warnes CA, Bradley E, et al, On behalf of the American Heart Association Council on Clinical Cardiology, Council on Arteriosclerosis, Thrombosis and Vascular Biology, Council on Cardiovascular and Stroke Nursing; and Stroke Council. Cardiovascular considerations in caring for pregnant patients: a scientific statement from the American heart association. Circulation 2020;141: e884–903.

39. Simon M, Korn K, Cho L, et al. Cardiac rehabilitation: a class 1 recommendation. Cleve Clin J Med 2018;85(7):551–8.

40. Corcoran JR, Herbsman JM, Bushnik T, et al. Early rehabilitation in the medical and surgical intensive care units for patients with and without mechanical ventilation: an interprofessional performance improvement project. Pharm Manag PM R 2017;9(2):113–9. Epub 2016 Jun 23. PMID: 27346093.

41. Kourek C, Dimopoulos S. Cardiac rehabilitation after cardiac surgery: an important underutilized treatment strategy. World J Cardiol 2024;16(2):67–72.

42. Taylor JL, Bonikowske AR, Olson TP. Optimizing outcomes in cardiac rehabilitation: the importance of exercise intensity. Front Cardiovasc Med 2021;8: 734278. Published 2021 Sep 3.

43. Williams MA. Exercise testing in cardiac rehabilitation. Exercise prescription and beyond. Cardiol Clin 2001;19(3):415–31.

44. Kramps K, Lane-Cordova A. High-intensity interval training in cardiac rehabilitation. Sport Sci Health 2021;17:269–78.

45. Khadanga S, Savage PD, Pecha A, et al. Optimizing training response for women in cardiac rehabilitation: a randomized clinical trial. JAMA Cardiol 2022;7(2): 215–8.

46. Dun Y, Smith JR, Liu S, et al. High-intensity interval training in cardiac rehabilitation. Clin Geriatr Med 2019;35(4):469–87.

47. Reed JL, Keast ML, Beanlands RA, et al. The effects of aerobic interval training and moderate-to-vigorous intensity continuous exercise on mental and physical health in women with heart disease. Eur J Prev Cardiol 2019;26(2):211–4.

48. Centers for Disease Control and Prevention. Cardiac Rehabilitation Change Package. Second Edition. Atlanta (GA): Centers for Disease Control and Prevention, US Department of Health and Human Services; 2023.

49. Bozkurt B, Fonarow GC, Goldberg LR, et al. Cardiac rehabilitation for patients with heart failure: JACC expert panel. J Am Coll Cardiol 2021;77(11):1454–69.

50. Bartels MN, Prince DZ. Acute medical conditions: cardiopulmonary disease, medical frailty, and renal failure. Braddom's Phys. Med. Rehabil 2021;511–34.e515.
51. Mola A, Lloyd M, Villegas-Pantoja M. A mixed method review of tobacco cessation for the cardiopulmonary rehabilitation clinician. J Cardpulm Rehabil Prev 2017;37(3):160–74.
52. Mampuya WM. Cardiac rehabilitation past, present and future: an overview. Cardiovasc Diagn Ther 2012;2(1):38–49.
53. Katrina L, Troiano RP, Ballard RM, et al. The physical activity guidelines for Americans. JAMA 2018;320(19):2020–8.
54. Mamataz T, Ghisi GLM, Pakosh M, et al. Nature, availability, and utilization of women-focused cardiac rehabilitation: a systematic review. BMC Cardiovasc Disord 2021;21(1):459.
55. Mathews L, Brewer LC. A review of disparities in cardiac rehabilitation: evidence, drivers, and solutions. J Cardiopulm Rehabil Prev 2021;41(6):375–82.
56. Beckstead JW, Pezzo MV, Beckie TM, et al. Physicians' tacit and stated policies for determining patient benefit and referral to cardiac rehabilitation. Med Decis Mak Int J Soc Med Decis Mak 2014;34(1):63–74.
57. Mochari H, Lee JR, Kligfield P, et al. Ethnic differences in barriers and referral to cardiac rehabilitation among women hospitalized with coronary heart disease. Prev Cardiol 2006;9(1):8–13.
58. Sawan MA, Calhoun AE, Fatade YA, et al. Cardiac rehabilitation in women, challenges and opportunities. Prog Cardiovasc Dis 2022;70:111–8.
59. Mathews L, Brewer LC. A review of disparities in cardiac rehabilitation: evidence, drivers, and solutions. J Cardiopulm Rehabil Prev 2021;41(6):375–82.
60. Beckie TM, Fletcher G, Groer MW, et al. Biopsychosocial health disparities among young women enrolled in cardiac rehabilitation. J Cardiopulm Rehabil Prev 2015;35(2):103–13.
61. Gardner JK, McConnell TR, Klinger TA, et al. Quality of life and self-efficacy: gender and diagnoses considerations for management during cardiac rehabilitation. J Cardpulm Rehabil 2003;23(4):299–306.
62. Way KL, Reed JL. Meeting the needs of women in cardiac rehabilitation. Circulation 2019;139(10):1247–8.
63. Moncion K, Rodrigues L, Wiley E, et al. Aerobic exercise interventions for promoting cardiovascular health and mobility after stroke: a systematic review with Bayesian network meta-analysis. Br J Sports Med 2024;58(7):392–400.
64. Way KL, Reed JL. Meeting the needs of women in cardiac rehabilitation. Circulation 2019;139(10):1247–8.
65. Daniels KM, Arena R, Lavie CJ, et al. Cardiac rehabilitation for women across the lifespan. Am J Med 2012;125(9):937.e1–7.
66. Ghisi GLM, Supervia M, Turk-Adawi K, et al. Women-focused cardiac rehabilitation delivery around the world and program enablers to support broader implementation. CJC Open 2023;6(2Part B):425–35. PMID: 38487061; PMCID: PMC10935990.

Rehabilitation Considerations in Women with Traumatic Brain Injury

Christine Greiss, DO*, Arielle Berkowitz, DO, Jessie P. Chan, MD, Ally Ferber, MD

KEYWORDS

- TBI women • Gender • Neuroinflammation • Estrogen • LGBTQIA+

KEY POINTS

- The physiologic/anatomic differences between men and women impact symptomatology, prognosis, and functional outcome following traumatic brain injury (TBI).
- Hormonal fluctuations over a woman's lifetime can impact TBI susceptibility/outcomes.
- Women have a higher prevalence of post-TBI depression, anxiety, and posttraumatic stress disorder compared to men.
- Women with TBI encounter unique challenges in regards to social/sexual intimacy, self-esteem, and relationships highlighting the necessary social support for successful reintegration into the community.
- It is important to consider domestic violence in the diagnosis and management of TBI in female individuals.

INTRODUCTION

Traumatic brain injury (TBI) poses a significant public health concern with unique challenges in both diagnosis and treatment. Female TBI survivors face distinct challenges and barriers, compared to their male counterparts, given the anatomic, hormonal, socioeconomic, and cultural differences. The goal of this study is to enhance the understanding of, and provide guidance for, a more effective/tailored approach to treatment and rehabilitation for the female TBI population.

PHYSIOLOGIC/HORMONAL CHANGES

Numerous physiologic changes occur after TBI, many of which may impact certain populations more than others. It has been postulated that estrogen has neuroprotective

Department of Physical Medicine and Rehabilitation, JFK Johnson Rehabilitation Institute, Hackensack Meridian Health, 65 James Street, Edison, NJ 08820, USA
* Corresponding author.
E-mail address: christine.greiss@hmhn.org

Phys Med Rehabil Clin N Am 36 (2025) 239–251
https://doi.org/10.1016/j.pmr.2024.11.002
1047-9651/25/© 2024 Elsevier Inc. All rights are reserved, including those for text and data mining, AI training, and similar technologies.

effects through the reduction of neuroinflammation and maintenance of the blood–brain barrier. In a study by Khaksari and colleagues,[1] exogenous estrogen administered after TBI decreased inflammation through reduction of proinflammatory cytokine tumor necrosis factor-alpha. In turn, reduced 17b-estradiol has been shown to contribute to increased brain damage.[2] Following TBI, women have higher levels of testosterone, which suggests an impaired conversion to estrogen. Men, who lack estradiol receptors, tend to show worse outcomes after TBI.[3]

Like estrogen, progesterone and its metabolites may have neuroprotective effects. Progesterone protects glial cells from brain edema, necrosis, apoptosis, and inflammation.[4,5] Nevertheless, women of childbearing age, when progesterone peaks, tend to have the worst outcomes compared to women of other age groups.[6] The significant changes in progesterone levels during a woman's menstrual cycle have been implicated as an explanation. The dramatic drop in progesterone following TBI, in addition to the luteal phase of menstruation, causes a noteworthy drop in progesterone leading to worse outcomes, known as the "withdrawal hypothesis."[7] From this, estrogen and progesterone appear to be influential in neuroprotection after TBI.

The Progesterone for Traumatic Brain Injury, Experimental Clinical Treatment double-blinded multicenter clinical trial presented exogenous progesterone to patients with moderate–severe TBI in an effort to improve outcomes. At 6 months after injury, there was no significant benefit in outcome identified with the use of the Glasgow Outcome Scale-Extended (GOSE), Disability Rating Scale, and/or patient mortality rates.[8]

Given the fluctuation of hormone levels throughout the female lifespan, it is crucial to consider the timing of TBI. In a study by Wunderle and colleagues,[7] reproductive-aged female individuals presenting to the emergency department within 4 hours after a mild TBI (mTBI) endorsed greater postconcussive symptoms 3 months after injury, suspected to be related to the disruption of endogenous sex hormone production. Injuries during the luteal phase of menses showed worse quality of life scores at 1 month compared to women injured during the follicular phase or on oral contraceptives (OCP). Women with high levels of progesterone during and after injury (taking OCPs) had outcomes that were similar to those injured during the follicular phase.[7]

The pregnant woman experiences hormonal and hematologic changes such as reduced progesterone and increased clotting factors. In addition, pregnancy leads to physiologic alterations including vasodilation, hemodilution, increased cardiac output, and greater oxygen demand, in an effort to support the growing fetus. Following TBI, pregnant women must be monitored for miscarriage, premature labor, and additional complications including deep vein thrombosis with careful use and consideration of medications.[9]

Menstrual irregularities are well recognized after TBI; however, it remains unclear if hormonal changes play a role in the potential trauma and stress response. In a study of 30 participants, 60% with severe TBI, there was a significant increase in missed cycles and dysmenorrhea after injury compared to preinjury. Although TBI severity had no correlation with amenorrhea duration, there was a significant correlation with posttraumatic amnesia (PTA). For every 1 day increase in PTA, there was a 2% increase in the duration of amenorrhea. Duration of amenorrhea was associated with worse Short Form 12-item Health Survey, GOSE, and Mayo-Portland Adaptability Inventory participation subscale scores (114–344 days) when controlling for severity of injury, age, and time after injury. Prolonged amenorrhea was associated with lower quality of life, global outcome, and community participation. There was no difference in preinjury and postinjury fertility; however, only 4 patients became pregnant.[10]

There is scarce literature on female fertility and pregnancy complications despite the known dysfunction of the gonadal pituitary axis. Anto-Ocrah and colleagues[11] identified a lower incidence of pregnancy among concussed female individuals 2 years after injury compared to orthopedic-injured controls, in addition to lower incidence of pregnancy in patients with menstrual disruption following TBI. Colantonio and colleagues[12] reported a lower percentage of attempted/successful pregnancy after severe TBI compared to matched controls but also monitored premenopausal women age 5 to 12 years after moderate–severe TBI and found no significant difference in fertility between women with TBI and controls. However, women with TBI had fewer children overall. This demonstrates the gap in knowledge of TBI's effects on fertility.

Interestingly, patients with TBI had higher rate of induction, use of operative vaginal deliveries, unplanned and elective cesarean sections, and were more likely to use epidural and spinal pain-reducing agents.[13,14] Patients with previous TBI had slightly increased preterm and low birth weight infants, thus putting the infants at risk for requiring intensive monitoring.[13] Adams and colleagues[14] found women with TBI were at a higher risk of placental abruption, infants large for gestational age, and a drastically higher risk of stillbirth. Additionally, there were postpregnancy complications such as pain, fatigue, depression, and cognitive disorder. These findings highlight the need for identifying history of TBI in a female's obstetric and gynecologic visits as crucial information could significantly impact pregnancy and deliveries. Research is needed to focus on long-term menstrual restoration, fertility, and other menstrual abnormalities, with differentiation between the stress response and direct trauma to the pituitary gland.[10]

Perimenopausal and menopausal women may be at higher risk of detrimental effects after TBI compared to their younger counterparts. Blaya and colleagues[15] observed worse somatic/cognitive symptoms after TBI in women aged 35 to 49 years compared to younger female individuals. This is possibly due to the loss of ovarian function with age causing a decline of estrogen and progesterone levels with resultant increase in chronic low-grade inflammation.[15] Perimenopause is thus an inflammatory state predisposing an exacerbation of neurologic symptoms and worsening secondary injury. Elderly female individuals have hormonal levels near that of male individuals, thus the difference in TBI outcomes in this age group is likely attributable to other factors, such as the increased risk of frailty and osteoporosis secondary to decreased estrogen after menopause.

In addition to hormonal fluctuations, it has been found that cerebral blood flow and neuroinflammation also differ based on sex and age following TBI. In a study by Wagner and colleagues,[16] women had fewer cerebrospinal fluid markers of excitotoxicity compared to male individuals. It was also noted that older women had higher markers of oxidative stress compared to younger women suggesting higher susceptibility to secondary brain damage. Women aged under 50 years had higher intracerebral pressures, brain swelling, and increased mortality at 6 months after injury compared to female individuals aged over 50 years.[17]

PSYCHOLOGICAL AND COGNITIVE CHANGES

Human behavior is a complex, multifaceted phenomenon that is impacted by nature and nurture. Following TBI, structural alterations to the brain, damage to the limbic system, changes to neurotransmitters (serotonin, dopamine, gamma-aminobutyric acid [GABA], glutamate, acetylcholine, and norepinephrine), and the psychological response to injury, place both men and women at an increased risk for neuropsychiatric disorders.[18]

Men and women experience unique clinical outcomes following TBI as a result of differing hormones, anatomy, and functionality of the brain at baseline.[19,20] Women tend to have more "bilateral representation of verbal abilities and performance IQ than men."[21] Despite these biologic/structural differences, women also tend to have a unique "growing environment, neurodevelopment, and sociologic attributes" leading to specific neuropsychological outcomes.[19] While gene expression can alter cell protein production through neurotransmitter signal cascades, our environment also has the capability to alter gene expression through the activation/silencing of histones in a phenomenon known as epigenetics.[22]

Mood Disorders

Depression in the general population has a prevalence of 8% to 10%, with a 70% increased likelihood of depression in women compared to men.[18,23] This higher risk of depression in women has been attributed to "gonadal hormones, early life stressors, reductions in brain volumes, and/or history of abuse in early life."[24] Of note, the (Diagnostic and Statistical Manual of Mental Illnesses 5 [DSM5]) used to diagnose neuropsychiatric disorders has also been postulated to be better geared toward detecting the depressive symptoms expressed by women.[18]

Within the first year following TBI, 25% to 65% of patients are diagnosed with depression. As this population faces new challenges and adapts to changes in professional life, family life, and the community, the apparent obstacles cause a rise in stress and depressive symptoms.[25] Along with depression comes the increased risk for social isolation, hostility, and cognitive decline that are only amplified by brain injury.[18] Almost a quarter (21-22%) of TBI survivors experience suicidal ideation (SI) placing them at an increased risk for suicide. Data suggests that following a severe TBI, patients have a 3 to 4 time higher relative risk of suicide compared to the general population. Decreased brain-derived neurotrophic factor functioning as well as serotonin/norepinephrine dysregulation has been hypothesized to play a role in depression/suicidality following TBI.[26]

Women with TBI are also more likely to have higher levels of depressive symptoms, perceived stress, and motor/cognitive/somatic symptoms, compared to men following a mild/moderate brain injury.[23,24] Women not only tend to report depressive symptoms more frequently than men following TBI but also report differing concerns to health care providers. Women report psychosomatic symptoms, including pain and sleep disturbance, whereas men tend to present with cognitive difficulties including concentration issues.[18,24]

Many differences have been attributed to the unique gender responsibilities and expectations of women. Women with TBI often endorse challenges including an "altered sense of self, issues with power, control, and isolation, as well as an alteration in caring and gender roles." Many women report feeling vulnerable and share a fear of feeling stigmatized." Fabricius and colleagues[27] discuss the consequences of no longer being able to "do gender" the way that they performed preinjury. There is "guilt and shame" of inadequately performing gender roles. This study also highlights difficulty in "navigating the health care system from a subordinate social position undermining self-advocacy and patient credibility." Despite these challenges, Oyesanya and colleagues[23] report that many women continue to care for themselves with little to no assistance, and often, receive poor self-care. Many women have poor long-term outcomes including return to work (RTW) with only 51% of women returning to work compared to 66% of men.

Women, regardless of TBI history, are 4 fold more likely than men to have an anxiety disorder. Generalized anxiety disorder (GAD) and posttraumatic stress disorder

(PTSD) are more commonly seen in the TBI population compared to the general public. Anxiety disorders following TBI have a prevalence of 19% to 50% and tend to emerge earlier following TBI than mood disorders.[25] Albicini and colleagues[28] reported that children who endured moderate/severe brain injuries, particularly female individuals, were more likely to experience psychological effects later in life compared to young male individuals with mild injuries. In this study, patients with a childhood TBI not only had a 5 fold increased likelihood of anxiety disorder later in life but also a 4 fold increased chance of panic attacks, specific phobias, and depression. Anxiety in patients with TBI has been linked to poor social interpersonal functioning, decline in independent living, and is a positive predictor of depression. Anxiety disorders frequently coincide with depression (75% of the time) as well as substance abuse, attention-deficit hyperactivity disorder (ADHD), bipolar disorder, pain disorders, and sleep disorders.[22,25]

PTSD following TBI is a consequence of the co-occurring psychological trauma of the injury rather than by the biomechanical force to the brain. TBI is a risk factor for the development of PTSD with a rate of 12% to 30% in mild, 15% to 27% in moderate, and 3% to 23% in severe TBI.[22] Patients with mTBI have an increased risk of PTSD by a factor of 1.23, and patients with moderate/severe TBI have an increased risk factor of 1.71. Other risks include lower education, black race, and young age. The lifetime prevalence of PTSD is 10% to 12% in women and 5% to 6% in men. Women seem to have higher subcluster scores for PTSD than men, which could be due to variations in the hypothalamuc-pituitary-adrenal (HPA) axis and oxytocin levels.[29]

Postinjury mania "elevated/expansive or irritable" mood with at least 4 of the following: "inflated self-esteem/grandiosity, increased goal directed activity or agitation, risk taking, decreased need for sleep, distractibility, pressured speech, and racing thoughts" is a less common mood disorder appearing in TBI approximately 1.7% to 9% of the time.[25] While mania is due to excess monoamine transmitters, both depression and mania can occur simultaneously.[22]

Affective Disorders

Affective disorders involve "emotional dyscontrol" and are "brief, discrete episodes of abnormal emotions" that last seconds to minutes. Emotional dyscontrol includes pseudobulbar affect (PBA), affective lability, and irritability. PBA is a form of emotional dyscontrol with "brief, stereotyped, intense, and uncontrollable episodes of laughing or crying." The prevalence of PBA in TBI has been reported to be 21.4%, 17.5%, and 15.5% at 3, 6, and 12 months, respectively, after injury. Women, and those with left-sided lesions, more commonly present with pathologic crying, whereas pathologic laughing may be more prevalent in men and those with right-sided lesions.[25] Affective lability, becoming "overcome by intense emotions in reaction to stimuli of personal or social import," has been seen in 28% of mTBI and 33% to 46% early postinjury, and 14% to 62% later postinjury in severe TBI. Irritability, becoming "impatient, annoyed, easily angered," increases following a TBI with approximately 63%, 69%, and 71% of patients with moderate to severe experiencing this at 3, 6, and 12 months.[25]

Cognition

In general, women perform better than men on verbal memory and perceptual motor speed tasks, whereas men tend to perform better in visual-spatial, mental rotation, and quantitative problem-solving tasks.[20] Following TBI, there is an increased risk of cognitive dysfunction including, but not limited to, attention, processing speed, verbal/working memory, and language/communication.[19] Worsening cognitive abilities result in an increased likelihood of worse social, emotional, physical, and mental health function. Pre-existing conditions including learning disabilities, ADHD, and prior brain trauma may contribute to these cognitive impairments following brain trauma.[25]

Liossi and colleagues[21] reported that women were significantly more impaired in verbal and visual memory following TBI than men. Hui-Ling Hsu and colleagues provided objective fMRI evidence of hypoactivation of the working memory circuit in women, compared to men, following mTBI. Women may have more ongoing working memory issues following TBI compared to men. Women in the study also had more difficulty performing the total digit span compared to men following brain injury.[30] Ma and colleagues[19] reported that men with TBI more commonly had better recovery of verbal tasks while women with TBI showed quicker advances in spatial positioning.

Sleep

In the discussion of mental health following TBI, the bidirectional impact of sleep on psychological/cognitive function is paramount. Following TBI, there is a 46% prevalence in sleep disturbance. Following an mTBI, there is an increased prevalence of insomnia (29%), sleep apnea (25%), hypersomnia (28%), and narcolepsy (4%). Patients with TBI are noted to have a longer sleep onset latency, shorter sleep duration, increased nighttime awakenings, and decreased rapid eye movement (REM) sleep. This poor quality/quantity of sleep leads to increased fatigue and worsened cognitive function/behavioral outcomes.[31]

SOCIAL AND INTIMATE RELATIONSHIPS
Socialization

Due to the effects on cognition and communication, TBI during adolescence and adulthood can result in difficulties with social relationships, leading to isolation. Social intimacy is a fundamental need met via physical and sexual intimacy, friendships, self-conceptualization, and communication. TBI can lead to difficulty with the interpretation of emotions, tones of voice, social cues, emotional lability, impulsivity, inappropriate affect, and slowed or impaired speech all of which can decrease one's ability to participate socially. Female patients with TBI report higher rates of loss of confidence, depression, anxiety, stress, and loss of trust leading to social isolation and increased risk of physical, sexual, and psychological abuse.[32] There is evidence that female gender confers an emotional recognition advantage following TBI. Pediatric female patients with TBI perform better on facial affect-recognition tasks following injury and improve faster over time as compared to pediatric male patients with TBI. Adult female individuals with TBI significantly outperform adult male individuals with TBI in dynamic emotional recognition tasks; differences in performance were not seen in non-TBI control groups and were not correlated with location of lesions.[33] This is bolstered by findings showing that women experience better social outcomes following TBI compared to men.[34]

With social media use, many individuals with TBI are utilizing technology to build relationships and community.[32] In related studies, participants aged under 65 years, especially those ages 18 to 29 years, were more likely to use social media.[32,35] There are benefits to incorporating social media and Internet education into therapies, to teach patients the nuances of Internet communication needed to build and maintain healthy social relationships online. Critically, gender-appropriate and developmentally appropriate training should be provided to patients and caretakers regarding online safety, privacy, cyberbullying, and overuse; this is especially important for girls and women with TBI who are at an increased risk of sexual exploitation through manipulative intimate relationships online.[32]

In the care of patients with TBI, it is also important to acknowledge the value of both genetically related and chosen families for social, physical, and emotional connection and support. Challenges in the care of lesbian, gay, bisexual, transsexual, queer/questioning, intersex, and asexual (LGBTQIA+) populations with TBI may arise if sexual orientation or an intimate partner was not known to family prior to injury. Partnerships without an established legal relationship have issues with legal or medical decision-making, leading to increased financial and insurance-related stressors.[36]

Sexual Dysfunction

The barriers to social communication following TBI also influence romantic and sexual relationships. Changes in fatigue, mood, mobility, sensation, and self-image can affect new or pre-existing intimate relationships.[37] Approximately 80% of people resume sexual activity following TBI but 33% report reduced sexual frequency, desire, and function. Women are more likely to report sexual dissatisfaction, dysfunction, and lowered self-esteem as compared to men following TBI.[37,38] These women commonly report anorgasmia and men report reduced sexual desire.[38] More men receive information about sexual activity after TBI compared to women, but there is no gender difference regarding interest in or perceived importance of sex and intimacy education. Ninety-seven percent of surveyed health care professionals reported that it is important to discuss sexual function following TBI, but only 36% addressed it with patients.[37]

Health care providers should provide education regarding intimacy and sexual activity following TBI. Resources suggest the permission (P), limited information (LI), specific suggestions (SS), and intensive therapy (IT) (PLISSIT) model to assess sexuality in brain injury rehabilitation; this model is commonly used in the field of sex therapy and offers a framework to evaluate and address sexual concerns (**Fig. 1**). In addition to specific concerns, providers can offer generalized education regarding anatomy, sexual function, sex and intimacy communication, sexuality, sexual and gender identity, relationships, and coping with changes and stressors.[37] In patients reporting sexual dysfunction, consider causes such as medication side effects and physical

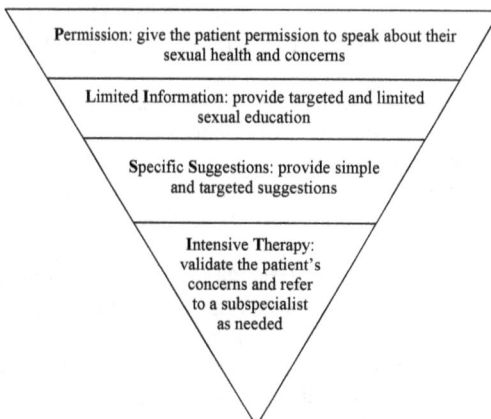

Permission: give the patient permission to speak about their sexual health and concerns

Limited Information: provide targeted and limited sexual education

Specific Suggestions: provide simple and targeted suggestions

Intensive Therapy: validate the patient's concerns and refer to a subspecialist as needed

Fig. 1. The PLISSIT model, an inverted pyramid framework to assess and address sexuality.

impairments.[38] Encourage patients to explore both solo and partnered sexual activity as they adjust to changes in mobility and sensation following TBI; women are more likely to be open to or have already tried sexual aids and toys at time of counseling.[37]

Divorce rates after TBI are estimated to be between 15% and 54%; longer duration of relationship prior to injury and older age were protective factors. Longer loss of consciousness was associated with higher divorce rates, but there was no association with duration of PTA. Divorce rates were higher in patients who experienced TBI secondary to physical violence. There was no statistically significant difference in divorce rate whether the brain injury survivor was the male or female partner in a heterosexual marriage.[39]

A major research gap regarding brain injury and intimate LGBTQIA+ relationships exists due to lack of advocacy in a health system that fails to fully meet their needs. LGBTQIA+ patients with TBI may fear discrimination or dismissal of sexual concerns from health care professionals. It is important not to assume heterosexuality or monogamy in patients and to provide the same level of care when providing sexuality and intimacy education. Additional considerations include differences in tools and resources for safe sex practices and adaptive positions for impaired mobility. Depending on local regulations, there may be legal issues surrounding postinjury sexual counseling and education in locations with laws against anal sex or lack of recognition of LGBTQIA+ couples.[36]

Domestic Violence

Intimate partner violence (IPV), a subset of domestic violence, is defined as "behaviors that are intended to exert power and control over another individual, including physical, sexual, verbal, emotional, and financial abuse, and/or stalking."[40] Girls and women between the ages of 18 and 34 years are at the greatest risk of IPV; approximately 44% of women in the general population experience IPV in their lifetime.[41,42] Additionally, TBI and IPV are intricately related risk factors for each other.[43] Female TBI survivors often suffer from cognitive impairments leading to impulsivity and compromised decision-making. They may be at an increased risk of sexual, physical, and psychological abuse.[32] In addition to women, thousands of heterosexual and homosexual men are victims of IPV each year.[44] Women who are military veterans, Native American, Black, or immigrant Asian are at an increased risk of IPV. The LGBTQIA+ community has increased rates of IPV compared to their cisgendered, heterosexual counterparts; this is attributed to minority stressors, reduced reporting due to fear of discrimination, mistreatment, and/or not being believed by police and health care workers.[43]

Symptoms of TBI in survivors of IPV are often missed during routine medical evaluation, especially when they resemble the effects of drugs and alcohol use.[43] They include headache, confusion, memory loss, emotional lability, posttraumatic wound infection, and genitourinary dysfunction such as vaginal infections and bleeding, sexually transmitted infections, pelvic pain, and urinary tract infections.[43,44] Among women who present with unverifiable injuries, the presence of head, neck, and face injuries increases the risk of IPV victimhood by 24%.[45] Strangulation is life-threatening, strongly associated with IPV, and approximately 50% of cases do present with any visible marks upon the neck.[46] Instead, survivors present with petechial hemorrhage, throat pain, voice hoarseness, painful swallowing, and mental status changes secondary to hypoxia.[46,47] Computed tomography and MRI of the head can detect maxillofacial injuries and large brain contusions or bleeds but are not useful for the detection of mTBI.[44]

VOCATIONAL/COMMUNITY REINTEGRATION
Vocational Rehabilitation

An estimated 18% to 60% of patients RTW after TBI.[48] Women with TBI who are unemployed prior to injury are less likely to be employed postinjury and also experience decreased economic quality of life postinjury, regardless of employment status.[49] The vast variability of RTW rates is due to different TBI severities, follow-up times, sample sizes, and definitions of RTW. Both personal and environmental factors emerged as hindrances to returning to work.[48]

One study of patients with mTBI without structured rehabilitation reported an RTW rate of 62% at 1 year after injury.[49] Several factors complicate the process of RTW, including postconcussion symptoms, demographic factors, preinjury occupational status, previous psychiatric history, and injury severity.[50,51] A National Institutes of Health consensus panel on TBI has suggested that women need more attention in the work setting, indicating that men and women experience different cognitive, emotional, and vocational outcomes following TBI.[49]

Vocational rehabilitation proved successful in establishing worker identity among participants; however, particular focus should be placed on the function-dysfunction continuum of the process of workplace integration to further develop and enhance sustainable RTW programs for women with TBI.[52] Results of a recent Science Direct study suggest that the Compensatory Cognitive Training-Supported Employment intervention might help patients with mild-to-moderate TBI who are still sick-listed 8 to 12 weeks after injury in an earlier return to stable employment.[53,54] Many included patients were female individuals (59%), most were highly educated, and most had an mTBI (94%).[55] Several studies evaluated differences in injury severity, demographics, neuropsychological abilities, and vocational and financial outcomes for 78 persons with TBI (55 male, 23 female) who received services from the state Vocational Rehabilitation Division (DVR). Despite similar injury severity, neuropsychological, and demographic characteristics, more men (43.6%) received maintenance services from DVR than women (21.7%). Of note, only 4.4% of the women were successfully employed through DVR, compared to 23.6% of the men. In addition, 73.9% of the women had services terminated after being accepted by DVR but before services were initiated, compared to 56.4% of the men. The significance of these results and their limitations are still in discussion, and further research is needed regarding this gender discrepancy.[56]

Community Integration

Community integration is an essential component for rehabilitation among TBI survivors, which yields positive outcomes in terms of social activities, community participation, and productive work. A factor that usually facilitates community integration among TBI survivors is social support, whereas physical environment and fatigue are most often found as barriers.[57]

SUMMARY

Rehabilitation in women with TBI necessitates a focused approach, encompassing hormonal changes, menstrual cycle, and reproductive lifespan. These factors can significantly influence mood, cognition, and recovery time. Additionally, financial stressors, along with psychosocial issues, can exacerbate recovery challenges. The return to vocational duties/community integration can often be difficult, necessitating specialized support and intervention. Therefore, a comprehensive rehabilitation plan for women with TBI should consider all of these significant aspects to improve outcomes.

CLINICS CARE POINTS

- It is important to consider the fluctuations in estrogen/progesterone levels throughout the female lifespan and to recognize these hormonal differences between the sexes, when providing treatment to patients following TBI.

- Following TBI, women are as likely as men to value, but less likely to receive, information regarding resuming sexual activity and navigating challenges with intimacy; health care providers should regularly incorporate sexual education and counseling as part of care.

- Differences in male versus female anatomy, hormones, and societal stressors contribute to differing outcomes in psychological/cognitive changes following TBI. Physicians should be aware of, and screen for, these clinical changes, and be able to provide support and appropriate medical care to these patients in an effort to improve mental health and quality of life.

- Community reintegration of women with TBI requires a multidisciplinary approach to address education, family involvement, and community resources to target concerns related to childcare, household management, vocational training, and ongoing cognitive support.

DISCLOSURE

The authors have no competing interests and will not gain financial benefit from this research. This research received no specific funding, grant, or equipment from any source in the public, commercial, or not-for-profit sectors.

REFERENCES

1. Khaksari M, Keshavarzi Z, Gholamhoseinian A, et al. The effect of female sexual hormones on the intestinal and serum cytokine response after traumatic brain injury: different roles for estrogen receptor subtypes. Can J Physiol Pharmacol 2013;91(9):700–7.
2. Roof RL, Hall ED. Estrogen-related gender difference in survival rate and cortical blood flow after impact-acceleration head injury in rats. J Neurotrauma 2000; 17(12):1155–69.
3. Garringer JA, Niyonkuru C, McCullough EH, et al. Impact of aromatase genetic variation on hormone levels and global outcome after severe TBI. J Neurotrauma 2013; 30(16):1415–25.
4. Shear DA, Galani R, Hoffman SW, et al. Progesterone protects against necrotic damage and behavioral abnormalities caused by traumatic brain injury. Exp Neurol 2002;178(1):59–67.
5. He J, Evans C, Hoffman S, et al. Progesterone and allopregnanolone reduce inflammatory cytokines after traumatic brain injury. Exp Neurol 2004;189(2):404–12.
6. Bazarian JJ, Blyth B, Mookerjee S, et al. Sex differences in outcome after mild traumatic brain injury. J Neurotrauma 2010;27(3):527–39.
7. Wunderle K, Hoeger KM, Wasserman E, et al. Menstrual phase as predictor of outcome after mild traumatic brain injury in women. J Head Trauma Rehabil 2014;29(5):E1–8.
8. Wright DW, Yeatts SD, Silbergleit R, et al. Very early administration of progesterone for acute traumatic brain injury. N Engl J Med 2014;371(26):2457–66.
9. Leach MR, Zammit CG. Traumatic brain injury in pregnancy. In: Handbook of clinical neurology172. Elsevier; 2020. p. 51–61.

10. Ripley DL, Harrison-Felix C, Sendroy-Terrill M, et al. The impact of female reproductive function on outcomes after traumatic brain injury. Arch Phys Med Rehabil 2008;89(6):1090–6.

11. Anto-Ocrah M, Cafferky V, Lewis V. Pregnancy after concussion: a clarion call for attention? J Head Trauma Rehabil 2022;37(4):E268–79.

12. Colantonio A, Mar W, Escobar M, et al. Women's health outcomes after traumatic brain injury. J Womens Health 2010;19(6):1109–16.

13. Vaajala M, Kuitunen I, Nyrhi L, et al. Pregnancy and delivery after traumatic brain injury: a nationwide population-based cohort study in Finland. J Matern Fetal Neonatal Med 2024;35(25):9709–16.

14. Adams RS, Akobirshoev I, Brenner LA, et al. Pregnancy, fetal, and neonatal outcomes among women with traumatic brain injury. J Head Trauma Rehabil 2023; 38(3):E167–76.

15. Blaya MO, Raval AP, Bramlett HM. Traumatic brain injury in women across lifespan. Neurobiol Dis 2022;164:105613.

16. Wagner AK, Bayir H, Ren D, et al. Relationships between cerebrospinal fluid markers of excitotoxicity, ischemia, and oxidative damage after severe TBI: the impact of gender, age, and hypothermia. J Neurotrauma 2004;21(2):125–36.

17. Czosnyka M, Radolovich D, Balestreri M, et al. Gender-related differences in intracranial hypertension and outcome after traumatic brain injury. In: Steiger HJ, editor. Acta neurochirurgica supplementum102. Vienna: Springer; 2008. p. 25–8.

18. Lavoie S, Sechrist S, Quach N, et al. Depression in men and women one year following traumatic brain injury (TBI): a TBI model systems study. Front Psychol 2017;8:634.

19. Ma C, Wu X, Shen X, et al. Sex differences in traumatic brain injury: a multidimensional exploration in genes, hormones, cells, individuals, and society. Chin Neurosurg J 2019;5(1):24.

20. Covassin T, Savage JL, Bretzin AC, et al. Sex differences in sport-related concussion long-term outcomes. Int J Psychophysiol 2018;132:9–13.

21. Liossi C, Wood RL. Gender as a moderator of cognitive and affective outcome after traumatic brain injury. J Neuropsychiatry Clin Neurosci 2009;21(1):43–51.

22. Stahl S. Stahl's essential psychopharmacology print and online bundle: neuroscientific basis and practical applications. 4th edition. Cambridge University Press; 2013.

23. Oyesanya TO, Ward EC. Mental health in women with traumatic brain injury: a systematic review on depression and hope. Health Care Women Int 2016; 37(1):45–74.

24. Bay E, Sikorskii A, Saint-Arnault D. Sex differences in depressive symptoms and their correlates after mild-to-moderate traumatic brain injury. J Neurosci Nurs 2009;41(6):298–309.

25. Zasler ND, Katz DI, Zafonte RD. Brain injury medicine. 3rd Edition. Springer Publishing Company; 2021. *Principles and Practice.*

26. Torregrossa W, Raciti L, Rifici C, et al. Behavioral and psychiatric symptoms in patients with severe traumatic brain injury: a comprehensive overview. Biomedicines 2023;11(5):1449.

27. Fabricius AM, D'Souza A, Amodio V, et al. Women's gendered experiences of traumatic brain injury. Qual Health Res 2020;30(7):1033–44.

28. Albicini M, McKinlay A. Anxiety disorders in adults with childhood traumatic brain injury: evidence of difficulties more than 10 Years postinjury. J Head Trauma Rehabil 2018;33(3):191–9.

29. Olff M. Sex and gender differences in post-traumatic stress disorder: an update. Eur J Psychotraumatology 2017;8(sup4):1351204.
30. Hsu HL, Yen-Ting Chen D, Tseng YC, et al. Sex differences in working memory after mild traumatic brain injury: a functional mr imaging study. Radiology 2016;280(2):653.
31. Aoun R, Rawal H, Attarian H, et al. Impact of traumatic brain injury on sleep: an overview. Nat Sci Sleep 2019;11:131–40.
32. Wiseman-Hakes C, Saleem M, Poulin V, et al. The development of intimate relationships in adolescent girls and women with traumatic brain injury: a framework to guide gender specific rehabilitation and enhance positive social outcomes. Disabil Rehabil 2020;42(24):3559–65.
33. Rigon A, Turkstra L, Mutlu B, et al. The female advantage: sex as a possible protective factor against emotion recognition impairment following traumatic brain injury. Cogn Affect Behav Neurosci 2016;16(5):866–75.
34. Farace E, Alves WM. Do women fare worse: a metaanalysis of gender differences in traumatic brain injury outcome. J Neurosurg 2000;93(4):539–45.
35. Baker-Sparr C, Hart T, Bergquist T, et al. Internet and social media use after traumatic brain injury: a traumatic brain injury model systems study. J Head Trauma Rehabil 2018;33(1):E9–17.
36. Moreno A, Laoch A, Zasler ND. Changing the culture of neurodisability through language and sensitivity of providers: creating a safe place for LGBTQIA+ people. In: Moreno A, Gan C, Zasler ND, editors. NeuroRehabilitation 2017;41(2): 375–93.
37. Ek AS, Holmström C, Elmerstig E. Unmet need for sexual rehabilitation after acquired brain injury (ABI): a cross-sectional study concerning sexual activity, sexual relationships, and sexual rehabilitation after ABI. Sex Disabil 2023;41(2): 387–410.
38. Vikan JK, Snekkevik H, Nilsson MI, et al. Sexual satisfaction and associated biopsychosocial factors in stroke patients admitted to specialized cognitive rehabilitation. Sex Med 2021;9(5):1.
39. Kreutzer JS, Marwitz JH, Hsu N, et al. Marital stability after brain injury: an investigation and analysis. In: Sander AM, editor. NeuroRehabilitation 2007;22(1):53–9.
40. Ivany AS, Bullock L, Schminkey D, et al. Living in fear and prioritizing safety: exploring women's lives after traumatic brain injury from intimate partner violence. Qual Health Res 2018;28(11):1708–18.
41. Thompson RS, Bonomi AE, Anderson M, et al. Intimate partner violence. Am J Prev Med 2006;30(6):447–57.
42. Shannan Catalano. Special report: intimate partner violence, 1993-2010. 2012. Available at: https://bjs.ojp.gov/content/pub/pdf/ipv9310.pdf.
43. Costello K, Greenwald BD. Update on domestic violence and traumatic brain injury: a narrative review. Brain Sci 2022;12(1):122.
44. Furlow B. Domestic violence. Radiol Technol 2010;82(2):133–53.
45. Wu V, Huff H, Bhandari M. Pattern of physical injury associated with intimate partner violence in women presenting to the emergency department: a systematic review and meta-analysis. Trauma Violence Abuse 2010;11(2):71–82.
46. Strack GB, McClane GE, Hawley D. A review of 300 attempted strangulation cases part i: criminal legal issues. J Emerg Med 2001;21(3):303–9.
47. McClane GE, Strack GB, Hawley D. A review of 300 attempted strangulation cases part II: clinical evaluation of the surviving victim. J Emerg Med 2001; 21(3):311–5.

48. Gormley M, Devanaboyina M, Andelic N, et al. Long-term employment outcomes following moderate to severe traumatic brain injury: a systematic review and meta-analysis. Brain Inj 2019;33(13–14):1567–80.
49. Røe C, Sveen U, Alvsåker K, et al. Post-concussion symptoms after mild traumatic brain injury: influence of demographic factors and injury severity in a 1-year cohort study. Disabil Rehabil 2009;31(15):1235–43.
50. Shames J, Treger I, Ring H, et al. Return to work following traumatic brain injury: trends and challenges. Disabil Rehabil 2007;29(17):1387–95.
51. Mani K, Cater B, Hudlikar A. Cognition and return to work after mild/moderate traumatic brain injury: a systematic review. Work Read Mass 2017;58(1):51–62.
52. Soeker MS, Darries Z. The experiences of women with traumatic brain injury about the barriers and facilitators experienced after vocational rehabilitation in the Western Cape Metropole, South Africa. Work Read Mass 2019;64(3):477–86.
53. Poritz JMP, Vos L, Ngan E, et al. Gender differences in employment and economic quality of life following traumatic brain injury. Rehabil Psychol 2019; 64(1):65–71.
54. Corrigan JD, Lineberry LA, Komaroff E, et al. Employment after traumatic brain injury: differences between men and women. Arch Phys Med Rehabil 2007; 88(11):1400–9.
55. Fure SCR, Howe EI, Andelic N, et al. Cognitive and vocational rehabilitation after mild-to-moderate traumatic brain injury: a randomised controlled trial. Ann Phys Rehabil Med 2021;64(5):101538.
56. Bounds TA, Schopp L, Johnstone B, et al. Gender differences in a sample of vocational rehabilitation clients with TBI. NeuroRehabilitation 2003;18(3):189–96.
57. Lama S, Damkliang J, Kitrungrote L. Community integration after traumatic brain injury and related factors: a study in the Nepalese context. SAGE Open Nurs 2020;6. 237796082098178.

The Role of Rehabilitation for Women with Cancer

Vishwa S. Raj, MD[a,b,c,*], Bhavesh D. Patel, DO[a,b,c],
Sarah Mullan, MS, OTR/L[b], Rebecca Hine, PT, DPT[d],
Page P. Mack, PT, MPT, CLT[b], Terrence Pugh, MD[a,b,c]

KEYWORDS

- Cancer pain • Cancer survivors • Function recovery • Lymphedema • Quality of life
- Rehabilitation • Survivorship

KEY POINTS

- Survivorship and rehabilitation are vital components of the oncological plan of care.
- Rehabilitation interventions improve the quality of life and function of women with cancer.
- Symptoms associated with cancer and its treatment are amenable to medical management.
- Rehabilitation services, including physiatry, physical therapy, occupational therapy, speech and language pathology, and neuropsychology, help improve cognitive and physical function.
- Treatments for psychological stress improve function and performance status.

INTRODUCTION

"Cancer rehabilitation is medical care that should be integrated throughout the oncology care continuum and delivered by trained rehabilitation professionals who have it within their scope of practice to diagnose and treat patients' physical, psychological, and cognitive impairments in an effort to maintain or restore function, reduce symptom burden, maximize independence and improve quality of life (QOL) in this medically complex population."[1] Within the United States, it is estimated that over 2 million new cases of cancer will be diagnosed in 2024, with women representing 48.6% of the total. Although breast represents the majority, women can develop a

[a] Department of Orthopaedics and Rehabilitation Medicine, Wake Forest University School of Medicine, Winston-Salem, NC 27101, USA; [b] Department of Supportive Care Section of Cancer Rehabilitation, Atrium Health Levine Cancer, Charlotte, NC 28204, USA; [c] Department of Physical Medicine and Rehabilitation, Carolinas Rehabilitation Atrium Health, Charlotte, NC 28203, USA; [d] Department of Inpatient Therapy, Carolinas Rehabilitation Atrium Health, Charlotte, NC 28203, USA
* Corresponding author. Carolinas Rehabilitation, Department of Physical Medicine and Rehabilitation, 1100 Blythe Boulevard, Charlotte, NC 28203.
E-mail address: vishwa.raj@atriumhealth.org

Phys Med Rehabil Clin N Am 36 (2025) 253–266
https://doi.org/10.1016/j.pmr.2024.11.007
pmr.theclinics.com

variety of malignancies specific to organ system and gender (**Fig. 1**).[2] The number of cancer survivors living in the United States is also increasing, due to improvements in early detection, treatment advances, and the growth and aging of the population (**Table 1**).[3] The scope of survivorship, especially when considering the wide range of experiences from time of initial diagnosis to end of life for different malignancies, is broad. Physical, emotional, social, and spiritual well-being, in the context of QOL, play important roles when optimizing survivorship care plans.[4] Understanding gender-specific cancer diagnoses and treatment effects is important to support the survivorship and rehabilitation needs for women.

ONCOLOGICAL PATHOLOGIES COMMON TO WOMEN
Breast Cancer

With an estimated incidence over 300,000 in 2024, breast cancer accounts for over 30% of all new cancer diagnoses in women.[2] It is the most common malignancy impacting women in the United States, with about 1 in 8 persons affected within their lifetime. According to the American Cancer Society (ACS), women between the ages of 40 and 44 years with average risk can consider yearly screening with a mammogram, and women aged 45 to 54 years should get a mandatory screening mammogram yearly.[5] After the age of 54 years, survivors can choose between annual or biennial testing. For those with a high risk of disease secondary to family history or genetic mutations, MRI should be used in addition to mammography.[5] Examples of genetic signatures include hormone receptor (HR) and human epidermal growth factor receptor 2 (HER2) activity, and they can be categorized as positive (+) or negative (−). The main subtypes ordered by prevalence are HR+/HER2-, HR-/HER2-, HR+/HER2+, and HR-/HER2+. With better screening, enhanced surveillance methods, and diminished toxicity profiles of treatment, the 5 year survival rate has improved to 90.8% as of 2019.[6]

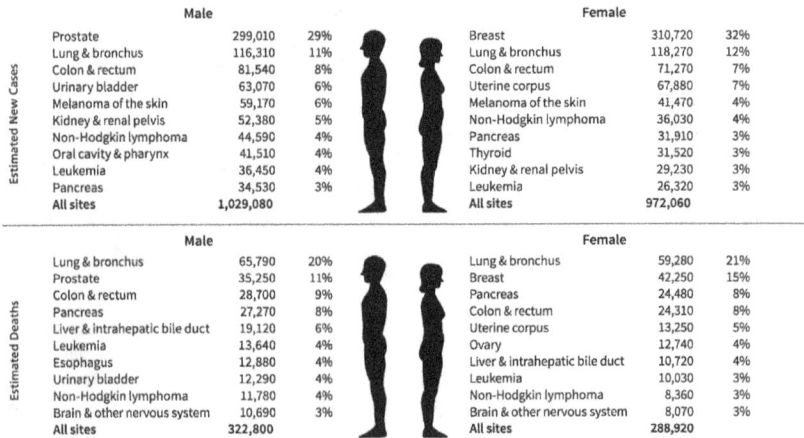

Estimated New Cases

Male				Female		
Prostate	299,010	29%		Breast	310,720	32%
Lung & bronchus	116,310	11%		Lung & bronchus	118,270	12%
Colon & rectum	81,540	8%		Colon & rectum	71,270	7%
Urinary bladder	63,070	6%		Uterine corpus	67,880	7%
Melanoma of the skin	59,170	6%		Melanoma of the skin	41,470	4%
Kidney & renal pelvis	52,380	5%		Non-Hodgkin lymphoma	36,030	4%
Non-Hodgkin lymphoma	44,590	4%		Pancreas	31,910	3%
Oral cavity & pharynx	41,510	4%		Thyroid	31,520	3%
Leukemia	36,450	4%		Kidney & renal pelvis	29,230	3%
Pancreas	34,530	3%		Leukemia	26,320	3%
All sites	1,029,080			All sites	972,060	

Estimated Deaths

Male				Female		
Lung & bronchus	65,790	20%		Lung & bronchus	59,280	21%
Prostate	35,250	11%		Breast	42,250	15%
Colon & rectum	28,700	9%		Pancreas	24,480	8%
Pancreas	27,270	8%		Colon & rectum	24,310	8%
Liver & intrahepatic bile duct	19,120	6%		Uterine corpus	13,250	5%
Leukemia	13,640	4%		Ovary	12,740	4%
Esophagus	12,880	4%		Liver & intrahepatic bile duct	10,720	4%
Urinary bladder	12,290	4%		Leukemia	10,030	3%
Non-Hodgkin lymphoma	11,780	4%		Non-Hodgkin lymphoma	8,360	3%
Brain & other nervous system	10,690	3%		Brain & other nervous system	8,070	3%
All sites	322,800			All sites	288,920	

Fig. 1. Estimated incidence and number of death of new cancer cases in the United States stratified by gender.[2] Estimates are rounded to the nearest 10, and cases exclude basal cell and squamous cell skin cancers and in situ carcinoma except urinary bladder. Estimates do not include Puerto Rico or other US territories. Ranking is based on modeled projections and may differ from the most recent observed data. ©2024, American Cancer Society, Inc., Surveillance and Health Equity Science.

Table 1

Estimated number of female cancer survivors in 2022[3]

Years Since Diagnosis	Number	Percent	Cumulative Percent
0 to <5	2,802,390	29	29
5 to <10	2,063,560	21	50
10 to <15	1,598,790	16	66
15 to <20	1,173,480	12	78
20 to <25	806,370	8	87
25 to <30	527,280	5	92
30+	767,040	8	100

Gynecologic Cancer

Human papillomavirus (HPV) is the primary cause of cervical cancer and is most often transmitted through skin-to-skin contact. Current ACS recommendations suggest all children between the ages of 9 and 12 years receive the HPV vaccine, with access available up until the age of 26 years. Screening every 3 to 5 years with the use of a primary HPV or Papanicolaou test (better known as Pap test or smear) should start at the age of 25 years and continue until the age of 65 years. No further evaluations are necessary for individuals with hysterectomy or aged 65 years with a 10 year history of negative testing. However, cervical pre-cancer assessments should continue for at least 25 years after initial diagnosis, regardless of age.[5] For 2023, cervical cancer accounted for 13,960 of new cases (0.7% of all new cancer cases) in the United States and had a 5 year survival rate of 67.2%.[7]

Endometrial cancer originates from the inner lining of the uterus. There are no specific screening tests for endometrial cancer, but addressable risk factors include excess body weight and lack of physical activity. Consideration should be made for individuals with early onset menstruation, late menopause, hormone replacement therapy, history of hereditary nonpolyposis colorectal cancer (Lynch syndrome), increasing age, and polycystic ovary syndrome as these are associated with higher risk of diagnosis. Women who have Lynch syndrome should be offered yearly testing, including endometrial biopsy from the age of 35 years.[5] There were an estimated 66,200 cases of uterine cancer in the United States (3.4% of all cancer cases in 2023) and a 5 year survival rate of 81.0%.[8] The risk of developing ovarian cancer also increases with age and Lynch syndrome, but additional factors include breast cancer 1 and 2 gene mutations, cigarette smoking, excess body weight, hormone replacement therapy, and history of breast or ovarian cancer.[8] Again, there are no available routine screening tests, but some women opt for preventative hysterectomy based on their medical profiles. Ovarian cancer incidence in 2023 was 19,710 (1.0% of all cases), but 5 year survival was lower at 50.8% due to diagnosis at time of increased severity of disease.[9]

Behavior Modification

Addressing specific behaviors may help decrease the chance of developing cancer in women, such as cessation of tobacco use and incorporation of a consistent physical activity program. The American College of Sports Medicine recommends 150 to 300 minutes per week of moderate intensity or 75 to 150 minutes per week of vigorous aerobic exercise with twice weekly strength training, which in addition to helping with performance status can potentially decrease the risk of breast, endometrial, and ovarian cancers.[10] Diets integrating more fruits, vegetables, and whole grains while limiting processed foods, red meat, refined grains, and sugary drinks can also play a role. Moderation of alcohol consumption to one drink per day for women, along with following appropriate screening guidelines, is also recommended.[5]

CONDITIONS ASSOCIATED WITH CANCER
Cancer Pain

Pain is one of the most common complaints of cancer survivors regardless of whether the tumor is localized or has spread beyond initial presentation.[11] Patients should be screened during each encounter to understand potential sources, including disease recurrence, new malignancy, or treatment effects from cancer itself. It is prudent to differentiate cancer-related pain and non-cancer pain as approaches can vary drastically for optimal management. For example, shoulder pain in breast cancer survivors can be due to underlying shoulder arthropathy or possible bony metastasis. If conservative measures and therapeutic interventions are not successful, opioids can be considered for cancer-related pain while utilizing adjuvant and non-opioid analgesics.[12] The World Health Organization Four-Step Ladder is a useful tool to determine the appropriate types of analgesic based on pain complaints (**Fig. 2**).[13] Several different agents can be considered when treating mild, moderate, and severe cancer pain (**Table 2**).[14]

If oral pharmaceutical agents are not sufficient or tolerated for adequate analgesic relief, interventional procedures with ultrasound or fluoroscopic guidance can also be utilized to manage pain. Intraarticular corticosteroid injections for adhesive capsulitis have been documented to be safe in populations with breast cancer who have active cancer or are undergoing active treatment.[15] Chemodenervation with botulinum toxin or phenol has been shown to relieve pain related to cervical dystonia or spasticity after radiation treatment.[16] Selective nerve blocks, such as pectoral or dorsal spinal, can successfully manage postmastectomy pain syndrome and increase QOL.[17] Additionally, selective stellate ganglion blocks show promise as an option for reducing pain in postmastectomy pain syndrome. Superior hypogastric plexus and ganglion impar

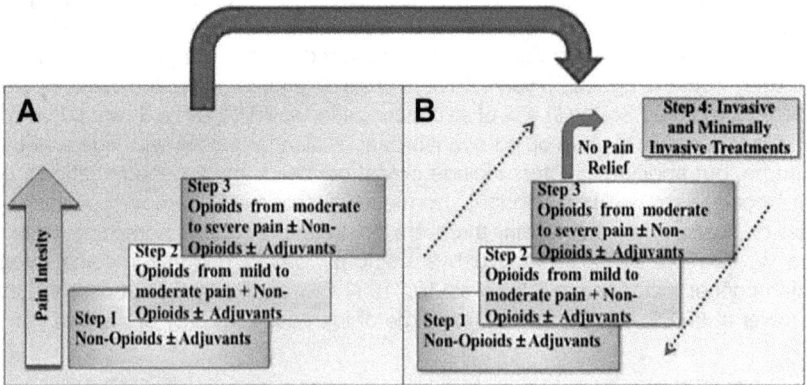

Fig. 2. WHO analgesic ladder.13 Transition from the original WHO 3 step analgesic ladder (*A*) to the revised WHO fourth-step form (*B*). The additional step 4 is an "interventional" step and includes invasive and minimally invasive techniques. This updated WHO ladder provides a bidirectional approach. (*With permission from* Dr. Marco Cascella, MD. Anekar AA, Hendrix JM, Cascella M. WHO Analgesic Ladder. Published April 2, 2023. Accessed April 22, 2024. In: StatPearls [Internet]. Treasure Island (FL): StatPearls Publishing; 2024 Jan-. Available from: https://www.ncbi.nlm.nih.gov/books/NBK554435/.)

Table 2
Common analgesics used to treat cancer pain[13]

	Types of Pain	
Mild	Mild to moderate	Moderate to severe
Non-opioids	Weak opioids (in combination	Strong opioids
• Paracetamol	with non-opioids)	• Buprenorphine
• Nonsteroidal	• Codeine	• Diamorphine
anti-inflammatories	• Dihydrocodeine	• Fentanyl
	• Tramadol	• Hydromorphone
	Low-dose strong opioids	• Morphine
Breakthrough	Bone	Cancer-related neuropathic
Immediate-release opioids	Bisphosphonates	Adjuvants
• Hydrocodone	Denosumab	• Duloxetine
• Oxycodone	Dexamethasone	• Gabapentin
	Radiation therapy	• Pregabalin
		• Tricyclic antidepressants
		Opioids (in combination
		with adjuvants)

blocks can also provide analgesia for visceral pain associated with uterine, ovarian, and cervical cancers.[18]

Malnutrition

Malnutrition in cancer is a result of increased inflammatory cytokines, metabolic alterations, and inadequate availability of nutrients due to anorexia from disease and its treatment effects.[19] Optimizing nutrition is a vital cornerstone in cancer survivorship to maintain QOL, support adequate treatment effects, and limit adverse clinical outcomes. Although enteral tube feeding and parental nutrition can be applied to patients with cancer, improvement of oral intake is the preferred method to address patient needs.[20] As part of a multidisciplinary therapeutic strategy, appetite stimulants can play a vital role in mitigating cancer-associated anorexia. Mirtazapine, a specific noradrenergic and serotonergic antidepressant, can increase appetite in patients with cancer-associated anorexia without depression.[20] Other agents such as the antipsychotic olanzapine, the cannabinoid dronabinol, and the progestin megestrol acetate have also shown benefit in increasing appetite.[21] However, the side effect profiles of these agents are more consequential than mirtazapine, especially megestrol acetate that can increase the risk of venous thromboembolisms.[22]

SEQUELAE OF CANCER TREATMENT
Cancer-Related Cognitive Impairment

Cancer-related cognitive impairment (CRCI) refers to changes in cognitive function in noncentral nervous system cancers that occur during or after cancer treatment. Up to 75% of survivors experience cognitive changes during and 60% after treatment, respectively.[23] Deficits are usually mild to moderate and can include challenges with attention, executive functions, processing speed, and short-term and working memory.[24] The duration of impairments varies, and although many resolve within 6 to 12 months of treatment, difficulties can persist for years or decades.[25] CRCI affects women with various malignancies, including breast, lung, colorectal, ovarian, leukemia and lymphoma.[26] Cognitive impairment can be affected by age, cancer diagnoses themselves, oncological treatments (such as chemotherapy, hormone therapies, and targeted therapies), and psychological factors. CRCI can negatively impact QOL, as cognitive function is related to independence in decision-making as well as instrumental activities of daily living (ADL), return to work, self-confidence, and social relationships.[22]

Rehabilitation professionals play a key role in assessing for and treating CRCI in women with cancer. Neuropsychological evaluation provides objective assessments of various cognitive domains and psychological factors (including anxiety, depression, and fatigue) that may affect cognitive function.[24] Integration of these into the care plan helps guide management and treatment interventions, including cognitive rehabilitation and behavioral therapies. Cognitive rehabilitation is typically completed by speech and language pathology (SLP), with focus on building metacognitive awareness, compensatory strategy training, environmental modifications, retraining of cognitive skills, and structured and functional tasks.[27] Behavioral therapies include counseling, mindfulness and meditation, and self-efficacy. Exercise therapy and pharmacologic interventions are also recommended; however, more research is needed to assess their effectiveness.[28] Evidence is lacking specifically regarding medication options for cognitive dysfunction.[29] However, considerations should be made given that cognitive dysfunction can lead to impairments in attention, concentration, memory, and multi-tasking.[30] In combination with rehabilitation interventions, pharmaceutical options can play a role in supporting patients' participation and progress. Stimulants, such as methylphenidate and modafinil, may aid in cancer-related cognitive changes.[31,32]

Cancer-Related Fatigue

Cancer-related fatigue (CRF) is defined as a distressing, persistent, and subjective sense of physical, emotional, or cognitive tiredness or exhaustion. It can result from cancer and its treatment. Symptoms often are not proportional or correlated to recent activity.[33] Factors associated with CRF include chemotherapy, depression, female gender, insomnia, neuroticism, pain, poor performance status, and radiation therapy.[34] CRF is frequently associated with breast cancer after chemotherapy or radiation, but when both interventions are combined, symptoms are far more significant.[35] In women, it can also impact cognitive, physical, and social functioning as well as QOL and self-confidence. Diagnosis is important given that prevalence is 1.4 times greater than that in men.[36]

Multidimensional assessment tools are necessary when evaluating CRF as it is known to have a combination of affective, cognitive, and physical domain impairments.[34] The Brief Fatigue Inventory and the European Organization for Research and Treatment of Cancer-QOL Questionnaire C30 are helpful to determine the impact of symptoms.[33] Evaluation should be initiated at the time of cancer diagnosis and continued during regular intervals within the treatment and posttreatment period. Cognitive behavioral therapy and physical activity are beneficial for CRF.[34] Specifically, for patients with breast cancer, yoga, as well as aerobic and resistance exercises, can improve symptoms.[37] Continued programs with vigorous and rhythmic exercise, such as aerobic resistance training, aerobic yoga, and traditional yoga, remain valuable after completion of oncological treatments for breast cancer.[36] Although there are no standard protocols to help with CRF, medications such as antidepressants, psychostimulants such as methylphenidate and modafinil, and steroids may be of helpful.[30,31,38]

Chemotherapy-Induced Peripheral Neuropathy

Chemotherapy-induced peripheral neuropathy (CIPN) is a toxic side effect from systemic treatment of malignancy. It is induced by specific types of treatments, including chemotherapy, targeted agents, and immunotherapy medications that are commonly used in breast and gynecologic cancers (**Table 3**). For women, CIPN was reported in up to 47% of individuals even after 6 years from completion of treatment.[39] It presents in a stocking and glove distribution with involvement of longer axons and is typically characterized as a sensory axonal peripheral neuropathy.[40] Symptoms include burning, cold sensitivity, impaired motor function of the hands or feet, numbness, pain, and tingling. Onset can occur anytime during or after chemotherapy treatment.[38]

Functional impairments are common in CIPN. Patients report difficulty with cooking, dressing, typing, and writing, which in turn may affect home and work roles. Occupational therapy (OT) is a valuable resource to address these needs, specifically with upper extremity symptoms. For the lower extremities, physical therapy (PT) can be valuable as survivors may have fall risk due to changes in balance and gait. Slower gait and increased disability can lead to 1.8 times increase in falls.[38] Both PT and OT can apply manual therapy techniques, such as soft tissue massage, to decrease pain and increase blood flow in affected areas. Supervised exercise programs may also be valuable to address motor weakness and range of motion deficits. For women receiving taxane-based treatments, exercise before and during treatment decreased symptoms of CIPN and improved health-related QOL.[41] Both compression and kinesiotape are useful to help with sensory symptoms. Burning, pain, and tingling may improve with proper application of modalities, including ultrasound and transcutaneous electrical nerve stimulation. Considerations for durable medical equipment, such as canes and walkers, and orthotics, including ankle foot orthoses, may be helpful for individuals experiencing motor symptoms and gait instability. Early intervention with therapy can help address and prevent functional decline. However, medical management may also help to alleviate symptoms.

Clinicians can treat neuropathic pain with adjuvant medications and adjust doses based on symptom severity and potential side effects.[42] Although topical agents such as capsaicin and menthol have shown some benefit, challenges may arise if large areas of the body require application. Gabapentinoids, such as gabapentin or pregabalin, are commonly utilized as first-line treatments. However, the selective serotonin and norepinephrine reuptake inhibitor duloxetine is one of the only pharmaceutical agents with evidence supporting clinical benefit.[43] It can also be used to help with musculoskeletal pain associated with aromatase inhibitors, commonly associated with the treatment of breast cancer.[44]

Lymphedema

Lymphedema is described as swelling secondary to dysfunction of the lymphatic system. Damage to the lymph nodes and collectors may be due to surgery and radiation for cancer treatment. For patients with breast cancer, the prevalence of lymphedema is 21.4% with increased risk secondary to higher body mass index and axillary lymph node dissection.[45,46] Lymphedema is also common within gynecologic and colorectal

---

Table 3
Common causes of chemotherapy-induced peripheral neuropathy[38]

Chemotherapy	Targeted therapy
Platinum-based Compounds	Bortezomib
• Carboplatin	Immunotherapy
• Cisplatin	Thalidomide
Taxanes	
• Taxol	
• Taxotere	
Vinca Alkaloids	
• Vinblastine	
Vincristine	

malignancies. Female survivors of ovarian, endometrial, and colorectal cancers, who met criteria for lymphedema, demonstrated point prevalences of 37%, 33%, and 31%, respectively.[47] Symptoms include achiness, heaviness, numbness and tingling, and swelling in the affected area causing difficulty with ADLs and mobility. Breast cancer-related lymphedema (BCRL) has become a significant financial burden on the health care system, and with 5 year survival rates of 90%, it can significantly impact QOL long term.[48]

The cornerstones for management of early-stage lymphedema include comprehensive multidisciplinary assessment at the time of initial diagnosis, early referral to therapy after surgery, and patient education regarding weight loss, skin changes, and nail care.[47] Treatment options can be broken down into nonsurgical and surgical options (**Table 4**).[49] Evaluation by a certified lymphedema therapist (CLT) can be helpful in creating the lymphedema plan of care. CLTs are either PT, OT, or SLP that assess skin condition, measure volume of swollen areas, and predict impact on function. Complete decongestive therapy remains the standard of care in BCRL and consists of manual lymphatic drainage (MLD), compression prescription, exercise, and skin care education to reduce the risk of cellulitis and progression of swelling. The application of MLD results in a sequenced and manual method to move fluid from an impaired area to a competent area in the body for improved lymphatic fluid distribution. Then compression with bandaging to reduce swelling in phase I followed by compression garments to maintain reduction in phase II result in sustainable volume reduction. Exercise is encouraged to facilitate muscle pumping action for further fluid decompression. The risk of cellulitis with skin breakdown can be addressed with further skin care education (**Fig. 3**). Additional treatment options may include intermittent pneumatic compression, nonpneumatic active compression devices, and low-level laser therapy.[50] For appropriate patients, lymphedema surgery may be considered, including vascularized lymph node transfer or lymphaticovenous anastomoses.[51]

Pelvic Floor Dysfunction

Pelvic floor dysfunction (PFD) refers to a wide range of disorders that affect the function of the pelvic floor musculature, leading to challenges with defecation, pelvic pain, pelvic organ prolapse, sexual dysfunction, and voiding.[52] It can occur in women with bladder, colorectal, and gynecologic malignancies, including cervical, endometrial, ovarian, uterine, vaginal, and vulval, and is typically due to radiation or surgery. Prevalence can vary widely between diagnoses and their treatments, but approximately 50% of colorectal cancer survivors experience anorectal, bowel, sexual, and urinary dysfunction after intervention.[53] With resection of rectal cancer, 37% to 90% experience low anterior resection syndrome and significant bowel dysfunction.[54] Other common symptoms in gynecologic cancers include dyspareunia, urinary incontinence, and fecal incontinence at rates of 7% to 58%, 4% to 76%, and 2% to 37%, respectively.[55]

Table 4
Nonsurgical and surgical options for treatment of lymphedema[48]

Nonsurgical Treatments	Surgical Treatments
Complete decongestive therapy	Reductive techniques
• Manual lymph drainage	• Direct excision
• Compression therapy	• Liposuction
• Exercise	Physiologic techniques
• Skin care	• Lymphatico-lymphatic bypass
• Compression garments	• Lymphatico-venous bypass
Advanced pneumatic compression therapy	• Lymph node transfer

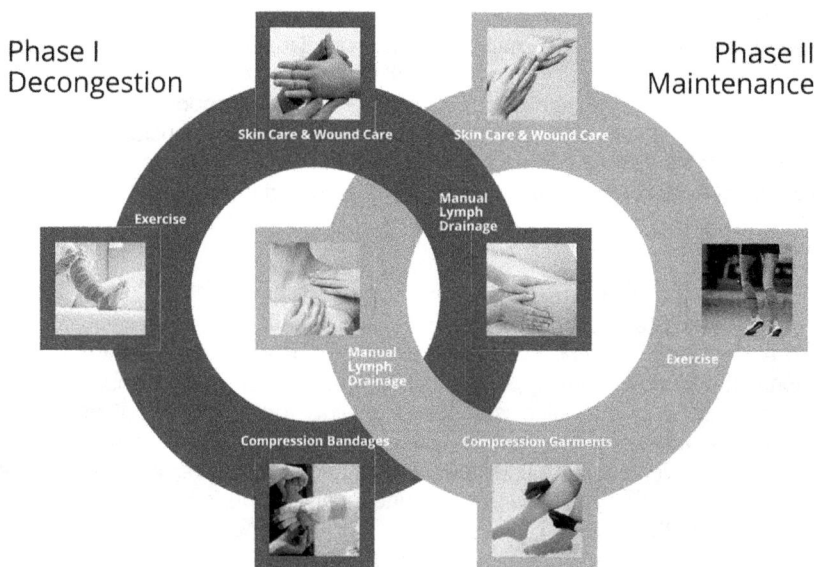

Fig. 3. Complex decongestive therapy.[68]

For women, PFD can negatively impact emotional, physical, psychological, and social well-being as well as QOL.[56] Pelvic floor rehabilitation is performed by PT and OT with specialized training. Interventions include biofeedback, dilator education and progression, joint mobilization, myofascial release, neuromuscular electrical stimulation, and trigger point massage.[57] Pelvic floor muscle training, which includes repetitive voluntary contraction of pelvic floor muscles, has been shown to have positive effects for many PFDs.[58] Bowel medications, including fiber supplements, stimulants, and osmotic laxatives, may be effective to treat constipation associated with PFD.[59]

Psychological Stress and Sexual Dysfunction

Women are at risk for psychological effects from cancer and its treatment. Conditions such as anxiety, depression, and impaired body image are common in breast cancer survivors and can present several years after initial diagnosis.[60,61] Prolonged and significant cancer-related impairments are associated with anxiety and depression in breast cancer as well. After treatment, concerns about breast symmetry or changes in skin texture and sensitivity could lead to impaired self-image. Early identification can lead to appropriate referrals to improve QOL and survival.[62] Cognitive-behavioral and psycho-educational therapies help to improve anxiety and depression, leading to better adjustment in terms of the survivor's diagnosis, mood, and QOL.[63] Addressing physical function through exercise is important as well, as psychological symptoms are predictive of impaired performance status.[64] Body perception exercises and relaxation techniques found in mindfulness-based cognitive therapy reduce stress levels.[62] Yoga has a role to improve anxiety, depression, and fatigue regardless of stage of diagnosis.[65] Selective-serotonin reuptake inhibitors and anxiolytics are also important in management.[66]

Sexual dysfunction is another common impairment and can occur in 30% to 80% of women with cancer.[60] Symptoms associated with sexual dysfunction include dyspareunia as well as decreased ability to orgasm, arousal, desire, and lubrication. Malignancies most often associated with these challenges are breast, cervical and endometrial. In addition, treatments such as chemotherapy, hormonal therapies, radiation, and surgery may exacerbate the condition. Treatment requires a multidisciplinary approach, especially with emphasis on PFD therapy to address health education and persistent symptom management. Social support groups also help to validate experiences and decrease associated stress.[60] Consideration can be made for over-the-counter moisturizers and lubricants, or prescription of estrogen versus selected estrogen receptor modulators based on the clinical diagnosis.[67]

SUMMARY

The impact of cancer on women is significant. With almost half of all new cases per year in the United States attributed to women, and continually increasing survival rates due to earlier diagnosis, improved treatments, and behavior modification, QOL and functional status are becoming priorities in the oncological care continuum. Rehabilitation intervention and medical management allow for application of rehabilitation principles to a variety of malignancies common in women. By addressing cognitive, physical, and psychological challenges associated with cancer and its treatment, women have the opportunity for better functional and performance status, which translates into better QOL.

CLINICS CARE POINTS

- Cancer rehabilitation treats physical, psychological, and cognitive impairments to maximize independence and QOL.
- Women with cancer have a wide range of experiences, based on the pathology and prognosis of malignancy and its subsequent impact on physical, emotional, social, and spiritual well-being.
- Conditions such as cancer pain and malnutrition benefit from medical management.
- Sequelae of cancer treatment (such as CRCI, CRF, CIPN, lymphedema, PFD, psychological stress, and sexual dysfunction) respond to rehabilitation interventions, including PT, OT, SLP, and psychology.
- Integration of rehabilitation and survivorship into the oncological plan of care is necessary for optimization of outcomes, including QOL and function.

DISCLOSURES

The authors have nothing to disclose.

REFERENCES

1. Silver JK, Raj VS, Fu JB, et al. Cancer rehabilitation and palliative care: critical components in the delivery of high-quality oncology services. Support Care Cancer 2015;23(12):3633–43.
2. Siegel RL, Giaquinto AN, Jemal A. Cancer statistics, 2024. CA Cancer J Clin 2024;74(1):12–49.
3. Miller KD, Nogueira L, Devasia T, et al. Cancer treatment and survivorship statistics, 2022. CA Cancer J Clin 2022;72(5):409–36.
4. American Cancer Society. Cancer treatment & survivorship facts & figures 2022-2024. Atlanta: American Cancer Society; 2022.

5. American Cancer Society. Cancer Facts for Women. Available at: https://www.cancer.org/cancer/risk-prevention/understanding-cancer-risk/cancer-facts/cancer-facts-for-women.html (Accessed 27 March 2024).

6. National Institutes of Health National Cancer Institute Surveillance, Epidemiology, and End Results Program. Cancer Stat Facts: Female Breast Cancer. Available at: https://seer.cancer.gov/statfacts/html/breast.html (Accessed 27 March 2024).

7. National Institutes of Health National Cancer Institute Surveillance, Epidemiology, and End Results Program. Cancer Stat Facts: Cervical Cancer. Available at: https://seer.cancer.gov/statfacts/html/cervix.html (Accessed 27 March 2024).

8. National Institutes of Health National Cancer Institute Surveillance, Epidemiology, and End Results Program. Cancer Stat Facts: Uterine Cancer. Available at: https://seer.cancer.gov/statfacts/html/corp.html (Accessed 15 April 2024).

9. National Institutes of Health National Cancer Institute Surveillance, Epidemiology, and End Results Program. Cancer Stat Facts: Ovarian Cancer. Available at: https://seer.cancer.gov/statfacts/html/ovary.html (Accessed 15 April 2024).

10. American College of Sports Medicine. Effects of exercise on health-related outcomes in those with cancer. Available at: https://www.acsm.org/docs/default-source/files-for-resource-library/cancer-infographic-sept-2022.pdf. Accessed April 15, 2024.

11. Snijders RAH, Brom L, Theunissen M, et al. Update on prevalence of pain in patients with cancer 2022: a systematic literature review and meta-analysis. Cancers (Basel) 2023;15(3):591. https://doi.org/10.3390/cancers15030591. Published 2023 Jan 18.

12. Paice JA, Portenoy R, Lacchetti C, et al. Management of chronic pain in survivors of adult cancers: American society of clinical oncology clinical practice guideline. J Clin Oncol 2016;34(27):3325–45.

13. Anekar AA, Hendrix JM, Cascella M. WHO analgesic ladder. In: StatPearls [internet]. Treasure Island (FL): StatPearls Publishing; 2024. Available at: https://www.ncbi.nlm.nih.gov/books/NBK554435/. Accessed April 22, 2024.

14. Fallon M, Giusti R, Aielli F, et al, ESMO Guidelines Committee. Management of cancer pain in adult patients: ESMO Clinical Practice Guidelines. Ann Oncol 2018;29(Suppl 4):iv166–91.

15. Leite VF, Padro-Guzman J. Intra-articular injections for musculoskeletal pain in a cancer rehabilitation clinic. Int J Physical Rehabil Med 2020;3(3):87–90.

16. Grenda T, Grenda A, Krawczyk P, et al. Botulinum toxin in cancer therapy-current perspectives and limitations. Appl Microbiol Biotechnol 2022;106(2):485–95.

17. Chappell AG, Yuksel S, Sasson DC, et al. Post-mastectomy pain syndrome: an up-to-date review of treatment outcomes. JPRAS Open 2021;30:97–109.

18. Hao D, Sidharthan S, Cotte J, et al. Interventional therapies for pain in cancer patients: a narrative review. Curr Pain Headache Rep 2021;25(7):44.

19. Barreira JV. The role of nutrition in cancer patients. Nutr Cancer 2021;73(11–12):2849–50.

20. National Institutes of Health National Cancer Institute. Nutrition in cancer care. Available at: https://www.cancer.gov/about-cancer/treatment/side-effects/appetite-loss/nutrition-pdq#_177. Accessed April 20, 2024.

21. Turcott JG, Zatarain-Barrón ZL, Cárdenas Fernández D, et al. Appetite stimulants for patients with cancer: current evidence for clinical practice. Nutr Rev 2022;80(4):857–73. https://doi.org/10.1093/nutrit/nuab045.

22. Bolen JC, Andersen RE, Bennett RG. Deep vein thrombosis as a complication of megestrol acetate therapy among nursing home residents. J Am Med Dir Assoc 2000;1(6):248–52.

23. Lange M, Joly F, Vardy J, et al. Cancer-related cognitive impairment: an update on state of the art, detection, and management strategies in cancer survivors. Ann Oncol 2019;30(12):1925–40.

24. Joly F, Giffard B, Rigal O, et al. Impact of cancer and its treatments on cognitive function: advances in research from the Paris international cognition and cancer task force symposium and update since 2012. J Pain Symptom Manage 2015; 50(6):830–41.

25. Pendergrass JC, Targum SD, Harrison JE. Cognitive impairment associated with cancer: a Brief review. Innov Clin Neurosci 2018;15(1–2):36–44.

26. Lv L, Mao S, Dong H, et al. Pathogenesis, assessments, and management of chemotherapy-related cognitive impairment (CRCI): an updated literature review. J Oncol 2020;2020:3942439.

27. Fernandes HA, Richard NM, Edelstein K. Cognitive rehabilitation for cancer-related cognitive dysfunction: a systematic review. Support Care Cancer 2019; 27(9):3253–79.

28. Mackenzie L, Marshall K. Effective non-pharmacological interventions for cancer related cognitive impairment in adults (excluding central nervous system or head and neck cancer): systematic review and meta-analysis. Eur J Phys Rehabil Med 2022;58(2):258–70.

29. Fleming B, Edison P, Kenny L. Cognitive impairment after cancer treatment: mechanisms, clinical characterization, and management. BMJ 2023;380: e071726.

30. Wefel JS, Witgert ME, Meyers CA. Neuropsychological sequelae of non-central nervous system cancer and cancer therapy. Neuropsychol Rev 2008;18(2): 121–31.

31. Thong MSY, van Noorden CJF, Steindorf K, et al. Cancer-related fatigue: causes and current treatment options [published correction appears in curr treat options oncol. 2022 mar;23(3):450-451]. Curr Treat Options Oncol 2020;21(2):17.

32. Asher A, Myers JS. The effect of cancer treatment on cognitive function. Clin Adv Hematol Oncol 2015;13(7):441–50.

33. Koh WJ, Abu-Rustum NR, Bean S, et al. Cervical cancer, version 3.2019, NCCN clinical practice guidelines in oncology. J Natl Compr Canc Netw 2019;17(1): 64–84.

34. Ma Y, He B, Jiang M, et al. Prevalence and risk factors of cancer-related fatigue: a systematic review and meta-analysis. Int J Nurs Stud 2020;111:103707.

35. Ruiz-Casado A, Álvarez-Bustos A, de Pedro CG, et al. Cancer-related fatigue in breast cancer survivors: a review. Clin Breast Cancer 2021;21(1):10–25.

36. Kang YE, Yoon JH, Park NH, et al. Prevalence of cancer-related fatigue based on severity: a systematic review and meta-analysis. Sci Rep 2023;13(1):12815.

37. Liu YC, Hung TT, Konara Mudiyanselage SP, et al. Beneficial exercises for cancer-related fatigue among women with breast cancer: a systematic review and network meta-analysis. Cancers (Basel) 2022;15(1):151.

38. National Institutes of Health National Cancer Institute. Cancer fatigue. Available at: https://www.cancer.gov/about-cancer/treatment/side-effects/fatigue#treating-cancer-fatigue. Accessed April 20, 2024.

39. Winters-Stone KM, Horak F, Jacobs PG, et al. Falls, functioning, and disability among women with persistent symptoms of chemotherapy-induced peripheral neuropathy. J Clin Oncol 2017;35(23):2604–12.

40. Starobova H, Vetter I. Pathophysiology of chemotherapy-induced peripheral neu-ropathy. Front Mol Neurosci 2017;10:174.

41.. Brownson-Smith R, Orange ST, Cresti N, et al. Effect of exercise before and/or during taxane-containing chemotherapy treatment on chemotherapy-induced peripheral neuropathy symptoms in women with breast cancer: systematic review and meta-analysis. J Cancer Surviv 2023. https://doi.org/10.1007/s11764-023-01450-w.

42. Edwards HL, Mulvey MR, Bennett MI. Cancer-related neuropathic pain. Cancers (Basel) 2019;11(3):373.

43. Burgess J, Ferdousi M, Gosal D, et al. Chemotherapy-induced peripheral neuropathy: epidemiology, pathomechanisms and treatment. Oncol Ther 2021;9(2):385–450.

44. Hyder T, Marino CC, Ahmad S, et al. Aromatase inhibitor-associated musculoskeletal syndrome: understanding mechanisms and management. Front Endocrinol (Lausanne) 2021;12:713700.

45. National Institute of Health National Cancer Institute. Lymphedema (PDQ)-Health professional version. AccessedAbout cancer-lymphedema. National Cancer Institute; 2023. Available at: https://www.cancer.gov/about-cancer/treatment/side-effects/lymphedema/lymphedema-hp-pdq. Accessed March 29, 2024.

46. Shen A, Qiang W, Zhang L, et al. Risk factors for breast cancer-related lymphedema: an umbrella review. Ann Surg Oncol 2024;31(1):284–302.

47. Zhang X, McLaughlin EM, Krok-Schoen JL, et al. Association of lower extremity lymphedema with physical functioning and activities of daily living among older survivors of colorectal, endometrial, and ovarian cancer. JAMA Netw Open 2022;5(3):e221671.

48. Tandra P, Kallam A, Krishnamurthy J. Identification and management of lymphedema in patients with breast cancer. J Oncol Pract 2019;15(5):255–62.

49. Kayıran O, De La Cruz C, Tane K, et al. Lymphedema: from diagnosis to treatment. Turk J Surg 2017;33(2):51–7.

50. Donahue PMC, MacKenzie A, Filipovic A, et al. Advances in the prevention and treatment of breast cancer-related lymphedema. Breast Cancer Res Treat 2023;200(1):1–14.

51. Granzow JW. Lymphedema surgery: the current state of the art. Clin Exp Metastasis 2018;35(5–6):553–8.

52. Riaz H, Nadeem H, Rathore FA. Recent advances in the pelvic floor assessment and rehabilitation of Women with Pelvic Floor Dysfunction. J Pak Med Assoc 2022;72(7):1456–9.

53. Zhu L, Li X, Zhou C, et al. Pelvic floor dysfunction after colorectal cancer treatment is related to physical and psychological health and body image: a cross-sectional study. Eur J Oncol Nurs 2023;67:102425.

54. Nocera F, Angehrn F, von Flüe M, et al. Optimising functional outcomes in rectal cancer surgery. Langenbeck's Arch Surg 2021;406(2):233–50.

55. Brennen R, Lin KY, Denehy L, et al. The effect of pelvic floor muscle interventions on pelvic floor dysfunction after gynecological cancer treatment: a systematic review. Phys Ther 2020;100(8):1357–71.

56. Peinado Molina RA, Hernández Martínez A, Martínez Vázquez S, et al. Influence of pelvic floor disorders on quality of life in women. Front Public Health 2023;11:1180907.

57. Roldan CJ, Thomas A, Samms N, et al. Non-invasive pelvic floor rehabilitation in cancer population: an incomplete cohort. Pain Physician 2022;25(7):E1115–20.

58. Cai L, Wu Y, Xu X, et al. Pelvic floor dysfunction in gynecologic cancer survivors. Eur J Obstet Gynecol Reprod Biol 2023;288:108–13.

59. Bharucha AE, Lacy BE. Mechanisms, evaluation, and management of chronic constipation. Gastroenterology 2020;158(5):1232–49.e3.
60. Carreira H, Williams R, Müller M, et al. Associations between breast cancer survivorship and adverse mental health outcomes: a systematic review. J Natl Cancer Inst 2018;110(12):1311–27.
61. Sousa Rodrigues Guedes T, Barbosa Otoni Gonçalves Guedes M, de Castro Santana R, et al. Sexual dysfunction in women with cancer: a systematic review of longitudinal studies. Int J Environ Res Public Health 2022;19(19):11921.
62. Tsaras K, Papathanasiou IV, Mitsi D, et al. Assessment of depression and anxiety in breast cancer patients: prevalence and associated factors. Asian Pac J Cancer Prev 2018;19(6):1661–9.
63. Guarino A, Polini C, Forte G, et al. The effectiveness of psychological treatments in women with breast cancer: a systematic review and meta-analysis. J Clin Med 2020;9(1):209.
64. Faller H, Strahl A, Richard M, et al. Symptoms of depression and anxiety as predictors of physical functioning in breast cancer patients. A prospective study using path analysis. Acta Oncol 2017;56(12):1677–81.
65. Cramer H, Lauche R, Klose P, et al. Yoga for improving health-related quality of life, mental health and cancer-related symptoms in women diagnosed with breast cancer. Cochrane Database Syst Rev 2017;1(1):CD010802.
66. Venkataramu VN, Ghotra HK, Chaturvedi SK. Management of psychiatric disorders in patients with cancer. Indian J Psychiatry 2022;64(Suppl 2):S458–72.
67. Del Pup L, Villa P, Amar ID, et al. Approach to sexual dysfunction in women with cancer. Int J Gynecol Cancer 2019;29(3):630–4.
68. National Lymphedema Network. Lymphedema therapy. Available at: https://lymphnet.org/lymphedema-therapy. Accessed April 19, 2024.

Rehabilitation Considerations for Women with Spinal Cord Injury

Jennifer Chui, MD[a,]*, Phillip Gordon, MD[b]

KEYWORDS

- Women • Rehabilitation • Spinal cord injury • Annual evaluation
- Neurogenic lower urinary tract dysfunction • Sexuality • Fertility • Pregnancy

KEY POINTS

- Women with spinal cord injury (SCI) have specific medical and rehabilitation needs.
- Women with SCI encounter barriers to accessing primary care and should be assessed for general health and SCI-specific issues.
- Bladder management for women with SCI depends on medical and functional ability with clinician guidance.
- Sexuality in women with SCI is often overlooked, but most patients can have rewarding experiences.
- Education on reproductive health for women after SCI is limited, and it is crucial for women and health care providers to understand potential complications.

INTRODUCTION

The World Health Organization estimates that there are over 15 million individuals globally living with a spinal cord injury (SCI),[1] and the incidence and prevalence have been increasing each year. Although men are more commonly affected than women, women account for approximately 20% of the SCI population.[2] However, guidelines for best care and management of these individuals are generally non-sex specific. Differences between men and women necessitate medical and rehabilitation considerations such as primary care annual evaluation for women with SCI, bladder management, and sexuality and reproductive health issues.

PRIMARY CARE/ANNUAL EVALUATIONS

There are many barriers to care for the general population and even more for individuals with SCI.[3,4] Studies have shown that women with SCI are less likely to receive the

[a] Department of Physical Medicine & Rehabilitation, Hackensack Meridian JFK Johnson Rehabilitation Institute, 65 James Street, Edison, NJ 08820, USA; [b] Department of Physical Medicine & Rehabilitation, Mount Sinai Hospital, New York, NY, USA
* Corresponding author.
E-mail address: jenniferm.chui@hmhn.org

Phys Med Rehabil Clin N Am 36 (2025) 267–278
https://doi.org/10.1016/j.pmr.2024.11.003
pmr.theclinics.com
1047-9651/25/© 2024 Elsevier Inc. All rights reserved, including those for text and data mining, AI training, and similar technologies.

recommended examinations.[5] Challenges specifically include but are not limited to inaccessibility (office space or office equipment), socioeconomic systemic issues (cost, transportation), or lack of knowledge by providers (conscious or unconscious biases).[3] Preventative care guidelines for women with SCI follow similar guidelines as the general population, including screening, evaluations of health risk and needs, counseling, and immunization, but annual evaluations should include a focus on SCI specific issues.[4]

Primary care annual examinations are based on age, medical or family history, and lifestyle and health behaviors.[3,4] General health evaluations can include blood pressure screening, monitoring for obesity and diabetes, folic acid supplementation, lipid screening, and unhealthy alcohol and drug use.[3] Individuals with SCI should be evaluated for routine immunizations including tetanus, influenza, pneumococcal, and human papilloma virus.[3,4] Along with colon cancer screenings, women with SCI should have breast and cervical cancer screenings at the same frequency as the general population.[5] However, women with SCI face logistical barriers that can impact obtaining testing at appropriate times such as inability to position for mammography and pelvic examinations, inaccessible clinician offices, or inability to transfer to examination tables for appropriate evaluations.[3,4]

Annual evaluation for genitourinary issues typically focuses on neurogenic lower urinary tract dysfunction (NLUTD) and bladder programs.[4,6] Bladder program and management refers to types of bladder emptying such as voiding (volitionally or spontaneously), clean intermittent catheterization (CIC), or use of indwelling catheters. Clinicians should evaluate for complications such as recurrent urinary tract infections (UTIs), nephrolithiasis or bladder lithiasis, or vesicoureteral reflux causing hydronephrosis and kidney dysfunction.[6] Women should follow closely with urology and should have renal imaging depending on the risk factors.[5–8] Urodynamic studies should optimally be completed within 3 months of new SCI and repeated with new symptoms or complications to adjust treatment strategies.[7,8] Cystoscopy can be used to evaluate the lower urinary tract but should not be routinely performed for screening or surveillance.[7,8]

The focus for gastrointestinal issues typically revolves around neurogenic bowel dysfunction and bowel programs. Bowel program and management refer to the activities that help a person with SCI achieve regular planned and time-limited bowel evacuation with sufficient stool volume and adequate consistency, and avoid complications and unplanned defecation. During evaluation, clinicians should take a detailed history including effectiveness, timing, diet, oral medication, rectal interventions, and complications.[9]

After SCI, there can be other cardiac issues such as autonomic dysfunction depending on level of injury. Adults with cervical- and thoracic-level injuries can present with orthostatic hypotension.[10] Individuals with SCI at T6 or above are at higher risk of autonomic dysreflexia (AD), with signs and symptoms of elevated systolic blood pressure 20 mm Hg above their usual baseline, headache, changes in heart rate, sweating or flushing of the skin, piloerection below level of injury, blurred vision, nasal congestion, and feelings of apprehension or anxiety.[10] Some individuals may not have symptoms other than elevated blood pressure. Common triggers are noxious stimuli related to bladder, bowel, and skin.[10] Specifically, women should be educated on AD caused by menses, pelvic floor dysfunction, stretching of vagina during sexual activity, and pregnancy.[10–12] Women who have AD episodes should be educated on typical management to alleviate these triggers and pharmacologic management when needed.[10–12]

Women with cervical SCIs are at a higher risk of pulmonary dysfunction because of impairments of innervation of the diaphragm and accessory breathing muscles.[4,13]

Women have proportionally smaller lungs and airways compared with men and lower absolute measures of resting pulmonary function.[14] Annual maintenance evaluations should include immunization,[3,4] surveillance for signs and symptoms of sleeping-disordered breathing, education of regular use of respiratory muscle training exercises, and consideration of pulmonary function testing.[4,13]

Hormone differences with testosterone and estrogen impact the structure of the skin. Male skin on average is 20% thicker than female skin and contains more collagen.[15] As individuals age, collagen content decreases and female skin is affected more after menopause.[16] Women with SCI have impaired sensation and mobility, which increase their risk of pressure injuries. Annual examination should assess risk factors for skin breakdown including nutrition and adequate support surfaces (wheelchair cushions, mattresses, commode chairs) and have a full skin examination. Any wounds should be documented regarding location, size, appearance of wound bed, wound edges, and staging.[17] Wound care plans should include an interdisciplinary approach and focus on control of infection, removal of necrotic or nonviable tissue, moisture management, and frequency of treatments.[4,17]

Although there are no specific guidelines regarding annual musculoskeletal issues, issues related to spasticity, overuse injuries, and heterotopic ossification should be evaluated, as complications can reduce function, cause pain, and decrease quality of life. Women tend to experience more overuse-related injuries compared with men and are more susceptible to shoulder laxity and rotator cuff tears.[18] Loss of range of motion and increased pain can interfere with position in wheelchairs, cause pressure injuries, and limit functional mobility such as transfers and wheelchair propulsions.[19]

Although osteoporosis screening begins at age 65 in women,[20] individuals with SCI have bone loss beginning immediately after injury, and this is the most severe in the next 2 years.[21,22] All parts of the skeleton below the level of injury are affected, and the amount of bone loss depends on incompleteness of motor function.[21] Assessment of fracture and fall risk should be evaluated on an annual basis. Bone health can be screened with laboratory testing, and postmenopausal women should have additional measurements of prolactin, follicle-stimulating hormone (FSH), luteinizing hormone (LH), and estradiol levels.[22] Newer guidelines recommend bone density testing with dual energy X-ray absorptiometry (DXA) of the total hip, proximal tibia, and distal femur as soon as medically stable.[22] However, implementation in clinical practice can be limited, as typical DXA screening is obtained for lumbar spine and hip. Vitamin D should be repleted if deficient, and calcium supplementation is recommended depending on age.[22] Rehabilitation therapy that can reduce bone mineral density decline includes passive standing protocols, functional electrical stimulation (FES), or neuromuscular electrical stimulation (NMES).[22] Discussion regarding risk-benefit ratio of pharmacology therapy is recommended, and women with low bone mass and moderate to high fracture risk should be offered medications.

Mental health issues such as depression and anxiety are typically screened during annual evaluations.[3–5] Women have twice the lifetime rate of depression and anxiety disorders compared with men, while men are more likely to abuse illicit drugs and alcohol. After SCI, individuals are at greater risk for mental health issues, and thus all individuals, especially women, should be screened for depression, anxiety, and substance abuse.[23]

Lastly, other issues to evaluate on an annual basis include adjustment to disability, community participation, educational and employment status, equipment status, medical and functional status, transportation, and social and caregiver support.[3,4]

BLADDER MANAGEMENT

Neurogenic lower urinary tract dysfunction (NLUTD) affects most individuals with SCI because of interruption of the communication between the pontine micturition center and the spinal cord.[6] Between the sexes, there are significant differences in the anatomy and physiology of the lower urinary tract that impact function and rehabilitation needs.[24]

Differences in internal anatomy include a shorter urethral length in women, positioning of the bladder anterior to vagina, presence of the prostate in men, and differing pelvic floor physiology.[24] Differences in external anatomy include opening of the urethra meatus at the glans of the penis in men compared with opening of the meatus below the clitoris and above the vagina in women.[25]

Medications for management of bladder target different receptors within the bladder wall, and there are differences in the distribution of the receptor subtypes between men and women.[25,26] Antimuscarinic medications can decrease detrusor muscle contractions and spasms.[27] Prior studies have shown that asymmetry in receptor expression results in reduced efficacy of antimuscarinic medications in women.[25] β-Adrenoceptors mediate relaxation of smooth muscle in the bladder and urethra. $\alpha1$-adrenoceptors may play a more prominent functional role in the bladder neck, and hence the regulations of bladder outlet resistance.[27] Men typically have more $\alpha1$-adrenoceptors located in the bladder and urethra near the prostate.[26]

In women with a new SCI, providing education of bladder management is an interdisciplinary task.[6] Conservative methods of emptying bladder include triggering the bladder reflex, bladder expression, CIC, or use of an indwelling transurethral catheter. More invasive methods include suprapubic catheter (SPC) or surgical bladder procedures such as sacral anterior root stimulation, incontinent urinary diversions such as ileal or colon conduit, or continent urinary diversions like catheterizeable pouches or channels (Mitrofanoff procedure).[27] Each method has pros and cons, and women should decide with clinician guidance which would be best for them. Factors in choosing a method include other medical comorbidities (skin, bowel, or kidney dysfunction), caregiver involvement, cost, and functional ability of the individual.[6]

Voiding of the bladder involves a coordination of detrusor muscle contraction and sphincter relaxation. Women with sacral and infrasacral lesions may safely use bladder expression with Crede (manually pressing down on the bladder) or Valsalva techniques (increasing pressure inside the abdomen by bearing down) to facilitate voiding.[27] Women with reflexive bladder can use the bladder reflex and trigger voiding using stretch receptors when repeatedly tapping on the bladder. However, there can be complications of using this technique, such as AD, vesicoureteral reflux, renal deterioration, UTI, lithiasis, and loss of bladder compliance.[27] Thus reflex voiding is commonly discouraged by SCI clinicians unless confirmed safe by urodynamics study.[27] Other factors to consider for voiding include functional ability. If a woman is continent and voiding volitionally, she would need to be able to transfer to a commode, manage clothing, and manage hygiene. If a woman is spontaneously voiding and incontinent, she would need incontinence undergarments or diapers as there are limited external catheters for women. Men can use external condom catheters, while in women, external catheters require suction, are positioned between legs, and typically are only used in hospital settings.[28] The constant moisture with spontaneous voiding can cause further complications with fungal infections and skin breakdown.[28]

CIC is regarded as best practice for preventing UTIs compared with other methods, as there is no indwelling long-term foreign body, and CIC allows for more natural bladder filling and voiding cycles.[6,27,29,30] While women do not have prostates that can obstruct CIC, other functional considerations must be considered. Men with C7-C8 lesions can possibly perform CIC with adaptive equipment; however, women typically require intact bilateral hand function in order to undergo CIC without complications.[31] Additionally, women require adequate sitting balance, ability to manage legs and clothing, and appropriate positioning to be able to self-catheterize. And even with intact hand function, body habitus and skin folds of the labia can make catheterization difficult. Mirrors can be used to assist in visualization, and women can also be taught the touch technique, which uses vaginal landmarks and the position to feel for the urethral meatus.

Women are more likely to have an indwelling catheter (transurethral or suprapubic catheter) at discharge from rehabilitation.[24] This is because of the level of injury, hand function, mobility, and caregiver involvement. Transurethral catheters follow the urethral anatomy and do not require special procedures for placement. However, there is an increased risk of UTI, kidney or bladder lithiasis, and urethral erosion and leakage with long-term use.[27] Suprapubic catheter (SPC) is another option, with the catheter directly placed through the abdominal wall and into the bladder. Advantages of the SPC are less urethra trauma or strictures, less risk of catheter-induced urethritis, lack of interference with sexual function, and less likelihood of contamination from bowel incontinence.[27] Both indwelling transurethral catheters and SPC have continuous drainage bags and remain in the body for several weeks before being exchanged. Thus, caregivers must perform hygiene and empty the bag when full, which may be logistically easier than CIC.

Surgical management of NLUTD may be required when conservative methods fail.[27] For example, because a woman's urethra is shorter in length and long-term use of an indwelling catheter can lead to erosion, the indwelling catheters may leak or become dislodged overtime. Level of injury and diagnostic testing must be considered for surgical planning and sacral neuromodulation, and urinary diversion may be considered.[6,27]

SEXUALITY

Studies regarding sexuality in SCI are largely limited to men, but there is growing research into understanding the sexual disorders of women with SCI.[32] Prior research confirms that individuals with SCI can have the same levels of sexual desire as those without SCI.[33] However, physical and mental barriers may limit postinjury sexual intercourse and hinder romantic or intimate relationships. Additionally, the degree of sexual dysfunction may vary with the level and completeness of injury.

After SCI, there can be impairment of genital sensation and vaginal lubrication.[34,35] Sympathetic cell bodies that control vaginal blood flow can be impacted and may inhibit genital lubrication. Psychogenic lubrication is associated with retained perception of light touch and pinprick.[34] However, when these individuals lack sensation, significant genital lubrication is not possible.[34] Reflexive lubrication may also be affected, with literature showing up to 25% of women with complete lower motor neuron injuries capable of achieving psychogenic lubrication but not reflex lubrication because of lack of an intact sacral reflex arc.[36] This impairment in genital lubrication can be treated with over-the-counter water-soluble gel.[35] Also, also genital sensation may be decreased, evidence shows that erogenous zones above the SCI level such as the head, neck, and back are commonly enhanced.[32,35]

The ability to orgasm in women with SCI may be diminished. Fifty percent of women with SCI can achieve orgasm with T12-L1 level injuries, and about 17% of women with S2-S5 injuries may achieve orgasm.[32] Of the women with SCI who can climax, more time and more intense genital stimulation may be required. The orgasm may also be reduced in intensity and be less enjoyable than before injury.[32] This orgasmic dysfunction in women with SCI may be improved through use of tools such as a clitoral vacuum suction device. This instrument increases the ability to achieve climax by raising clitoral blood flow through suction. The resulting clitoral engorgement increases vaginal lubrication and boosts the chances for orgasm.[37]

Changes in bowel and bladder incontinence can also create barriers to physical intimacy. It is important to encourage people with SCI to perform urinary and intestinal care before sexual activity to prevent episodes of incontinence.[35,37,38] Although preventing urinary incontinence is possible, it can be incredibly distressing for individuals with SCI.[38] Catheterization and decreasing fluid intake prior to intercourse may reduce the risk of urinary incontinence during coitus. Washing and repeat catheterization immediately after intercourse reduces the risk of UTI; however, it is noted to have a negative impact on the subjective sexual experience.[35]

Control of stool or flatulence is more difficult than that of urine.[35] For individuals with lower motor neuron injury, elevated abdominal pressure caused by penetration may cause expulsion of stool. This risk may be further increased by certain positions such as knees to abdomen. Strategies such as digital rectal evacuation of the stool, restraining food intake before coitus, and a regular bowel routine can improve intestinal control. Although the anxiety of fecal incontinence may remain, employing these techniques regularly has been shown to reduce the frequency of fecal incontinence.[35,37]

Some evidence suggests that because sexuality has a large psychosocial component, sexual activity may be limited more by mental barriers rather than physical impairments.[35] Damage to self-esteem and body image, as well as lack of support during rehabilitation regarding changes in sexuality have been associated with limited postinjury sexual activity.

Anxieties regarding intercourse are common after SCI. Individuals may have concerns about body image, possible incontinence, risk of injury, and the ability to satisfy their partner. Weight and shape changes, scarring, and medical devices have been associated with an overall reduction in satisfaction with body image.[35]

Moreover, as the SCI partner becomes more dependent on the noninjured partner, the change in power dynamics of the relationship may create a barrier to intimacy.[38] Individuals with tetraplegia may note a rise in frustration and guilt for depending completely on their partner to coordinate the physical aspects of intercourse. The presence of a health aide nearby or knowing that caregivers might be aware of sexual activity is another barrier to physical intimacy.[35] Overall, women with SCI who are more independent and rely less on their uninjured partners for caregiving are more likely to have successful sexual lives after injury.

Support from the significant other has been shown to help with confidence and self-esteem issues for individuals after SCI.[35] Women with SCI have a greater chance of successful sexual adjustment if their noninjured partner has a better understanding of postinjury sexual needs.[38] Women with SCI have been noted to value sex as a positive, rewarding experience even when orgasm is unobtainable because of the emotional component increasing in significance.[35]

FERTILITY

About 60% of women with SCI experience an initial period of amenorrhea for an average of 5 to 6 months following SCI.[12,37,39] After this interval, it is possible for these women to successfully conceive and carry a child to delivery.[12] Although long-term fertility is unaffected and the desire to have children after injury is unchanged, women with SCI often face alterations in menses and new complications during pregnancy and childbirth.[12,37,40,41] Unfortunately, there is often little information given to women with SCI regarding pregnancy after injury.[40]

Menstruation length does not change following SCI. However, women after injury may have greater premenstrual and menstrual symptoms such as dysmenorrhea and cramping compared with women in the general population. These complaints can be treated with anti-inflammatory agents. Women with SCI may also encounter greater SCI-related complaints during these premenstrual and menstrual phases, including autonomic dysfunction, increased bladder spasms, and increased spasticity.[37,39]

Education regarding the return of menses should occur before discharge from acute inpatient rehabilitation and should include information on the application and use of feminine hygiene products. Some women may benefit from the use of mirrors to confirm placement of feminine products, splinting or adaptive equipment for better hand function, or instruction on how to best guide caregivers for assistance.[37]

Contraception is an important subject to discuss with women following an SCI. Prior literature shows that more than 70% of women with SCI use birth control, with condoms being the most common choice.[37] Oral contraceptive pills are another preferred method of birth control but should not be prescribed to women who are smokers, are within 1 year of injury, or have a history of cardiovascular problems because of increased risk of arterial and venous thrombosis.[37] Caution should be given to prescribing depot medroxyprogesterone acetate (DPMA) injections or subdermal implants, as they may exacerbate post-SCI bone loss.[37] Alternatives such as the barrier method (eg, intrauterine devices) are used less frequently because of an association with pelvic inflammatory disease. This is especially relevant to women with SCI, as they are already more prone to pelvic inflammatory disease because of their increased risk of UTIs and reduced pain sensation.[37] Other commonly used barriers such as diaphragms, cervical caps, and vaginal sponges may cause vaginal wall breakdown because of prolonged pressure.

In regards to menopause, literature shows that women with SCI experience similar symptoms as their noninjured counterparts.[42] However, there have been noted clinical observations that women with incomplete injuries report more frequent night sweats than those with complete injuries and women with paraplegia have increased bleeding than those with tetraplegia.[37]

When preparing for pregnancy, a woman with SCI should first undergo a thorough physical, psychological, and emotional evaluation that includes a discussion of the risks and benefits of bearing a child while having an SCI.[11,12,37] A multidisciplinary team should be assembled for comprehensive care of chronic medical conditions and changes during the pregnancy. This team may include but is not limited to an obstetrician with experience in caring for women with disabilities, maternal-fetal medicine physicians, SCI specialists, physiotherapists, and neonatologists.[11,12] Antenatal care visits should occur at a similar routine as women without SCI with specialist-specific visits as necessary.[12]

PREGNANCY

Many women of childbearing age with SCI will pursue a pregnancy sometime after the first year from injury.[12] There is no evidence to suggest a higher chance of adverse overall pregnancy outcomes,[12] but problems do exist that are unique to the pregnant SCI population.

Prior studies[11,12] have shown that the most common problems for pregnant women with SCI are urinary complications, with UTI and pyelonephritis being the most common reason for antenatal hospitalization. These individuals are also at increased risk of renal calculi because of incomplete bladder voiding, catheterization, and postinjury immobilization hypercalcemia.[12]

As the pregnancy develops, women with SCI will have worsening immobility and progressive difficulty with transfers. Despite the elevated risk immediately following injury, women with SCI have a similar chance of venous thromboembolism during pregnancy as the general population, when this increased immobility is accounted for. This congruence is because of the vessel remodeling and physiologic adaptation that occurs over time below the spinal level of injury.[12]

Skin care routines to prevent pressure injuries may need to be adjusted as the gestation age progresses. Weight gain, increased tissue edema, and the increased immobility during pregnancy can worsen the risk of women with SCI to develop decubitus ulcers. Overall, about 6% to 15% of pregnant women with SCI will develop decubital ulcers.[11,43] Therefore, there should be greater attention to skin care, use of pressure-relieving support surfaces, and appropriate weight shifting, especially in the postpartum phase and in any inpatient admission during pregnancy.[12]

Spasticity may be another challenge for women with SCI carrying a child. Prior evidence shows a 12% incidence of worsening spasms during pregnancy in this population.[12,44] Although treatment can include medications like baclofen, tizanidine, or benzodiazepines, these drugs are not recommended during pregnancy, as they can cause neonatal withdrawal symptoms.[12] Spasticity management during pregnancy may rely more heavily on regular stretching routines and occasional adjustments to medical equipment to account for the changes in mobility.[12]

In women with spinal cord lesions above the T4 level, there may progressive difficulty breathing because of weakened muscles of ventilation.[12] These can necessitate chest physiotherapy, continuous positive airway pressure, or even mechanical ventilation as the pregnancy develops. It is important for physicians to acquire baseline pulmonary function testing and look for signs of nocturnal hypercapnia that may predict impending ventilatory failure.[12]

Preterm birth is common for women with SCI.[11,12,39,40] Some evidence suggests this may in part be caused by the higher rates of infection including UTI.[39] As delivery approaches, it is vital that women with SCI have good communication with the delivery unit.[11,12] Because pain in the first stage of labor is innervated by the T10 to L1 spinal segments,[45] women with injuries at the T10 level or higher may be unaware of uterine contractions because of decreased labor pain. Instead, these individuals may experience other symptoms controlled by the sympathetic nervous system such as leg spasms, increased spasticity, or shortness of breath.[11] In order to minimize risk, it is important to instruct women how to recognize these atypical symptoms of labor and how to perform uterine palpation techniques to detect contractions.[11]

The most serious complication that can happen in women with SCIs is autonomic dysreflexia, which occurs in 85% of individuals with lesions at the T6 level or higher.[11,12] It is most likely to occur during labor but is possible during any phase of pregnancy. AD may be distinguished from pre-eclampsia by several differences including hypertension present only during labor contractions and the lack of proteinuria as seen in pre-eclampsia.[12] AD must be treated quickly, as this complication can result in serious complications such as hypertensive encephalopathy, cerebrovascular accidents, intraventricular hemorrhage, retinal hemorrhage, and death.[11]

Although women with injuries at or above the T10 level may have diminished pain perception, appropriate use of anesthesia is still necessary as labor begins. Some women may be concerned about further injuring their spinal cord during the administration of an epidural. Determining the success of an epidural block is not possible in women with complete SCI; however, a block height of T8-T10 is typically adequate, and the lack of subsequent AD is a good indication of efficacy.[12]

Women with SCI may give birth vaginally, but if autonomic dysreflexia occurs during the second stage of labor, forceps or vacuum-assisted delivery may be necessary to expedite delivery. If an episode of autonomic dysreflexia cannot be controlled, then a cesarean birth may be required.[12] Previous literature has shown significantly elevated rates of cesarean births (up to 69% in women with SCI).[11,39,43,46]

Regardless of delivery type, women with SCI tend to have longer hospitalization stays. This may be because of physicians attempting to confirm that individuals are able to balance care of the infants and themselves within their specific mobility restrictions and that sufficient education and care needs are arranged before discharge.[11,39] It is also important to examine any perineal wounds or cesarean incisions because of delayed wound healing.[39] Counseling should be provided to women regarding postpartum medications and procedures, such as fundal massage, that raise the risk of autonomic dysreflexia.

Breast feeding may be difficult in these individuals as injuries may suppress breast feeding and are associated with shorter breastfeeding times.[11] There is also some evidence that oxybutynin, which is used for bladder spasms, may also impede lactation. It is important for providers to adequately review this information and medications with women with SCI and to consult lactation specialists as needed.[12]

Screening for maternal mental health disorders is particularly critical in women with SCI, as they have been shown to have increased rates of depression, alcoholism, and suicide.[12,39,47] Some studies report a six- to ninefold increase in postpartum depression rehospitalization,[48] while another study showed the most common postpartum complication as depression.[39,40,48]

Additional complications exist for women who experience SCI during pregnancy. Some evidence shows an association between these individuals and higher risk of fetal loss and fetal malformation, possibly because of the period of hypoxia during spinal shock.[12,49,50] However, this risk is reduced if blood pressure and oxygenation are maintained properly and if the SCI occurs toward the end of pregnancy.[12,50] It is important to note that surgery on an unstable spine is not contraindicated by concomitant pregnancy.[12,51]

SUMMARY

Women with SCI have specific medical and rehabilitation needs compared with men. Primary care annual evaluation, bladder management, and sexuality and reproductive health issues for women with SCI are often overlooked, as most guidelines are non-sex specific. Clinicians caring for women with SCI must understand these differences and work with interdisciplinary teams for best outcomes and improve quality of life and function.

CLINICS CARE POINTS

- Primary care evaluations for women with SCI should follow the general population for screening, evaluations of health risk and needs, counseling, and immunizations.
- Multisystem SCI issue evaluations specific for women should be addressed on annual basis.

- Anatomic differences between men and women result in different rehabilitation needs, equipment, education, and functional status after SCI for bladder management.
- Physical and mental barriers may limit postinjury sexual intercourse and hinder romantic or intimate relationships.
- Reproduction and fertility after injury are unaffected after injury; however, functional difference can cause barriers for care.
- Pregnancy in women with SCI has medical and rehabilitation considerations, and interdisciplinary teams are needed to avoid complications.

DISCLOSURE

The authors have nothing to disclose.

REFERENCES

1. World Health Organization. Spinal cord injury. 2024. Available at: https://www.who.int/news-room/fact-sheets/detail/spinal-cord-injury. Accessed May 1, 2024.
2. National Spinal Cord Injury Statistical Center. Traumatic spinal cord injury facts and figures at a glance. Birmingham, Alabama: University of Alabama at Birmingham; 2024.
3. Milligan J, Burns S, Groah S, et al. A primary care provider's guide to preventive health after spinal cord injury. Top Spinal Cord Inj Rehabil 2020;26(3): 209–19.
4. Gibson-Gill C, Mingo T. Primary care in the spinal cord injury population: things to consider in the ongoing discussion. Curr Phys Med Rehabil Rep 2023;11(1): 74–85.
5. Slocum C, Halloran M, Unser C. A primary care provider's guide to clinical needs of women with spinal cord injury. Top Spinal Cord Inj Rehabil 2020;26(3):166–71.
6. Consortium for Spinal Cord. Bladder management for adults with spinal cord injury: a clinical practice guideline for health-care providers. J Spinal Cord Med 2006;29(5):527–73.
7. Ginsberg DA, Boone TB, Cameron AP, et al. The AUA/SUFU guideline on adult neurogenic lower urinary tract dysfunction: diagnosis and evaluation. J Urol 2021;206(5):1097–105.
8. Ginsberg DA, Boone TB, Cameron AP, et al. The AUA/SUFU guideline on adult neurogenic lower urinary tract dysfunction: treatment and follow-up. J Urol 2021;206(5):1106–13.
9. Johns J, Krogh K, Rodriguez GM, et al. Management of neurogenic bowel dysfunction in adults after spinal cord injury: clinical practice guideline for health care providers. Top Spinal Cord Inj Rehabil 2021;27(2):75–151.
10. Consortium for Spinal Cord M. Acute management of autonomic dysreflexia: individuals with spinal cord injury presenting to health-care facilities. J Spinal Cord Med 2002;25(Suppl 1):S67–88.
11. Obstetric management of patients with spinal cord injuries: ACOG Committee opinion, number 808. Obstet Gynecol 2020;135(5):e230–6.
12. Robertson K, Ashworth F. Spinal cord injury and pregnancy. Obstet Med 2022; 15(2):99–103.
13. Galeiras Vazquez R, Rascado Sedes P, Mourelo Farina M, et al. Respiratory management in the patient with spinal cord injury. BioMed Res Int 2013;2013:168757.

14. Mann LM, Angus SA, Doherty CJ, et al. Evaluation of sex-based differences in airway size and the physiological implications. Eur J Appl Physiol 2021; 121(11):2957–66.

15. Rahrovan S, Fanian F, Mehryan P, et al. Male versus female skin: what dermatologists and cosmeticians should know. Int J Womens Dermatol 2018;4(3):122–30.

16. Calleja-Agius J, Brincat M. The effect of menopause on the skin and other connective tissues. Gynecol Endocrinol 2012;28(4):273–7.

17. Kottner J, Cuddigan J, Carville K, et al. Prevention and treatment of pressure ulcers/injuries: the protocol for the second update of the international Clinical Practice Guideline 2019. J Tissue Viability 2019;28(2):51–8.

18. Wright CL, Patel J, Hettrich CM. Sports-related shoulder injuries among female athletes. Curr Rev Musculoskelet Med 2022;15(6):637–44.

19. Wellisch M, Lovett K, Harrold M, et al. Treatment of shoulder pain in people with spinal cord injury who use manual wheelchairs: a systematic review and meta-analysis. Spinal Cord 2022;60(2):107–14.

20. LeBoff MS, Greenspan SL, Insogna KL, et al. The clinician's guide to prevention and treatment of osteoporosis. Osteoporos Int 2022;33(10):2049–102.

21. Bauman WA, Cardozo CP. Osteoporosis in individuals with spinal cord injury. Pharm Manag PM R 2015;7(2):188–201, quiz 201.

22.. Consortium for Spinal Cord Medicine. Bone health and osteoporosis management in individuals with spinal cord injury: clinical practice guideline for health care providers. Paralyzed Veterans of America 2022;2–7.

23. Consortium for Spinal Cord M. Management of mental health disorders, substance use disorders, and suicide in adults with spinal cord injury. Paralyzed Veterans of America; 2020.

24. Anderson CE, Birkhauser V, Liechti MD, et al. Sex differences in urological management during spinal cord injury rehabilitation: results from a prospective multicenter longitudinal cohort study. Spinal Cord 2023;61(1):43–50.

25. Patra PB, Patra S. Sex differences in the physiology and pharmacology of the lower urinary tract. Curr Urol 2013;6(4):179–88.

26. Michel MC, Vrydag W. Alpha1-alpha2- and beta-adrenoceptors in the urinary bladder, urethra and prostate. Br J Pharmacol 2006;147(Suppl 2):S88–119.

27.. Perez NE, Godbole NP, Amin K, et al. Neurogenic bladder physiology, pathogenesis, and management after spinal cord injury. J Pers Med 2022;12(6):968.

28. Beeson T, Davis C. Urinary management with an external female collection device. J Wound, Ostomy Cont Nurs 2018;45(2):187–9.

29. Unger CA, Tunitsky-Bitton E, Muffly T, et al. Neuroanatomy, neurophysiology, and dysfunction of the female lower urinary tract: a review. Female Pelvic Med Reconstr Surg 2014;20(2):65–75.

30. Panicker JN. Neurogenic bladder: epidemiology, diagnosis, and management. Semin Neurol 2020;40(5):569–79.

31.. Consortium for Spinal Cord M. Outcomes following traumatic spinal cord injury: clinical practice guidelines for health-care professionals. Paralyzed Veterans of America 1999;12–9.

32. Otero-Villaverde S, Ferreiro-Velasco ME, Montoto-Marques A, et al. Sexual satisfaction in women with spinal cord injuries. Spinal Cord 2015;53(7):557–60.

33. Zizzo J, Gater DR, Hough S, et al. Sexuality, intimacy, and reproductive health after spinal cord injury. J Personalized Med 2022;12(12).

34. Sipski ML, Alexander CJ, Rosen RC. Physiologic parameters associated with sexual arousal in women with incomplete spinal cord injuries. Arch Phys Med Rehabil 1997;78(3):305–13.

35. Thrussell H, Coggrave M, Graham A, et al. Women's experiences of sexuality after spinal cord injury: a UK perspective. Spinal Cord 2018;56(11):1084–94.

36. Sipski ML, Alexander CJ, Rosen R. Sexual arousal and orgasm in women: effects of spinal cord injury. Ann Neurol 2001;49(1):35–44.

37. Consortium for Spinal Cord. Sexuality and reproductive health in adults with spinal cord injury: a clinical practice guideline for health-care professionals. J Spinal Cord Med 2010;33(3):281–336.

38. Forsythe E, Horsewell JE. Sexual rehabilitation of women with a spinal cord injury. Spinal Cord 2006;44(4):234–41.

39. Crane DA, Doody DR, Schiff MA, et al. Pregnancy outcomes in women with spinal cord injuries: a population-based study. Pharm Manag PM R 2019;11(8): 795–806.

40. Ghidini A, Healey A, Andreani M, et al. Pregnancy and women with spinal cord injuries. Acta Obstet Gynecol Scand 2008;87(10):1006–10.

41. Hocaloski S, Elliott S, Hodge K, et al. Perinatal care for women with spinal cord injuries: a collaborative workshop for consensus on care in Canada. Top Spinal Cord Inj Rehabil 2017;23(4):386–96.

42. Dannels A, Charlifue S. The perimenopause experience for women with spinal cord injuries. Sci Nurs 2004;21(1):9–13.

43. Le Liepvre H, Dinh A, Idiard-Chamois B, et al. Pregnancy in spinal cord-injured women, a cohort study of 37 pregnancies in 25 women. Spinal Cord 2017; 55(2):167–71.

44. Jackson AB, Wadley V. A multicenter study of women's self-reported reproductive health after spinal cord injury. Arch Phys Med Rehabil 1999;80(11):1420–8.

45. Labor S, Maguire S. The pain of labour. Rev Pain 2008;2(2):15–9.

46. Bertschy S, Bostan C, Meyer T, et al. Medical complications during pregnancy and childbirth in women with SCI in Switzerland. Spinal Cord 2016;54(3):183–7.

47. Cesario SK. Spinal cord injuries. Nurses can help affected women & their families achieve pregnancy birth. AWHONN Lifelines 2002;6(3):224–32.

48. Mitra M, Iezzoni LI, Zhang J, et al. Prevalence and risk factors for postpartum depression symptoms among women with disabilities. Matern Child Health J 2015;19(2):362–72.

49. Baranovic S, Maldini B, Cengic T, et al. Anesthetic management of acute cervical spinal cord injury in pregnancy. Acta Clin Croat 2014;53(1):98–101.

50. Engel S, Ferrara G. Obstetric outcomes in women who sustained a spinal cord injury during pregnancy. Spinal Cord 2013;51(2):170–1.

51. Gotfryd AO, Franzin FJ, Poletto PR, et al. Fracture-dislocation of the thoracic spine during second trimester of pregnancy: case report and literature review. Rev Bras Ortop 2012;47(4):521–5.

Considerations for the Rehabilitation Management of the Female Athlete

Allison N. Schroeder, MD[a,b,1,*], Crystal Graff, MD[c,2],
Maura Guyler, BA[b,3]

KEYWORDS

• Female athlete • Rehabilitation • Injury • Performance

KEY POINTS

- Increased participation of females in sport has led to an increase in injuries and the need for rehabilitation protocols targeting the unique characteristics of female athletes.
- A paradigm shift is required to understand the physiologic, anatomic, and hormonal factors that impact a female athlete's predisposition to and recovery from injury.
- Female athletes' physiology fluctuates depending on age, life circumstances (eg, pregnancy), and their menstrual cycle; therefore, rehabilitation considerations must evolve through a female athlete's lifespan.
- Rehabilitation of injuries for female athletes often involves a multidisciplinary approach that incorporates strength training, nutrition, and psychological readiness.

INTRODUCTION/BACKGROUND

Since the passing of Title IX in 1972, female participation in sport has grown at an exponentially large rate.[1] In marathon and ultramarathon events, female participation has increased by at least 50% over the past 40 years with females surpassing males in some age groups.[2] In the 2022 to 2023 school year, 3,328,180 females participated in high school sports in the United States.[3] For collegiate athletics, in 2023, the number of female athletes increased to 226,212, compared with approximately 30,000 in

[a] Department of Physical Medicine and Rehabilitation, MetroHealth Rehabilitation Institute and Case Western Reserve University, Cleveland, OH, USA; [b] Case Western University School of Medicine, Cleveland, OH, USA; [c] Department of Orthopedics and Rehabilitation, University of Iowa Sports Medicine, Iowa City, IA, USA
[1] Present address: 16609 Ernadale Avenue, Cleveland, OH 44111.
[2] Present address: 2275 Willenbrock Circle, Iowa City, IA 52245.
[3] Present address: 12201 Larchmere Boulevard, Apartment 423, Cleveland, OH 44120.
* Corresponding author. Department of Physical Medicine and Rehabilitation, MetroHealth Rehabilitation Institute, 2500 MetroHealth Drive, Cleveland, OH 44109.
E-mail address: Aschroe1@alumni.nd.edu

Phys Med Rehabil Clin N Am 36 (2025) 279–295
https://doi.org/10.1016/j.pmr.2024.11.012
1047-9651/25/© 2024 Elsevier Inc. All rights are reserved, including those for text and data mining, AI training, and similar technologies.
pmr.theclinics.com

Abbreviations	
ACL	anterior cruciate ligament
BMD	bone mineral density
BSI	bone stress injury
LEA	low energy availability
PFPS	patellofemoral pain syndrome
RED-S	relative energy deficiency in sport

1972.[4] Female athletes are more likely than male athletes to specialize in and undertake a high competition volume, both of which predispose them to overuse injuries.[5] As the trend of increased female participation in sports continues, it is imperative that medical professionals have a thorough understanding of the health considerations unique to female athletes.

This article will discuss the anatomic, physiologic, hormonal, and psychosocial factors unique to the female athlete, review considerations unique to different stages of life in the female athlete, provide a current assessment on injury prevalence, and discuss specific considerations for the rehabilitation of several common conditions to identify how an understanding of characteristics unique to female athletes can guide optimization of rehabilitation protocols.

GENDER DIFFERENCES AFFECTING PERFORMANCE AND REHABILITATION
Anatomic/Mechanical

The differences in female musculoskeletal anatomy compared with males can affect the performance and rehabilitation outcomes (Table 1).[6,7] Notably, female's reduced height and center of gravity confer an advantage in sports requiring balance.[7] The differences of greatest impact are those related to a higher risk of injury in females compared with males (see specific injuries later).

Physiologic

There are several physiologic parameters to consider when treating and rehabilitating the female athlete (see Table 1).[6–9] The overall reduced blood volume, reduced vital capacity, and reduced Vo_{2max} in females lends to a lower ceiling on their aerobic capacity compared with males.[6,7,9] The differences in energy metabolism also has implications for how to adequately fuel female athletes compared with males.[6,8]

Neuromuscular

There are several sex differences related to neuromuscular control of joints, which are thought to relate to injury incidence and prevalence (see Table 1).[10–13] Neuromuscular training programs targeting these deficits are important to be considered in the rehabilitation of the female athlete.

Hormonal

Hormonal control and secretion play an intricate role in the functioning of the neuromusculoskeletal system. Sex hormones, in particular estrogen, progesterone, and testosterone, affect several parts of this system both in basal secretion and related to the female menstrual cycle and reproduction (Tables 2 and 3).[6,9,14] Other important players in this system include the hormones relaxin, growth hormone, and insulin-like growth factor 1. Important factors to keep in mind when planning the rehabilitation of a female athlete include estrogen's effect on bone density, ligamentous laxity, and reduced tendon stiffness.[14]

Table 1
Anatomic, physiologic, and neuromuscular gender difference affecting performance and rehabilitation

	Females Compared with Males	Injury and Rehabilitation Implications
Anatomic/Mechanical	• ↓ height • ↓ limb length • Wider pelvis • Narrower shoulders • ↑ percentage of subcutaneous fat • ↑ breast tissue • ↓ muscle mass • ↑ joint/ligamentous laxity • ↓ heart size • ↓ chest cavity size	• ↓ height → ↓ center of gravity → improved balance • ↑ fat→ greater buoyancy • ↑ joint/ligamentous laxity → ↑ joint dislocations, joint laxity, ligamentous sprains/tears
Physiologic	• ↓ sympathetic tone and systemic vascular resistance • ↓ stroke volume and cardiac output • ↓ blood volume and hemoglobin • ↓ total lung volume and vital capacity • ↓ Vo_{2max} • ↑ fat metabolism during exercise • ↑ thermoregulation	• ↓ Vo_2 max → ↓ aerobic capacity
Neuromuscular	• ↑ valgus knee angle with initial contact and landing • ↓ quadriceps and hamstring torque • ↑ quadriceps to hamstring strength ratio • ↓ core stability with landing	• Lack of neuromuscular control leads to higher injury rates in ACL tears, patellofemoral syndrome and ankle sprains. • Rehab efforts specifically targeting neuromuscular control, integrating balance, agility, and strength are effective.

Abbreviation: ACL, anterior cruciate ligament.
Data from Citations: [6,7](anatomy); [6–9](physiology); [10–13](neuromuscular).

Table 2
Hormonal gender difference affecting performance and rehabilitation

Hormone	Estrogen	Progesterone	Testosterone
Effects on the female body	• Modulates cardiac contractility • ↓ sympathetic tone ↓ blood pressure ↓ systemic vascular resistance • ↑ bone mass • ↑ muscle strength and lean muscle • ↑ ligamentous laxity • ↓ tendon stiffness	• ↑ body temperature and sweating • Enhances muscle growth • Inhibits neurons	• ↑ lean muscle

Data from Citations.[6,9,14]

Menstrual cycle

Female athletes must uniquely consider the hormonal fluctuations that accompany the menstrual cycle. The effect that the eumenorrheic menstrual cycle has on female athlete performance, injury risk, and rehabilitation potential is still being fully elucidated, but it seems that injury burden is higher in the late follicular and ovulatory phases (**Fig. 1**, see **Table 3**).[15–21]

Perturbations in the menstrual cycle, commonly due to relative energy deficiency in sport (RED-S) and low energy availability (LEA), lead to oligomenorrhea or amenorrhea. Menstrual dysfunction often impacts injury severity, sexual function, fertility, bone health, cognitive function, and mood.[7,22] There are a paucity of studies investigating how menstrual dysfunction affects healing and recovery from exercise and injury, except as it relates to bone stress injuries (BSIs).[22,23]

RELATIVE ENERGY DEFICIENCY IN SPORT AND LOW ENERGY AVAILABILITY

Historically, LEA was classified under the diagnosis of Female Athlete Triad, which encompasses a syndrome of (1) disordered eating, (2) reduced bone mineral density (BMD), and (3) menstrual dysfunction.[23,24] LEA has now been found to affect other body systems and terminology has transitioned to that of RED-S to better encompass the comprehensive and multisystem effects of energy deficiency. Most often RED-S is associated with menstrual dysfunction and impaired bone health but additionally has "other endocrine and metabolic effects, growth and development disruptions, cardiovascular system disturbances, gastrointestinal slowing, hematological and immunologic adaptions, and mental health disorders."[25]

Regardless of syndrome naming, RED-S and LEA are very common among female athletes. In a cohort of elite female athletes between ages 15 and 32, 40% exhibited at least 2 symptoms of RED-S.[26] Disordered eating among female athletes is as high as 62% with an up to 5 times greater prevalence than male athletes.[27–29] RED-S and LEA more often affect athletes who participate in "lean" or "weight-sensitive sports," like dance, gymnastics, running, and figure skating.[27] It is important to optimize energy availability during the rehabilitation of female athletes as RED-S and LEA may curtail injury healing efforts.

MENTAL HEALTH CONSIDERATIONS

Competing in sport presents a unique set of psychological challenges for the female athlete, including risk of suffering from anxiety, depression, body image issues, and interpersonal violence. Anxiety and depressive disorders are higher among female versus male athletes and show an equal or greater prevalence compared with nonathlete females.[28,30,31] Specific review of body image dissatisfaction reveals a higher trend among female athletes, particularly in leanness or esthetic-based sports, as they balance the pressure of aspiring to the "ideal" body for healthy sport participation versus per societal standards.[28,32,33] Athletes also experience pressure from social media and societal influences that often present a curated version of the "ideal" body.[32,33] Additionally, sport-related abuse, also known as interpersonal violence, comes in many forms, including psychological, sexual, physical, financial, and neglect types.[34,35] Female athletes experience abuse at higher rates compared with male athletes, with sexual violence estimated to be 4 times as common.[27]

It is furthermore important to consider minoritized female populations based on race, ethnicity, disability, and socioeconomic status who are especially vulnerable to psychological stressors on and off the field.[27,36] Greater psychological distress among female athletes is exacerbated by factors such as injury, performance

Table 3
Effects on the female body with menstruation

Stage	Premenstruation	Menstruation	Late Follicular/ Ovulation (Higher Estrogen)	Mid-Luteal (Lower Estrogen)
Effects on the female body	• Symptom burden affects training schedules and competitive performance	• ↑ impulsivity	• ↑ ligamentous and joint laxity • ↑ muscle stiffness • ↓ neuromuscular control • ? reduced performance in early follicular phase	• ↓ muscle power/ strength • Delayed recovery from high-intensity exercise

Data from Citations.[15–21]

pressure, financial hardship, gender inequality, sexual abuse, interpersonal violence, media sexualization and social media abuse, body image concerns, and family planning.[28,30,31,36] An especially important stressor for physicians to consider is the negative effect that injury has on athlete's mental health.[27,37] Therefore, it is important to ensure that the mental health of an athlete is optimized and that an athlete feels psychologically safe throughout the rehabilitation process. The medical team should consider psychological readiness in the return to play decision and can help in supporting positive factors like self-esteem, internal locus of control, and athletic identity while disbanding negative factors like kinesiophobia and fear of reinjury.[27] Rehabilitation from pelvic floor dysfunction may be a necessary part of the treatment of female athletes who have experienced abuse.[38]

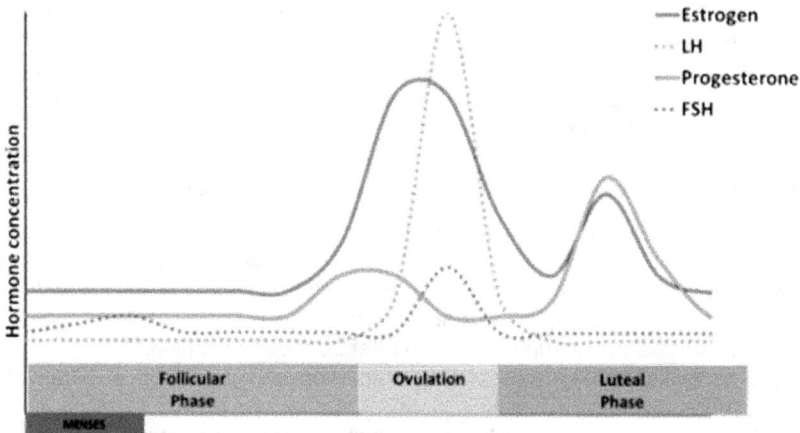

Fig. 1. Hormonal fluctuations in the female menstrual cycle. (*From* Golan E, Lopez MT, Wright V. Chapter 3 - Anterior Cruciate Ligament Injuries: Sex-Based Differences. In: Frank RM, ed. The Female Athlete. Elsevier; 2022.)

FEMALE ATHLETES BY AGE/STAGE OF LIFE
Pediatric/Adolescent

Youth athletes are participating in sports at an earlier age and with greater intensity than ever before.[39] Much research involving young athletes has revolved around the detrimental effects of early sport specialization, which is more common in females.[40] Risk of injury is higher in female athletes who specialize earlier on, likely due in part to the development of motor and coordination deficits with changes in center of gravity and limb length during puberty.[41] This highlights the importance of integrating early strength training and neuromuscular control programs for this population to reduce future injury burden.[42] Detecting menstrual cycle irregularities in female youth athletes is crucial, but it may be difficult to elicit irregularities in those who are around pubertal age. Menstrual irregularities affecting bone density accrual are particularly problematic in this population, as they may lead to lower bone density in adulthood.[43]

Recommendations for treating and rehabilitating pediatric/adolescent female athletes:

- Maintain a regular sleep-wake cycle—goal of around 9 to 10 hours of sleep per night reduces injury and improves performance.[44]
- Optimize nutrition (fuel to maintain menses)—adequate carbohydrates, protein, and fat, as well as micronutrients like calcium, Vitamin D, and iron are essential.[44]
- Delay sport specialization (until after puberty)—maintain 1 to 2 nonpractice days weekly and 3 months per year free of organized sport.[39,44]
- Participate in regular resistance training program fitted to biological age and psychosocial maturity.[42]
- Supervise rehabilitation and strength training programs—to ensure proper technique and safe progression.[42]

Pregnancy

The female body undergoes several anatomic and physiologic changes during pregnancy which increase the risk of musculoskeletal injury and affect their ability to remain active. Remaining physically active during pregnancy is highly recommended, although modifications may be necessary for the health of the mother and fetus.[45] Pregnant females experience soft tissue edema, ligamentous laxity, weight gain, and a shift in center of gravity leading to greater lumbar lordosis and stress on the low back and peripheral joints.[45,46] As a result, pregnant athletes often experience nonspecific low back pain and pelvic girdle pain, including sacroiliac joint and pubic symphysis dysfunction, hip pain, and compression-related peripheral neuropathies.[46]

Recommendations for treating and rehabilitating pregnant athletes:

- Perform both regular aerobic and anaerobic exercises as long as there are no contraindications (contraindications include: persistent bleeding, cardiovascular disease, restrictive lung disease, multiple gestation, cervical insufficiency, preeclampsia, and premature contractions).[47]
- Avoid exercise in the supine position after 20-week gestation.[45]
- Avoid activities with the risk of falling or collision, at high altitude, in extreme heat, and scuba diving.[47]
- Optimize pelvic floor strength to prevent urinary incontinence and low back pain.[48]
- Consider use of a sacroiliac joint belt and/or acupuncture for the treatment of pelvic girdle pain.[49,50]

Postpartum

Following childbirth, the postpartum period of a female's life poses its own unique chal-lenges regarding rehabilitation and return to activity. Physiologic changes of pregnancy may persist for up to 6 weeks postpartum and, subsequently, females often experience similar musculoskeletal complaints as during pregnancy.[45,46] Most recommend pelvic floor strengthening (Kegel exercises and core strengthening) begin immediately post-partum.[45,48] Early return to sport may be associated with an increased risk of sustaining ligamentous and/or bony injury, particularly sacral stress fractures, and breastfeeding re-quires extra nutritional energy that can predispose to the development of LEA and RED-S.[51] It is also important to note other social factors that may impede return to sport and in-crease injury risk postpartum, including access to childcare, lack of sleep, lack of maternal leave benefit, and loss of financial earnings through missed work/competition.[52]

Recommendations for treating and rehabilitating postpartum athletes:

- There is no specific guideline for timing to return to activity and it should be indi-vidualized and gradual.[53] Return to running postpartum should be guided by passing medical and impact screening milestones, healing completely from birth injuries, obtaining an adequate duration and quality of sleep, having adequate breast support, and being mentally ready for the task.[54,55]
- Optimize pelvic floor and core strength to prevent urinary incontinence, pelvic floor dysfunction, low back pain, and diastasis recti.[48,53]
- Optimize hip and knee stabilizer strength to prevent musculoskeletal injury related to return to activity.[55]
- Maintain adequate nutrition and hydration, particularly calcium intake, to poten-tially reduce risk of BSI with increasing exercise.[51,53,56]

Postmenopausal

Postmenopausal female athletes face similar considerations to those that are preg-nant and postpartum in that hormonal fluctuations affect exercise abilities and injury risk. This period is associated with reductions in bone mass, lean muscle mass and strength, and flexibility, as well as weight gain and increase in fat percentage due in part to reduced metabolic rate and proportion of type II muscle fibers.[57,58] The reduc-tion in bone mass is especially pertinent given the accompanying withdrawal in estro-gen with menopause.[59] Of particular importance is the risk of LEA and BSI in this population given an already hypo-estrogenic state and lack of ability to use loss of menstruation as a detection tool for RED-S and LEA.[60] To lessen performance decline and prevent injury, some propose a greater emphasis on nutritional intake for the mas-ters athlete, particularly a higher protein diet and considering timing of nutrient intake.[61,62] It is also important to consider that nutrient deficiencies are more common in older females, particularly Vitamin D, Vitamin B6 and B12, iron, and calcium.[61,62]

Recommendations for treating and rehabilitating postmenopausal athletes:

- Nutritional history and counseling is especially important in this population as their requirements for protein, Vitamin D, and omega 3 fatty acids are higher.[62]
- Consider the use of hormone replacement therapy for prevention and treatment of low BMD and chronic tendinopathies.[59,63,64]

REHABILITATION CONSIDERATIONS FOR INJURIES COMMON IN FEMALE ATHLETES
Anterior Cruciate Ligament Tear

Anterior cruciate ligament (ACL) tears are 10 times more likely in females, and females are between 2 and 8 times more likely tear their ACL through a "noncontact"

Table 4 Sex differences in risk factors for anterior cruciate ligament tears		
	Risk Factors in Females Compared with Males	**Implications for ACL Tear**
Anatomic	• ↑ pelvic width, → ↑ femoral anteversion, ↑ Q-angle, ↑ genu valgum, ↑ external tibial torsion • ↑ joint laxity • ↓ ligament size • ↓ intercondylar notch • ↑ posterior tibial plateau and meniscal slope • Shallower trochlear groove • ↑ BMI • ↓ hamstring stiffness • ↓ core strength	Increased Q-angle leads to lateral pull of the quadriceps putting greater stress on the ACL
Biomechanical (with landing)	• ↓ knee proprioception • Quadriceps dominant contraction • ↑ time to generate peak hamstring torque • ↓ hip and knee flexion	Reliance on quadriceps leads to weakening of the hamstrings that stabilize the knee and anterior movement of the tibia on the femur adding stress to the ACL
Hormonal	• ↑ estrogen → ↑ ligament laxity	ACL tears more frequently occur in the follicular and preovulatory phases of the menstrual cycle due to higher estrogen and relaxin levels

Abbreviation: ACL, anterior cruciate ligament. BMI, body mass index.
   Data from Citations.[6,24,65]

mechanism of injury when compared with males.[6,24] Inherent anatomic, biomechanical, and hormonal factors unique to female athletes contribute to their increased risk of ACL injury (**Table 4**).[6,24,65] Preventative rehabilitation that is individualized, sport-specific, and encompasses a combination of strengthening, plyometrics, proximal control, and balance/neuromuscular control exercises are beneficial but adherence is often poor.[66,67]

Treatment for ACL tears continues to rely on surgical reconstruction versus rehabilitation alone, especially for athletes experiencing symptoms of instability and engaging in sports reliant on jumping, cutting, and pivoting.[68] Presurgical rehabilitation to restore flexion and extension range of motion (ROM), reduce effusion, and improve quadriceps strength, as well as postsurgical rehabilitation focused on quadriceps and neuromuscular training, neuromuscular electrical stimulation, and open versus closed chain kinetic exercises for rehabilitation is recommended.[69,70] Following rehabilitation, female athletes display greater quadriceps strength asymmetry when compared with males suggesting that female's rehabilitation should focus more heavily on isolated quadriceps strengthening.[71]

Female athletes report a lower subjective function following ACL reconstruction, have a lower return to sport rate, and report declining performance compared with males; however, objective measures recorded between sexes are not significantly different, owing to the potential interplay of psychological readiness (fear avoidance or kinesiophobia, self-efficacy, stress, and social support).[27,71,72] Athletes with ACL injuries have reported symptoms of depression and post-traumatic stress disorder with females reporting a higher severity of symptoms.[27,30,73] Sustaining an ACL tear leads to increased risk of developing knee osteoarthritis and females who undergo ACL reconstruction surgery are more likely to eventually undergo total knee arthroplasty.[74,75]

Patellofemoral

Patellofemoral pain syndrome (PFPS) refers to anterior knee pain around the patella, and females are at least twice as likely to experience it as males.[76,77] There are several anatomic, biomechanical, and hormonal factors unique to female athletes that contribute to their increased risk of developing PFPS (**Table 5**).[78–80] In most cases of PFPS, there is no isolated anatomic or biomechanical cause, and it is often attributed to previous trauma, overuse, and drastic acute or chronic changes in training load.[77]

Understanding the factors that predispose females to develop PFPS helps inform rehabilitation and prevention efforts. It is important to properly identify, educate, and treat female athletes with PFPS as the development of PFPS may impact athletes' career longevity as there is a greater likelihood of developing patellofemoral joint osteoarthritis.[76] It can additionally have deleterious consequences on athletes' quality of life and mental health as it often recurs and is resistant to treatment.[81,82] Rehabilitation protocols should include a combination of strengthening, flexibility, proprioception, endurance, and functional training.[77] Strengthening focuses on targeting the muscles surrounding both the hip and knee joints, including core musculature.[76,83] However, current research does not support one unifying protocol for all patients. Other adjunctive interventions with mixed support include the use of patellar taping (McConnell or Kinesio), bracing (patellar sleeve or patellar stabilizing), foot orthoses, manual therapy, dry needling, blood flow restriction therapy, and gait retraining.[76,84] Patient education with the addition of mindfulness practice and other psychologically informed interventions are also effective.[81,85]

Bone Stress Injury

BSIs are overuse injuries resulting from repeated and sustained microtrauma and can be classified into 2 types, fatigue (too much load on normal bone) and insufficiency (normal load on weakened bone). In both sexes, BSIs comprise approximately 20% of all sports injuries and are more common in esthetic sports.[23,24] Females are twice as likely develop BSIs than males.[23] As part of the treatment and rehabilitation of BSIs, extrinsic and intrinsic risk factors, many of which are more common in females, should be addressed (**Table 6**).[23,86–89]

Following a BSI, rest/offloading of the affected joint should be combined with an assessment of risks of BSIs, which should be addressed prior to a gradual progression of loading/strengthening before full return to activity. RED-S and LEA and their subsequent complications are commonly cited intrinsic risk factors for the development of BSIs and should be addressed as part of the rehabilitation process.[86] Optimization of the hypothalamic-pituitary-gonadal access is important in the management of BSIs, as chronic hypoestrogenism leads to a loss of bone density, akin to what is seen in older females going through menopause, due to suppression of osteoblast function.[90] Athletes with oligomenorrhea and/or secondary amenorrhea due to RED-S and LEA experienced BSIs 2 to 4 times more frequently than female athletes without menstrual irregularities and have greater severity of injury according to MRI staging.[91] Unfortunately, athletes who lose bone mass because of secondary amenorrhea may never recover the lost bone mass and may develop premenopausal osteoporosis.[90]

Table 5
Sex differences in risk factors for patellofemoral pain syndrome

	Risk Factors in Females Compared with Males	Implications for Patellofemoral Syndrome
Anatomic	• ↑ femoral neck anteversion • ↑ genu valgus • ↑ trochlear dysplasia • ↑ patella alta • Tighter lateral retinaculum and iliotibial band • ↑ quadriceps weakness • Vastus lateralis > vastus medialis strength. *Conflicting evidence on the contribution of the static Q-angle and rearfoot pronation.	Anatomic differences lend to the patella tracking more laterally within the trochlear groove leading to greater symptoms and increased risk of dislocation.
Biomechanical	• ↑ dynamic medial femoral translation and rotation • Lagging activation time of vastus medialis vs vastus lateralis • ↑ dynamic Q-angle (and knee valgus moment) • ↑ knee and lower leg stiffness in landing and deep squat. *Conflicting evidence on whether greater or lesser hip abduction and external rotation strength contributes.	These biomechanical alterations lead to greater pull of the patella laterally during dynamic movements such as running, jumping, and squatting.
Hormonal	• ↑ knee joint laxity • ↑ body mass and longer joints following puberty	Leads to greater patellar mobility and alteration in biomechanics without adequate strength to compensate

* Indicates conflicting evidence.
Data from Citations.[78–80]

Table 6
Risk factors for bone stress injuries

Intrinsic Factors	Extrinsic Factors
• Prior BSI • Low energy availability • ↓ mean muscle mass • ↓ overall bone density • ↓ calf circumference • ↑ tibial free moment • ↑ peak hip adduction • Hindfoot eversion	• Rapid change in activity • Early sport specialization • Repetitive loading • Higher amount of time spent in sport • Corticosteroid use • High NSAID intake • Low Vitamin D and Calcium intake *Conflicting evidence on the influence of footwear and training surface, oral contraceptive use, BMI.

Abbreviation: BSI, bone stress injury. NSAID, nonsteroidal anti-inflammatory drugs.
* Indicates conflicting evidence.
Data from Citations.[23,86–89]

DISCUSSION

This review highlights important considerations unique to the female athlete as their participation in sport increases. These considerations relate to several intrinsic factors associated with underlying differences in the anatomy and physiology of the female body, largely relating to the menstrual cycle and hormonal fluctuations. Female athletes are at higher risk of certain injuries such as ACL tears, PFPS, and BSIs. Additionally, often female athletes do not return to sport at the same rate as male athletes following injury, which can have life-long implications on participation in physical activity. Furthermore, females interested in starting a family must consider the influence that family planning, pregnancy, breastfeeding, and the postpartum period have on their athletic endeavors. Experts in the field of female athletes through the International Olympic Committee convened in 2020 to establish 10 primary health domains unique to female athletes to guide future research.[92] In this consensus statement, they highlighted considering different stages of a female athlete's lifespan and issues that specifically ail female athletes.[92]

It is also important to highlight extrinsic factors that create undue psychological stress for female athletes. Inequity of opportunity continues to mark female athlete's careers in issues ranging from lower financial compensation to limited female representation as coaches or leaders of sporting bodies.[27,36] Female athletes hoping to start a family are often presented with the choice of either continuing their athletic career or starting a family, and, more frequently than male athletes, end their career prematurely to accommodate family obligations.[36] The continued practice of sexualizing female athletes via social media has wide-ranging effects on the public's perception of them and their perception of themselves, as well as on younger females who may be looking to them for inspiration.[36,93] All of these factors can affect an athlete's path to recovery from injury and must be considered during the rehabilitation (and prevention) of injury in female athletes.

SUMMARY

In summary, there is much work to be done to better understand and support female athletes to optimize their health, quality of life, and ability to recover from injury to continue to participate in sport. This narrative review covers considerations unique to the rehabilitation of female athletes. Health care professionals play a vital role in the care of these athletes and are well poised to continue advocating for them as patients and people alike.

CLINICS CARE POINTS

- Rehabilitation considerations for female athletes must account for their unique neuromuscular, anatomic, physiologic, and hormonal factors.
- Physiologic changes and external stressors and life events outside of sport, such as family planning, pregnancy, and breastfeeding must be considered when developing rehabilitation strategies for female athletes.
- Anterior cruciate ligament tears and patellofemoral pain syndrome are more common in female athletes compared with males, and rehabilitation should focus on hip and knee stabilizer strengthening and neuromuscular training and incorporate a psychological readiness assessment prior to return to sport.
- The relationship between bone stress injuries and relative energy deficiency in sport underscores the importance of assessment of risk factors such as low bone mineral density

and a comprehensive and multidisciplinary rehabilitation approach that includes nutritional and mental health resources and support.

- Support for mental health concerns, body image stress, abuse, and other psychological stressors should be readily available during the rehabilitation process and incorporated into the culture of female athletics.

DISCLOSURE

The authors have nothing to disclose.

REFERENCES

1. NCAA. Title IX 50th Anniversary: The state of women in college sports. 2022.
2. Nesburg RA, Mason AP, Fitzsimmons B, et al. Sex differences in marathon running: physiology and participation. Exercise, Sport, and Movement 2023;1(3):e00010.
3. NFHS. High school sports participation continues rebound toward pre-pandemic levels. 2023. Available at: https://www.nfhs.org/articles/high-school-sports-partic ipation-continues-rebound-toward-pre-pandemic-levels/. Accessed October 3, 2024.
4. McGuire C. A look at trends for women in college sports. 2023. Available at: https://www.ncaa.org/news/2023/3/1/media-center-a-look-at-trends-for-women-in-college-sports.aspx. Accessed October 3, 2024.
5. Tanaka MJ, LiBrizzi CL, Rivenburgh DW, et al. Changes in U.S. girls' participation in high school sports: implications for injury awareness. Phys Sportsmed 2021; 49(4):450–4.
6. Bassett AJ, Ahlmen A, Rosendorf JM, et al. The biology of sex and sport. JBJS Rev 2020;8(3):e0140.
7. Hecht SS, Arendt E. Training the female athlete. In: Handbook of sports medicine and science. 2014. p. 1–8.
8. Tarnopolsky MA. Gender differences in metabolism; nutrition and supplements. J Sci Med Sport 2000;3(3):287–98.
9. Hunter SK, S SA, Bhargava A, et al. The biological basis of sex differences in athletic performance: consensus statement for the American college of sports medicine. Med Sci Sports Exerc 2023;55(12):2328–60.
10. Hewett TE, Myer GD, Ford KR. Decrease in neuromuscular control about the knee with maturation in female athletes. J Bone Joint Surg Am 2004;86(8):1601–8.
11. Female athlete issues for the team physician: a consensus statement-2017 update. Med Sci Sports Exerc 2018;50(5):1113–22.
12. Ford KR, Myer GD, Hewett TE. Increased trunk motion in female athletes compared to males during single leg landing: 821: June 1 8:45 AM - 9:00 AM. Med Sci Sports Exerc 2007;39(5):39.
13. Emery CA, Roy TO, Whittaker JL, et al. Neuromuscular training injury prevention strategies in youth sport: a systematic review and meta-analysis. Br J Sports Med 2015;49(13):865–70.
14. Caldwell M, Casey E, Powell B, et al. Sex hormones. In: Casey E, Rho M, Press J, editors. Sex Differences in Sports Medicine. New York: Springer Publishing Company; 2016. p. 1–30.
15. Maruyama S, Yamazaki T, Sato Y, et al. Relationship between anterior knee laxity and general joint laxity during the menstrual cycle. Orthop J Sports Med 2021; 9(3). 2325967121993045.

16. Herzberg SD, Motu'apuaka ML, Lambert W, et al. The effect of menstrual cycle and contraceptives on ACL injuries and laxity: a systematic review and meta-analysis. Orthop J Sports Med 2017;5(7). 2325967117718781.

17. Martínez-Fortuny N, Alonso-Calvete A, Da Cuña-Carrera I, et al. Menstrual cycle and sport injuries: a systematic review. Int J Environ Res Public Health 2023; 20(4):3264.

18. Sung ES, Kim JH. The difference effect of estrogen on muscle tone of medial and lateral thigh muscle during ovulation. J Exerc Rehabil 2018;14(3):419–23.

19. McNulty KL, Elliott-Sale KJ, Dolan E, et al. The effects of menstrual cycle phase on exercise performance in eumenorrheic women: a systematic review and meta-analysis. Sports Med 2020;50(10):1813–27.

20. Benito PJ, Alfaro-Magallanes VM, Rael B, et al. Effect of menstrual cycle phase on the recovery process of high-intensity interval exercise-A cross-sectional observational study. Int J Environ Res Public Health 2023;20(4):3266.

21. Prado RCR, Willett HN, Takito MY, et al. Impact of premenstrual syndrome symptoms on sport routines in nonelite athlete participants of summer olympic sports. Int J Sports Physiol Perform 2023;18(2):142–7.

22. Thein-Nissenbaum JM, Rauh MJ, Carr KE, et al. Menstrual irregularity and musculoskeletal injury in female high school athletes. J Athl Train 2012;47(1): 74–82.

23. Abbott A, Bird ML, Wild E, et al. Part I: epidemiology and risk factors for stress fractures in female athletes. Phys Sportsmed 2020;48(1):17–24.

24. Lin CY, Casey E, Herman DC, et al. Sex differences in common sports injuries. PMR 2018;10(10):1073–82.

25. Mountjoy M, Ackerman KE, Bailey DM, et al. 2023 international olympic committee's (IOC) consensus statement on relative energy deficiency in sport (REDs). Br J Sports Med 2023;57(17):1073–97.

26. Rogers MA, Appaneal RN, Hughes D, et al. Prevalence of impaired physiological function consistent with Relative Energy Deficiency in Sport (RED-S): an Australian elite and pre-elite cohort. Br J Sports Med 2021;55(1):38–45.

27. van Niekerk M, Matzkin E, Christino MA. Psychological aspects of return to sport for the female athlete. Arthrosc Sports Med Rehabil 2023;5(4):100738.

28. McManama O'Brien KH, Rowan M, Willoughby K, et al. Psychological resilience in young female athletes. Int J Environ Res Public Health 2021;18(16):8668.

29. Martinsen M, Sundgot-Borgen J. Higher prevalence of eating disorders among adolescent elite athletes than controls. Med Sci Sports Exerc 2013;45(6): 1188–97.

30. Wolanin A, Gross M, Hong E. Depression in athletes: prevalence and risk factors. Curr Sports Med Rep 2015;14(1):56–60.

31. Walton CC, Rice S, Gao CX, et al. Gender differences in mental health symptoms and risk factors in Australian elite athletes. BMJ Open Sport Exerc Med 2021; 7(1):e000984.

32. Jagim AR, Fields J, Magee MK, et al. Contributing factors to low energy availability in female athletes: a narrative review of energy availability, training demands, nutrition barriers, body image, and disordered eating. Nutrients 2022;14(5):986.

33. Wasserfurth P, Palmowski J, Hahn A, et al. Reasons for and consequences of low energy availability in female and male athletes: social environment, adaptations, and prevention. Sports Med Open 2020;6(1):44.

34. Mountjoy M, Brackenridge C, Arrington M, et al. International Olympic Committee consensus statement: harassment and abuse (non-accidental violence) in sport. Br J Sports Med 2016;50(17):1019–29.

35. Zogg CK, Runquist EB 3rd, Amick M, et al. Experiences of interpersonal violence in sport and perceived coaching style among college athletes. JAMA Netw Open 2024;7(1):e2350248.

36. Pascoe M, Pankowiak A, Woessner M, et al. Gender-specific psychosocial stressors influencing mental health among women elite and semielite athletes: a narrative review. Br J Sports Med 2022;56(23):1381–7.

37. Marconcin P, Silva AL, Flôres F, et al. Association between musculoskeletal injuries and depressive symptoms among athletes: a systematic review. Int J Environ Res Public Health 2023;20(12):6130.

38. Joy EA, Herring SA, Nelson C, et al. Sexual violence in sport: expanding awareness and knowledge for sports medicine providers. Curr Sports Med Rep 2021; 20(10):531–9.

39. Jayanthi NA, Post EG, Laury TC, et al. Health consequences of youth sport specialization. J Athl Train 2019;54(10):1040–9.

40. Jayanthi NA, Dugas LR. The risks of sports specialization in the adolescent female athlete. Strength Condit J 2017;39(2):20–6.

41. Jayanthi N, Schley S, Cumming SP, et al. Developmental training model for the sport specialized youth athlete: a dynamic strategy for individualizing load-response during maturation. Sports Health 2022;14(1):142–53.

42. Lloyd RS, Faigenbaum AD, Stone MH, et al. Position statement on youth resistance training: the 2014 International Consensus. Br J Sports Med 2014;48(7): 498–505.

43. Temm DA, Standing RJ, Best R. Training, wellbeing and recovery load monitoring in female youth athletes. Int J Environ Res Public Health 2022;19(18):11463.

44. Watkins RA, Guillen RV. Primary care considerations for the pediatric endurance athlete. Curr Rev Musculoskelet Med 2024;17(3):76–82.

45. Physical activity and exercise during pregnancy and the postpartum period: ACOG committee opinion, number 804. Obstet Gynecol 2020;135(4):e178–88.

46. Borg-Stein J, Dugan SA. Musculoskeletal disorders of pregnancy, delivery and postpartum. Phys Med Rehabil Clin N Am 2007;18(3):459–76, ix.

47. Bø K, Artal R, Barakat R, et al. Exercise and pregnancy in recreational and elite athletes: 2016/2017 evidence summary from the IOC expert group meeting, Lausanne. Part 5. Recommendations for health professionals and active women. Br J Sports Med 2018;52(17):1080–5.

48. Woodley SJ, Lawrenson P, Boyle R, et al. Pelvic floor muscle training for preventing and treating urinary and faecal incontinence in antenatal and postnatal women. Cochrane Database Syst Rev 2020;5(5):Cd007471.

49. Fitzgerald CM, Bennis S, Marcotte ML, et al. The impact of a sacroiliac joint belt on function and pain using the active straight leg raise in pregnancy-related pelvic girdle pain. PMR 2022;14(1):19–29.

50. Yang J, Wang Y, Xu J, et al. Acupuncture for low back and/or pelvic pain during pregnancy: a systematic review and meta-analysis of randomised controlled trials. BMJ Open 2022;12(12):e056878.

51. Kimber ML, Meyer S, McHugh TL, et al. Health outcomes after pregnancy in elite athletes: a systematic review and meta-analysis. Med Sci Sports Exerc 2021; 53(8):1739–47.

52. Tighe BJ, Williams SL, Porter C, et al. Barriers and enablers influencing female athlete return-to-sport postpartum: a scoping review. Br J Sports Med 2023; 57(22):1450–6.

53. Bø K, Artal R, Barakat R, et al. Exercise and pregnancy in recreational and elite athletes: 2016/17 evidence summary from the IOC Expert Group Meeting,

Lausanne. Part 3—exercise in the postpartum period. Br J Sports Med 2017; 51(21):1516–25.

54. Christopher SM, Donnelly G, Brockwell E, et al. Clinical and exercise professional opinion of return-to-running readiness after childbirth: an international Delphi study and consensus statement. Br J Sports Med 2023;58(6):299–312.

55. Rita ED, Gráinne MD, Emma B, et al. Clinical and exercise professional opinion on designing a postpartum return-to-running training programme: an international Delphi study and consensus statement. Br J Sports Med 2024;58(4):183.

56. Afifi T, Barrack MT, Casey E, et al. Infographic. Head to toe considerations for the postpartum endurance athlete. Br J Sports Med 2024;58(11):630–2.

57. Grindler NM, Santoro NF. Menopause and exercise. Menopause 2015;22(12): 1351–8.

58. Hulteen RM, Marlatt KL, Allerton TD, et al. Detrimental changes in health during menopause: the role of physical activity. Int J Sports Med 2023;44(6):389–96.

59. Raiser SN, Schroeder AN, Lawley RJ, et al. Bone health and the masters runner. Pm r 2024;16(4):363–73.

60. Folscher LL, Grant CC, Fletcher L, et al. Ultra-marathon athletes at risk for the female athlete Triad. Sports Med Open 2015;1(1):29.

61. Rothschild CE, Collingwood TG. Maximizing running participation and performance through menopause. J Womens Pelvic Health Physical Therapy 2023; 47(2):133–43.

62. Strasser B, Pesta D, Rittweger J, et al. Nutrition for older athletes: focus on sex-differences. Nutrients 2021;13(5):1409.

63. Jonely H, Jayaseelan DJ, Rieke M. Tendinopathy and aging: a review of literature and considerations for older adult athletes. Top Geriatr Rehabil 2016;32(1): E1–12.

64. Rodriguez-Santiago B, Castillo B, Baerga-Varela L, et al. Rehabilitation management of rotator cuff injuries in the master athlete. Curr Sports Med Rep 2019; 18(9):330–7.

65. Parker KM, Hagen MS. Chapter 1 - knee anatomy and biomechanics. In: Frank RM, editor. The female athlete. St. Louis, MO: Elsevier; 2022. p. 1–11.

66. Arundale AJH, Silvers-Granelli HJ, Myklebust G. ACL injury prevention: where have we come from and where are we going? J Orthop Res 2022;40(1):43–54.

67. Benjaminse A, Verhagen E. Implementing ACL injury prevention in daily sports practice-it's not just the program: let's build together, involve the context, and improve the content. Sports Med 2021;51(12):2461–7.

68. Diermeier TA, Rothrauff BB, Engebretsen L, et al. Treatment after ACL injury: panther symposium ACL treatment consensus group. Br J Sports Med 2021; 55(1):14–22.

69. Brinlee AW, Dickenson SB, Hunter-Giordano A, et al. ACL reconstruction rehabilitation: clinical data, biologic healing, and criterion-based milestones to inform a return-to-sport guideline. Sports Health 2022;14(5):770–9.

70. Culvenor AG, Girdwood MA, Juhl CB, et al. Rehabilitation after anterior cruciate ligament and meniscal injuries: a best-evidence synthesis of systematic reviews for the OPTIKNEE consensus. Br J Sports Med 2022;56(24):1445–53.

71. Branche K, Bradsell HL, Lencioni A, et al. Sex-based differences in adult ACL reconstruction outcomes. Curr Rev Musculoskelet Med 2022;15(6):645–50.

72. Webster KE, Nagelli CV, Hewett TE, et al. Factors associated with psychological readiness to return to sport after anterior cruciate ligament reconstruction surgery. Am J Sports Med 2018;46(7):1545–50.

73. Padaki AS, Noticewala MS, Levine WN, et al. Prevalence of posttraumatic stress disorder symptoms among young athletes after anterior cruciate ligament rupture. Orthop J Sports Med 2018;6(7). 2325967118787159.

74. Allen MM, Pareek A, Krych AJ, et al. Are female soccer players at an increased risk of second anterior cruciate ligament injury compared with their athletic peers? Am J Sports Med 2016;44(10):2492–8.

75. Leroux T, Ogilvie-Harris D, Dwyer T, et al. The risk of knee arthroplasty following cruciate ligament reconstruction: a population-based matched cohort study. J Bone Joint Surg Am 2014;96(1):2–10.

76. Collins NJ, Barton CJ, van Middelkoop M, et al. 2018 Consensus statement on exercise therapy and physical interventions (orthoses, taping and manual therapy) to treat patellofemoral pain: recommendations from the 5th International Patellofemoral Pain Research Retreat, Gold Coast, Australia, 2017. Br J Sports Med 2018;52(18):1170–8.

77. Vora M, Curry E, Chipman A, et al. Patellofemoral pain syndrome in female athletes: a review of diagnoses, etiology and treatment options. Orthop Rev (Pavia) 2017;9(4):7281.

78. Herbst KA, Barber Foss KD, Fader L, et al. Hip strength is greater in athletes who subsequently develop patellofemoral pain. Am J Sports Med 2015;43(11):2747–52.

79. Boling MC, Nguyen AD, Padua DA, et al. Gender-specific risk factor profiles for patellofemoral pain. Clin J Sport Med 2021;31(1):49–56.

80. Powers CM, Witvrouw E, Davis IS, et al. Evidence-based framework for a pathomechanical model of patellofemoral pain: 2017 patellofemoral pain consensus statement from the 4th International Patellofemoral Pain Research Retreat, Manchester, UK: part 3. Br J Sports Med 2017;51(24):1713–23.

81. Selhorst M, Fernandez-Fernandez A, Schmitt L, et al. Effect of a psychologically informed intervention to treat adolescents with patellofemoral pain: a randomized controlled trial. Arch Phys Med Rehabil 2021;102(7):1267–73.

82. Rathleff MS, Rathleff CR, Olesen JL, et al. Is knee pain during adolescence a self-limiting condition? Prognosis of patellofemoral pain and other types of knee pain. Am J Sports Med 2016;44(5):1165–71.

83. Hansen R, Brushøj C, Rathleff MS, et al. Quadriceps or hip exercises for patellofemoral pain? A randomised controlled equivalence trial. Br J Sports Med 2023;57(20):1287–94.

84. Sisk D, Fredericson M. Taping, bracing, and injection treatment for patellofemoral pain and patellar tendinopathy. Curr Rev Musculoskelet Med 2020;13(4):537–44.

85. Rathleff MS, Thomsen JL, Barton CJ. Patient education in patellofemoral pain: potentially potent and essential, but under-researched. Br J Sports Med 2018;52(10):623–4.

86. Hoenig T, Ackerman KE, Beck BR, et al. Bone stress injuries. Nat Rev Dis Primers 2022;8(1):26.

87. Chen YT, Tenforde AS, Fredericson M. Update on stress fractures in female athletes: epidemiology, treatment, and prevention. Curr Rev Musculoskelet Med 2013;6(2):173–81.

88. Beck BR, Rudolph K, Matheson GO, et al. Risk factors for tibial stress injuries: a case-control study. Clin J Sport Med 2015;25(3):230–6.

89. Cobb KL, Bachrach LK, Sowers M, et al. The effect of oral contraceptives on bone mass and stress fractures in female runners. Med Sci Sports Exerc 2007;39(9):1464–73.

90. Barrack MT, Van Loan MD, Rauh MJ, et al. Body mass, training, menses, and bone in adolescent runners: a 3-yr follow-up. Med Sci Sports Exerc 2011;43(6): 959–66.
91. Nattiv A, Kennedy G, Barrack MT, et al. Correlation of MRI grading of bone stress injuries with clinical risk factors and return to play: a 5-year prospective study in collegiate track and field athletes. Am J Sports Med 2013;41(8):1930–41.
92. Moore IS, Crossley KM, Bo K, et al. Female athlete health domains: a supplement to the International Olympic Committee consensus statement on methods for recording and reporting epidemiological data on injury and illness in sport. Br J Sports Med 2023;57(18):1164–74.
93. Dominguez EO. As women's sports continue to grow, mental health care for female athletes remains years behind. Boston Globe; 2023. Available at: https://www.bostonglobe.com/2023/08/04/metro/womens-sports-continues-grow-mental-health-care-female-athletes-remains-years-behind/#: ~ :text=Female%20athletes%20are%20prone%20to,well%20as%20sports-related%20injuries. Accessed October 3, 2024.

Common Pain Disorders in Women

Diagnosis, Treatment, and Rehabilitation Management

Alexander Shustorovich, DO[a,b,c,]*, Michael Bova, MD[c],
Laurent V. Delavaux, MD[a,b,c]

KEYWORDS

- Pain disorders • Women • Migraine • Fibromyalgia • Endometriosis
- Interstitial cystitis • Temporomandibular disorders • Osteoarthritis

KEY POINTS

- Men and women experience pain stimuli and pain states differently.
- Some of the most common women pain disorders are migraine headache, fibromyalgia, endometriosis, interstitial cystitis, temporomandibular joint disorder, and osteoarthritis.
- Treatment of any pain syndrome requires careful consideration of multiple factors, including gender, as well as the development of a multidisciplinary treatment plan.

INTRODUCTION/BACKGROUND/HISTORY

Epidemiologic data suggest that women are at higher risk for several clinical pain conditions in relation to their male counterparts.[1] Studies have suggested that sex differences exist in pain perception and pain tolerance to different painful stimuli, with women in particular exhibiting lower tolerance to certain stimuli.[2,3] Several hypotheses have been advanced to explain these gender disparities, including sex hormone differences as well as genetic or reproductive factors, but none of these have amounted to strong evidence on their own.[1] Historically, it has been accepted that women-specific pain issues have often gone undertreated, have not been well understood, or have been outright ignored.[4] To foster health-equity regarding sex differences, this brief review sheds light on a small group of "most common" clinical pain disorders among a larger subset. This article reviews the diagnoses of migraine, fibromyalgia, endometriosis, temporomandibular disorder (TMD), interstitial cystitis (IC), and osteoarthritis.

[a] Hackensack Meridian School of Medicine; [b] Rutgers- Robert Wood Johnson Medical School; [c] Department of Physical Medicine & Rehabilitation, JFK Johnson Rehabilitation Institute, 65 James Street, Edison, NJ 08820, USA
* Corresponding author. Department of Physical Medicine & Rehabilitation, 65 James Street, Edison, NJ 08820.
E-mail address: Alex.shustorovich@gmail.com

Phys Med Rehabil Clin N Am 36 (2025) 297–310
https://doi.org/10.1016/j.pmr.2024.11.011
1047-9651/25/© 2024 Elsevier Inc. All rights are reserved, including those for text and data mining, AI training, and similar technologies.

Abbreviations	
CBT	cognitive behavioral therapy
CNS	central nervous system
IASP	International Association for the Study of Pain
IBS	irritable bowel syndrome
IC	interstitial cystitis
PREEMPT	Phase 3 Research Evaluating Migraine Prophylaxis Therapy
TMD	temporomandibular disorder
TMJ	temporomandibular joint

Section 1: Migraines

Definition and pathophysiology

Migraines are a genetically influenced, complex subcategory of headaches with distinctive features. Migraines are broadly categorized as those with and without aura. An aura usually precedes the migraine attack and is characterized by a reversible neurologic disturbance manifesting in changes in vision, sensation, speech, motor, and brainstem functions. Acute migraine attacks generally last between 4 and 72 hours. The diagnosis of migraine is based on the International Classification of Headache Disorders criteria.[5] Chronic migraine is defined as headaches occurring on 15 or more days per month for greater than 3 months, with migraine features on at least 8 days per month. The prevailing and most widely accepted pathophysiologic mechanism of migraine is the theory of cortical spreading depression, where neuronal depolarizations are followed by activity suppression, resulting in changes to cortical blood flow. Other proposed mechanisms include the neurovascular and vascular theories.[6]

Prevalence and sex differences

Because of the difficulties in making accurate diagnoses, the prevalence of migraine headaches is difficult to precisely measure. The estimated prevalence of migraines worldwide is rising and currently stands at 14% to 15%, with a higher prevalence in women at nearly 19%.[7] While many theories have been proposed regarding the sex differences in migraine prevalence, many lack robust supportive evidence. Two such theories include higher pain thresholds in women compared with men, as well as sex-variable pharmacokinetic and pharmacodynamic responses to analgesics. The most likely proposed mechanism, based on available evidence, is that of hormone differences: fluctuations in estrogen, progesterone, and androgens have been shown to have variable effects on the risk of migraine attacks.[8–10] For example, premenstrual changes in hormone concentrations are associated with a higher risk of migraine attacks, whereas rates tend to improve during pregnancy, a time when hormone levels remain relatively stable.[1]

Symptoms

Migraines present as unilateral throbbing or pulsatile pain, moderate to severe intensity, and frequently include a combination of nausea, vomiting, sensitivity to light and sound, and a preceding aura. Symptoms tend to worsen with physical activity. Migraine attacks in women tend to be of longer duration, increased intensity, and with more frequent photophobia, phonophobia, nausea, and vomiting compared with men.[11] However, men tend to experience aura more frequently than women.[11]

Causes

Broadly speaking, migraine triggers can fall into 5 categories: emotional stress, hormone related, sleep disturbance, food and alcohol, and weather changes.[12] The most common triggers, in order, include stress, hormonal changes (premenstruation), fasting, weather fluctuations, and sleep disturbances.[13]

Treatment and rehabilitation

The goal of treatment and rehabilitation is to reduce/decrease the frequency of migraines, pain, and improve quality of life. Treatment strategies span from patient education on lifestyle changes and trigger avoidance to abortive and prophylactic interventions. Identifying and managing known triggers is a crucial first step in the management of migraines. While sleep disturbance is not the most common trigger for migraines, it serves as a fundamental aspect of one's health with many deleterious effects when compromised, and therefore must be prioritized. The mainstay of acute, abortive treatment includes non-steroidal anti-inflammatory drugs (NSAIDs), triptans, and newer medications such as calcitonin gene-related protein (cGRP) receptor antagonists.[1] The effectiveness of abortive treatments is highly correlative with earlier administration after initial symptom onset. Preventative medications should be tailored to the individual patient and can include beta-blockers, antidepressants, and antiepileptic medications. Additionally, the use of botulinum toxin type via the Phase 3 Research Evaluating Migraine Prophylaxis Therapy (PREEMPT) protocol has shown significant efficacy in chronic migraine prevention.[14] As previously discussed, there is a lack of evidence proving a differing or variable effectiveness of migraine treatments in women compared with men.[1]

Section 2: Fibromyalgia

Definition and pathophysiology

Fibromyalgia is a disorder characterized by widespread musculoskeletal pain. Patients with fibromyalgia display an increased sensitivity to a range of sensory stimuli which in a healthy individual would not usually evoke a pain response.[15] Evidence suggests that these changes in the perception of nonpainful stimuli as painful ones are mediated through neurochemical changes in the dorsal horn of the spinal cord and in the central nervous system (CNS).[16,17] The International Association for the Study of Pain (IASP) refers to this type of pain as nociplastic pain, explained as pain that "arises from altered nociception despite no clear evidence of actual or threatened tissue damage causing the activation of peripheral nociceptors or evidence for disease or lesion of the somatosensory system causing the pain."[18]

Prevalence and sex differences

The overall prevalence of fibromyalgia is between 6% and 7% in the United States, with European and South American studies showing a broader range of 3.3% to 8.3%.[19] Fibromyalgia is more prevalent in women than men; in the United States, one study found the prevalence to be 7.7% in women and 4.9% in men,[20] while a larger systematic review found that fibromyalgia is 8 to 9 times more common in women than in men.[21] A large study of German patients concluded that women reported more symptoms, more generalized pain, and the same study also suggested a linear relationship between being female and the presence and severity of fibromyalgia.[22]

Symptoms

Patients with fibromyalgia may often complain of accompanying symptoms including sleep disturbances, depression, cognitive disorders, gastrointestinal symptoms, poorly localized tingling sensations in the trunk or limbs, or morning stiffness.[23,24] It is not uncommon for these patients to also present with chronic fatigue syndrome, tension-type or migraine headaches, irritable bowel syndrome (IBS), or mood disorders.[24] Prolonged pain and sleep disturbances inherent to this disorder can be associated with "fibro fog" manifesting as memory impairment and impaired focus or attention to tasks. These issues can contribute to fatigue, anxiety, catastrophizing, as well as reported work and/or family life challenges.[1] These patients may present with overlapping pain conditions; most commonly chronic low back pain, interstial cystitis (IC), or temporomandibular joint (TMJ) disorder.[25] The diagnostic criteria for fibromyalgia as put forth by the American College of Rheumatology require exclusion of any other diagnoses that would explain the patient's pain, symptomatology of a consistent level lasting at least 3 months, and the use of both widespread pain index and symptom severity score of specific minimums.[26]

Causes
Fibromyalgia is considered a stress-related disorder and has been linked to alterations in cortisol suppression, with patients studied showing overall higher levels of plasma cortisol.[27] This suggests that these patients might be more susceptible to traumatic experiences which would cause cortisol elevations and potentially contribute to this disease state.[27] Fibromyalgia can be grouped into a family of affective spectrum disorders, including rheumatoid arthritis and major depressive disorder, which all appear to share a common genetic heritage, with first degree family members showing enhanced sensitivity to pain, but without clear elucidation of the genes responsible.[28]

Treatments
The mainstay of recommended treatments for fibromyalgia is centered around physical therapy and lifestyle changes with emphasis on aerobic exercise and improving sleep. Patients often struggle to persist with exercise and/or physical therapy interventions secondary to fatigue and pain, requiring a measured approach and encouragement. Several medications have been suggested as possible adjunctive therapies to these mainstays. These include but are not limited to serotonin-norepinephrine reuptake inhibitors (duloxetine, milnacipran), anticonvulsants (gabapentin, pregabalin), nonsteroidal anti-inflammatory drugs, tricyclic antidepressants (amitriptyline, desipramine), and muscle relaxants (cyclobenzaprine, methocarbamol). In general, these medications show "weak evidence" at best in treating fibromyalgia.[29] Optimization of nutrition to address any deficiencies may be a promising avenue.[24] Cognitive behavioral therapy (CBT), meditation, and/or mindfulness approaches to treating fibromyalgia are commonly employed despite also showing weak evidence and may be beneficial in addressing patient's common comorbid mood disorders.[29]

Rehabilitation
The gentle initiation of a physical therapy regimen is useful in helping patients establish their own successful home exercise routine. This is also done to foster resilience and to strengthen positive coping mechanisms. Rehabilitation of this nature has been shown to expand patients' coping repertoire by offering new symptom management options as well as fostering confidence in using said options on a more consistent basis. Patients should also be encouraged to learn stress reduction techniques and may be formally referred for such training with psychology or other professional counselors.[1]

Section 3: Endometriosis

Definition and pathophysiology
Endometriosis is a chronic inflammatory disease in which endometrial-like tissue grows outside the uterus.[30] There are immunologic, genetic, and hormonal factors

that may lead or increase risk of developing endometriosis. In many patients, this disorder is associated with chronic pelvic and/or abdominal pain often associated with infertility.[31] Location of the ectopic tissue may vary and includes superficial peritoneal, ovarian, deep, extra-abdominal, and iatrogenic (eg, after cesarean section) endometriosis.[32]

Prevalence in women
Endometriosis affects approximately 190 million women and patients who are female gender at birth worldwide.[30] Unfortunately, the time to diagnosis in almost 60% of affected patients is delayed. Females will see 3 or more clinicians over an average of 7 years for evaluation and treatment before an appropriate diagnosis of endometriosis is made.[33] Like other chronic conditions, women will lose on average 11 hours of work per week due to their endometriosis-related symptoms.[34] Patients with endometriosis have an increased risk by 2-fold for infertility compared with patients without endometriosis.[31]

Symptoms
Endometriosis includes a range of painful symptoms such as, chronic pelvic pain (cyclical and noncyclical), menstrual irregularities, dyspareunia, dysuria, painful defecation, and infertility.[30] Severity of pain symptoms are variable and do not necessarily correlate with the "severity" of the anatomic disease.

Causes
The most probable cause of endometriosis is reflux of endometrial tissue cells and protein rich fluid through the fallopian tubes into the pelvis during menstruation. However, this does not fully explain etiology as many women experience retrograde menstruation and do not develop this disease process.[35] The eutopic endometrial tissue in a patient with endometriosis has a different immune profile compared with individual without it. Yet, it remains unclear if this is the cause or effect of endometriosis. Shed endometrial tissue has pro-inflammatory cytokines, proteases, and immune cells (eg, tumor necrosis factor [TNF]-alpha, interleukin [IL]-1B, and nerve growth factor) that may trigger endometrial lesions.[30] Although chronic pelvic pain is a primary presenting symptom, patients with endometriosis have higher associated risk for comorbid pain conditions such a fibromyalgia, migraines, rheumatological disorders, and osteoarthritis.[30] Almost half of patients with IC have endometriosis.[36] Similarly, patients with IBS are at risk of co-occurring endometriosis. These conditions may share a common cause owing to environmental and genetic factors.[30]

Treatments
Ultrasound and MRI can be used to diagnose endometriosis preoperatively, but diagnostic laparoscopy with potential excision of lesions is often required.[37] Hormonal contraceptives, gonadotropin-releasing hormone agonists and antagonists, and progestin therapy are commonly used for the treatment of this disease process.[30] Untreated pelvic pain caused by endometriosis can lead to central sensitization, a phenomenon which results in a chronic pain syndrome due to a "wind-up" of their CNS. This leads to refractory symptoms despite conservative and surgical treatment stressing the importance of early diagnosis and treatment.[38] Timely referral to a pelvic pain specialist for a comprehensive, multidisciplinary pain management program, including consideration of sympathetic blockade (eg, hypogastric and/or ganglion impar blocks), peripheral nerve blocks, and trigger point injections can help patients improve symptoms and regain function.[39,40]

Rehabilitation

Regular exercise and stress management techniques can help manage endometriosis. Pelvic floor physical therapy is a mainstay of treatment of chronic pelvic pain syndrome. A recent study demonstrated the benefit of a comprehensive treatment protocol utilizing a full course of pelvic floor physical therapy (PT) combined with ultrasound-guided nerve blocks and trigger points injections.[40]

Section 4: Interstitial Cystitis

Definition and pathophysiology

IC is a chronic condition (>6 weeks) causing bladder pressure and bladder pain that is refractory to treatment.[41] It is characterized by chronic inflammation of the urinary tract, which is not due to infection or other identifiable causes.[42] The mechanism is not well understood and often is misdiagnosed or diagnosed late, especially in men. Pathogenesis is most likely multifactorial. Cystoscopy in patients with IC shows submucosal inflammation with glomerulations (Hunner's lesions).[41]

Prevalence in women

The most common prevalence is in women between 50 and 59 years of age and men between 56 and 74 years of age.[42] It is significantly more common in females than males, with 1 study noting a 5:1 ratio predominance in females.[43]

Symptoms

IC symptoms include chronic pelvic pain, a persistent urge to urinate, and frequent urination. Patients may describe pain in the bladder or suprapubic region, with severe urinary urgency. Dyspareunia in women and ejaculatory pain in men may occur. Symptoms are often refractory to standard treatment for overactive bladder therapy. Patients may develop chronic pelvic pain that significantly impacts wellbeing and quality of life.[44]

Causes

Left untreated, chronic inflammation of the urothelium can lead to chronic pelvic pain syndrome. Large groups of mast cells are frequently present that stimulate afferent sensory fibers causing afferent hyperactivity and nociceptive upregulation. Loss of tight junction and adhesive junction proteins cause a "leaky urothelium" associated with submucosal microvascular abnormalities and lack of normal bladder epithelial cell growth.[42] IC has been closely associated with autoimmune diseases such as Hashimoto's thyroiditis, rheumatoid arthritis, ankylosing spondylitis, IBS, fibromyalgia, chronic fatigue, and especially Sjogren syndrome.[41]

Treatments

Initial treatment for IC should be based on dietary and lifestyle modifications, specifically in reducing common irritants. Common bladder irritants include alcohol, benzyl alcohol, caffeine, carbonated beverages, coffee, chili, spices, sweeteners, tomato-based products, and vinegar. Pain management with a multimodal approach is recommended. This may include oral analgesics (nonopioid preferred) and bladder instillations (cocktail of medications ranging from lidocaine, corticosteroids, dimethyl sulfoxide, heparin, hyaluronic acid, and misoprostol).[42] Botox injections for overactive detrusor muscle have also been employed and supported in the literature.[42] In refractory cases, neuromodulation with sacral or dorsal root ganglion stimulator can be considered. There is some evidence for tibial nerve stimulation for the treatment of IC.[42,45] Surgical intervention is a last resort but may provide relief for up to 75% of patients.[42]

Rehabilitation

Myofascial release, physical therapy with relaxation exercises, and pelvic floor trigger point manual therapy provided by a skilled practitioner have shown significant symptom relief in 70% of patients.[46] Interestingly enough, standard pelvic floor PT in isolation is not recommended as it may worsen symptoms.[47] Stress reduction activities like yoga, meditation, and massage can help manage IC.[42]

Section 5: Temporomandibular Disorders

Definition and pathophysiology

TMDs are a group of orofacial pain conditions involving either the masticatory muscles and/or the TMJ. Myofascial TMD involves the muscles of mastication becoming overused, fatigued, and painful, developing potential trigger points. Causation is multifactorial but can include bruxism, increased stress levels or anxiety, mechanical or postural abnormalities, autoimmune disease, or fibromyalgia.[48] The most involved muscles are the 4 primary muscles of mastication: temporalis, medial pterygoid, lateral pterygoid, and masseter.[49] Articular TMD is caused by derangement of the TMJ articulation formed between the glenoid fossa of temporal bone and the mandibular condyle. Within this joint, an articular disc splits the joint into 2 synovial cavities (superior and inferior) with 2 distinctive movements characterized: translatory side to side movement in the superior portion and hinge movement of the jaw in the inferior portion.[50] A slew of mechanical, traumatic, inflammatory issues can cause joint pain, with displacement of the articular disc being the most common etiology of TMJ-based pain.[48]

Prevalence in women

The global prevalence of TMD has a large range. A recent systematic review of TMD epidemiology suggests that the prevalence of "severe" TMD overall is about 10% most common to occur between the ages of 25 to 45.[51] Almost every study included in the same review suggested that prevalence is higher in women as compared with men, with one large study suggesting that TMD prevalence for women was nearly 4 times higher than men. This considerable gender difference combined with the common age range during "reproductive years" has led to hypotheses about the roles that the reproductive hormones may have on this condition.[51]

Symptoms

TMD is a clinical diagnosis, and therefore requires a careful history and examination to correctly identify it as the most likely diagnosis. Patients often complain of pain at the TMJ or mandible as the primary symptom, with pain sometimes radiating to the head or neck. Pain is usually exacerbated by mastication, yawning, or prolonged talking,[52] and patients may report clicking, popping, crepitus, and even locking or difficulty opening/closing the mouth. Orofacial pain not associated with jaw movement is suggestive of a diagnosis besides TMD.[53] Tension-type headaches can be associated with TMD, and some patients may also report otalgia, tinnitus, vertigo, and even hearing impairment as well.[54]

Causes

The cause of TMD is often multifactorial. Etiologies of TMD can be grossly divided into myofascially derived pain versus intraarticular disorders of the TMJ. Certain behaviors, such as bruxism (grinding, clenching, or gnashing of the teeth) as well as psychological factors like stress and anxiety, can be linked to muscular pain.[55] Certain diagnoses such as depression, anxiety, autoimmune disorders, and fibromyalgia share associations with TMD.[56] Derangements of the TMJ itself may be linked to osteoarthritis, hypermobility, or trauma. The most likely inflammatory causes of TMJ pain are rheumatoid arthritis and ankylosing spondylitis.[54]

Treatments

Forty percent of patients with TMD will have spontaneous resolution of symptoms, and one long-term study determined that between 50% and 90% of patients had pain relief after conservative care.[57] Patient history and physical examination suggestive of trauma, dislocation, infection, or abscess warrant imaging (eg, X ray or computed tomography [CT]) and referral to a dentist or surgeon. Otherwise, treatment should be focused on resolving pain and restoring function. First-line agents are often NSAIDs. Muscle relaxants, antidepressants, or gabapentinoids have some support for pain reduction and are offered as adjuncts. CBT has level B evidence for improving short-term and long-term pain in TMD.[57] Diagnostic trigger point injections can be done in the suspected musculature involved. Intraarticular injection is indicated for pain control and improved function in severe TMJ but should be done with caution to prevent further degradation of articular cartilage. Surgical referral should be reserved for patients with clear acute indications above or those who have failed conservative treatment. Referral to a dentist should be considered in cases of poor dental health, caries, and suspected grinding that might be amenable to occlusal splinting.[58]

Rehabilitation

Physical therapy is a commonly used treatment for TMD with various treatments focused on decreasing neck and jaw pain, improving range of motion, and promoting home exercise habits. Exercises of the muscles of mastication as well as musculature of the neck can be combined with manual therapy and other passive modalities. However, a large systematic review of therapeutic exercise and manual therapy for TMD did not show high-level evidence for these interventions citing tremendous heterogeneity in treatment types and regimens.[59]

Section 6: Osteoarthritis

Definition

Osteoarthritis is a degenerative joint disease characterized by the progressive breakdown of the joint. The disease manifests first as a molecular derangement of normal joint metabolism and is followed closely by anatomic and physiologic derangements characterized by cartilage degradation, bone remodeling, osteophyte formation, joint inflammation, and maladaptive joint functioning.[60]

Epidemiology

Osteoarthritis is the most common form of arthritis. The global prevalence of osteoarthritis is roughly 528 million, 60% of which are women.[61] Prevalence of osteoarthritis increases with age, affecting roughly 10% of men and 18% of women aged 60 and older.[62] Rates also vary by affected joint, with women being affected more with hand and knee osteoarthritis while men are affected more by hip osteoarthritis.[63,64]

Symptoms

Osteoarthritis is characterized by pain and stiffness in the affected joints. Stiffness is worse in the morning or after prolonged inactivity and tends to improve within 30 minutes of initial activity, contrasting that of inflammatory arthritis where stiffness tends to remain for longer than 1 hour. On examination, osteoarthritis is usually associated with either absent or small effusions (such as in the knees), reduced range of motion with crepitus, and bony enlargement (such as Heberden's nodes). The classic radiographic triad of osteoarthritis includes joint space narrowing, osteophyte formation, and subchondral sclerosis.[65]

Pathophysiology

The pathophysiology of osteoarthritis involves a complex interplay of mechanical, biochemical, and genetic factors affecting cartilage, bone, synovium, ligaments, periarticular fat, and muscle. A classic example of how abnormalities in biomechanical alignment contribute to the development of osteoarthritis can be observed in the elevated rates of knee osteoarthritis in women. In general, the relatively wider hips seen in women create a greater Q-angle and resultant knee valgus alignment which can asymmetrically load the lateral knee compartment and contribute to knee osteoarthritis.[65] While there have been numerous papers devoted to addressing the question of whether hormones (including estrogen) play a role in the development or prevention of osteoarthritis, there is currently no definitive, clinically meaningful conclusion regarding this topic.[66–69]

Rehabilitation and treatment

The mainstay of osteoarthritis prevention includes optimizing fat-free body mass by promoting muscle development, increasing flexibility, improving metabolic health, and avoiding joint trauma and biomechanical inequalities. In treating symptomatic osteoarthritis, physician-directed exercise programs and formal physical and occupational therapy are the best first approaches to treatment and are aimed at addressing the previously stated elements of disease prevention. Durable medical equipment such as heel wedges, orthotics, braces, and splints can be used to correct causative biomechanical asymmetries. Initial pharmacologic treatments should include the use of short courses of acetaminophen, oral and topical NSAIDs, as well as ice, heat, lidocaine patches, and menthol-containing lotions. Adjunctive medications such as serotonin-norepinephrine reuptake inhibitors (eg, duloxetine) and anticonvulsants (eg, gabapentin) can be considered for more chronic cases of symptomatic osteoarthritis. Should these initial steps fail, the use of corticosteroids, hyaluronic acid, platelet-rich plasma injections, and genicular nerve blocks/ablations can be considered prior to consideration of more invasive treatments such as joint replacements.[65]

Discussion

The 6 pain disorders chosen for this review demonstrate the stark differences in prevalence among the sexes and serve to highlight the important role that rehabilitation physicians play when diagnosing and treating women patients. The prevalence of several painful clinical diagnoses is higher for women as compared with men, and among patients with chronic pain conditions who are admitted to rehabilitation units, more are women than men.[1] Exercise has been implicated as an intervention with high level of evidence for fibromyalgia, helping to improve symptoms, function, and decrease fatigue.[70] Physical therapy and exercise are also mainstays of treatment for TMD, chronic pelvic pain (in setting of endometriosis and/or IC), and osteoarthritis.[46,52,53,59,65,71,72] However, it is not well understood which therapeutic exercises or modalities are best suited to treat each sex, and further research is required. Patients with chronic pain conditions benefit most from evaluation by a multidisciplinary team comprising physicians, psychologists, nurses, physical and occupational therapists.[71] Each individual patient may benefit from disease-specific referral to a specialist, for early evaluation and targeted medical care. Much remains to be elucidated about sex differences in pain syndromes and how these differences might best be considered when planning evidence-based care for optimal patient outcomes.

SUMMARY

There is ample evidence to suggest that certain pain conditions affect women to a greater extent and in varying ways compared with men. The underlying pathophysiologic mechanisms, while hypothesized, remain largely inconclusive. Six of the more common pain conditions affecting women include migraine headache, fibromyalgia, endometriosis, IC, TMJ disorder, and osteoarthritis. Future research should address the underlying sex-specific mechanisms of these disorders, with particular attention given to pharmacologic, interventional, and rehabilitative treatment options that will allow physicians to provide the highest standard of care for women.

CLINICS CARE POINTS

- Aerobic exercise has the strongest evidence for the treatment of fibromyalgia.
- Exercise and physical therapy are mainstay modalities for treatment of temporomandibular disorder and osteoarthritis.
- Interstitial cystitis and endometriosis can contribute to chronic pelvic pain syndrome.
- Botox for migraines is an established treatment, but overall migraine management requires a multidisciplinary approach.
- Men and women experience pain stimuli and pain states differently, and therefore sex and gender should be considered in tailoring treatment for each patient.

DISCLOSURE

A. Shustorovich is part of the Speakers Program for Averitas. L.V. Delavaux and M. Bova have nothing to disclose.

REFERENCES

1. Casale R, Atzeni F, Bazzichi L, et al. Pain in women: a perspective review on a relevant clinical issue that deserves prioritization. Pain Ther 2021;10(1):287–314.
2. Racine M, Tousignant-Laflamme Y, Kloda LA, et al, A systematic literature review of 10 years of research on sex/gender and experimental pain perception – Part 1: are there really differences between women and men?, *Pain*, 153 (3), 2012, Available at: https://journals.lww.com/pain/fulltext/2012/03000/a_systematic_literature_review_of_10_years_of.16.aspx (Accessed 7 July 2024).
3. Bartley EJ, Fillingim RB. Sex differences in pain: a brief review of clinical and experimental findings. Br J Anaesth 2013;111(1):52–8.
4. Hoffmann DE, Tarzian AJ. The girl who cried pain: a bias against women in the treatment of pain. J Law Med Ethics 2001;29(1):13–27.
5. Headache Classification Committee of the International Headache Society (IHS). The international classification of headache disorders, 3rd edition. Cephalalgia 2018;38(1):1–211.
6.. Cuccurullo SJ. Physical medicine and rehabilitation board review. 4th edition. New York, NY: Demos Medical Publishing; 2020.
7. Steiner TJ, Stovner LJ. Global epidemiology of migraine and its implications for public health and health policy. Nat Rev Neurol 2023;19(2):109–17.
8. Brandes JL. The influence of estrogen on migraine. JAMA 2006;295(15):1824.
9. Reddy N, Desai MN, Schoenbrunner A, et al. The complex relationship between estrogen and migraines: a scoping review. Syst Rev 2021;10(1):72.

10. Sacco S, Ricci S, Degan D, et al. Migraine in women: the role of hormones and their impact on vascular diseases. J Headache Pain 2012;13(3):177–89.

11. Verhagen IE, van der Arend BWH, van Casteren DS, et al. Sex differences in migraine attack characteristics: a longitudinal E-diary study. Headache J Head Face Pain 2023;63(3):333–41.

12. Kesserwani H. Migraine triggers: an overview of the pharmacology, biochemistry, atmospherics, and their effects on neural networks. Cureus 2021. https://doi.org/10.7759/cureus.14243.

13. Kelman L. The triggers or precipitants of the acute migraine attack. Cephalalgia 2007;27(5):394–402.

14. Frank F, Ulmer H, Sidoroff V, et al. CGRP-antibodies, topiramate and botulinum toxin type A in episodic and chronic migraine: a systematic review and meta-analysis. Cephalalgia 2021;41(11–12):1222–39.

15. Carli G, Suman AL, Biasi G, et al. Reactivity to superficial and deep stimuli in patients with chronic musculoskeletal pain. Pain 2002;100(3):259–69.

16. Nielsen LA, Henriksson KG. Pathophysiological mechanisms in chronic musculoskeletal pain (fibromyalgia): the role of central and peripheral sensitization and pain disinhibition. Best Pract Res Clin Rheumatol 2007;21(3):465–80.

17. Watkins LR, Milligan ED, Maier SF. Glial activation: a driving force for pathological pain. Trends Neurosci 2001;24(8):450–5.

18. Trouvin AP, Perrot S. New concepts of pain. Best Pract Res Clin Rheumatol 2019; 33(3):101415.

19. Jones GT, Atzeni F, Beasley M, et al. The prevalence of fibromyalgia in the general population: a comparison of the American College of Rheumatology 1990, 2010, and modified 2010 classification criteria. Arthritis Rheumatol 2015;67(2): 568–75.

20. Vincent A, Lahr BD, Wolfe F, et al. Prevalence of fibromyalgia: a population-based study in olmsted county, Minnesota, utilizing the rochester epidemiology project. Arthritis Care Res (Hoboken) 2013;65(5):786–92.

21. Heidari F, Afshari M, Moosazadeh M. Prevalence of fibromyalgia in general population and patients, a systematic review and meta-analysis. Rheumatol Int 2017; 37(9):1527–39.

22. Wolfe F, Walitt B, Perrot S, et al. Fibromyalgia diagnosis and biased assessment: sex, prevalence and bias. PLoS One 2018;13(9):e0203755.

23. Marques AP, Santo ASDE, Berssaneti AA, et al. Prevalence of fibromyalgia: literature review update. Rev Bras Reumatol 2017;57(4):356–63.

24. Bjørklund G, Dadar M, Chirumbolo S, et al. Fibromyalgia and nutrition: therapeutic possibilities? Biomed Pharmacother 2018;103:531–8.

25. Maixner W, Fillingim RB, Williams DA, et al. Overlapping chronic pain conditions: implications for diagnosis and classification. J Pain 2016;17(9):T93–107.

26. Wolfe F, Clauw DJ, Fitzcharles M, et al. The American College of Rheumatology preliminary diagnostic criteria for fibromyalgia and measurement of symptom severity. Arthritis Care Res (Hoboken) 2010;62(5):600–10.

27. McCain GA, Tilbe KS. Diurnal hormone variation in fibromyalgia syndrome: a comparison with rheumatoid arthritis. J Rheumatol Suppl 1989;19:154–7.

28. Bradley LA. Pathophysiology of fibromyalgia. Am J Med 2009;122(12):S22–30.

29. Macfarlane GJ, Kronisch C, Dean LE, et al. EULAR revised recommendations for the management of fibromyalgia. Ann Rheum Dis 2017;76(2):318–28.

30. Horne AW, Missmer SA. Pathophysiology, diagnosis, and management of endometriosis. BMJ 2022;e070750. https://doi.org/10.1136/bmj-2022-070750.

31. Prescott J, Farland LV, Tobias DK, et al. A prospective cohort study of endometriosis and subsequent risk of infertility. Hum Reprod 2016;31(7):1475–82.

32. Tomassetti C, Johnson NP, Petrozza J, et al. An international terminology for endometriosis, 2021. Hum Reprod Open 2021;2021(4). https://doi.org/10.1093/hropen/hoab029.

33. Greene R, Stratton P, Cleary SD, et al. Diagnostic experience among 4,334 women reporting surgically diagnosed endometriosis. Fertil Steril 2009;91(1):32–9.

34. Simoens S, Hummelshoj L, D'Hooghe T. Endometriosis: cost estimates and methodological perspective. Hum Reprod Update 2007;13(4):395–404.

35. Halme J, Hammond MG, Hulka JF, et al. Retrograde menstruation in healthy women and in patients with endometriosis. Obstet Gynecol 1984;64(2):151–4.

36. Tirlapur SA, Kuhrt K, Chaliha C, et al. The 'evil twin syndrome' in chronic pelvic pain: a systematic review of prevalence studies of bladder pain syndrome and endometriosis. Int J Surg 2013;11(3):233–7.

37. Buck Louis GM, Hediger ML, Peterson CM, et al. Incidence of endometriosis by study population and diagnostic method: the ENDO study. Fertil Steril 2011;96(2):360–5.

38. McNamara HC, Frawley HC, Donoghue JF, et al. Peripheral, central, and cross sensitization in endometriosis-associated pain and comorbid pain syndromes. Frontiers in Reproductive Health 2021;3. Available at: https://www.frontiersin.org/articles/10.3389/frph.2021.729642.

39. Khodaverdi S, Alebouyeh MR, Sadegi K, et al. Superior hypogastric plexus block as an effective treatment method for endometriosis-related chronic pelvic pain: an open-label pilot clinical trial. J Obstet Gynaecol (Lahore) 2021;41(6):966–71.

40. Patil S, Daniel G, Vyas R, et al. Neuromuscular treatment approach for women with chronic pelvic pain syndrome improving pelvic pain and functionality. Neurourol Urodyn 2022;41(1):220–8.

41. Hanno PM, Burks DA, Clemens JQ, et al. AUA guideline for the diagnosis and treatment of interstitial cystitis/bladder pain syndrome. J Urol 2011;185(6):2162–70.

42. Lim YLSOS. Interstitial cystitis/bladder pain syndrome. StatPearls [Internet]; 2024.

43. Clemens JQ, Meenan RT, Rosetti MCO, et al. Prevalence of interstitial cystitis symptoms in a managed care population. J Urol 2005;174(2):576–80.

44. Bogart LM, Berry SH, Clemens JQ. Symptoms of interstitial cystitis, painful bladder syndrome and similar diseases in women: a systematic review. J Urol 2007;177(2):450–6.

45. Padilla-Fernández B, Hernández-Hernández D, Castro-Díaz DM. Current role of neuromodulation in bladder pain syndrome/interstitial cystitis. Ther Adv Urol 2022;14. 17562872221135940.

46. FitzGerald MP, Payne CK, Lukacz ES, et al. Randomized multicenter clinical trial of myofascial physical therapy in women with interstitial cystitis/painful bladder syndrome and pelvic floor tenderness. J Urol 2012;187(6):2113–8.

47. Clemens JQ, Erickson DR, Varela NP, et al. Diagnosis and treatment of interstitial cystitis/bladder pain syndrome. J Urol 2022;208(1):34–42.

48. Lomas J, Gurgenci T, Jackson C, et al. Temporomandibular dysfunction. Aust J Gen Pract 2018;47(4):212–5.

49. Alomar X, Medrano J, Cabratosa J, et al. Anatomy of the temporomandibular joint. Seminars Ultrasound, CT MRI 2007;28(3):170–83.

50. Sharma S, Gupta DS, Pal US, et al. Etiological factors of temporomandibular joint disorders. Natl J Maxillofac Surg 2011;2(2):116–9.
51. Ryan J, Akhter R, Hassan N, et al. Epidemiology of temporomandibular disorder in the general population: a systematic review. Advances in Dentistry & Oral Health 2019;10(3). https://doi.org/10.19080/ADOH.2019.10.555787.
52. Rodriguez-Lopez MJ, Fernandez-Baena M, Aldaya-Valverde C. Management of pain secondary to temporomandibular joint syndrome with peripheral nerve stimulation. Pain Physician 2015;18(2):E229–36.
53. Gauer RL, Semidey MJ. Diagnosis and treatment of temporomandibular disorders. Am Fam Physician 2015;91(6):378–86.
54. Ramirez LM, Ballesteros LE, Sandoval GP. Topical review: temporomandibular disorders in an integral otic symptom model. Int J Audiol 2008;47(4):215–27.
55. Reiter S, Goldsmith C, Emodi-Perlman A, et al. Masticatory muscle disorders diagnostic criteria: the American Academy of Orofacial Pain versus the research diagnostic criteria/temporomandibular disorders (RDC/TMD). J Oral Rehabil 2012;39(12):941–7.
56. Scrivani SJ, Keith DA, Kaban LB. Temporomandibular disorders. N Engl J Med 2008;359(25):2693–705.
57. La Touche R, Goddard G, De-la-Hoz JL, et al. Acupuncture in the treatment of pain in temporomandibular disorders: a systematic review and meta-analysis of randomized controlled trials. Clin J Pain 2010;26(6):541–50.
58. Al-Ani MZ, Davies SJ, Gray RJM, et al. Stabilisation splint therapy for temporomandibular pain dysfunction syndrome. Cochrane Database Syst Rev 2004;1: CD002778.
59. Armijo-Olivo S, Pitance L, Singh V, et al. Effectiveness of manual therapy and therapeutic exercise for temporomandibular disorders: systematic review and meta-analysis. Phys Ther 2016;96(1):9–25.
60. Kraus VB, Blanco FJ, Englund M, et al. Call for standardized definitions of osteoarthritis and risk stratification for clinical trials and clinical use. Osteoarthritis Cartilage 2015;23(8):1233–41.
61. Vos T, Lim SS, Abbafati C, et al. Global burden of 369 diseases and injuries in 204 countries and territories, 1990–2019: a systematic analysis for the Global Burden of Disease Study 2019. Lancet 2020;396(10258):1204–22.
62. Allen KD, Thoma LM, Golightly YM. Epidemiology of osteoarthritis. Osteoarthritis Cartilage 2022;30(2):184–95.
63. Segal NA, Nilges JM, Oo WM. Sex differences in osteoarthritis prevalence, pain perception, physical function and therapeutics. Osteoarthritis Cartilage 2024. https://doi.org/10.1016/j.joca.2024.04.002.
64. Lespasio MJ, Sultan AA, Piuzzi NS, et al. Hip osteoarthritis: a primer. Perm J 2018;22(1). https://doi.org/10.7812/TPP/17-084.
65. Katz JN, Arant KR, Loeser RF. Diagnosis and treatment of hip and knee osteoarthritis: a review. JAMA 2021;325(6):568–78.
66. Dennison EM. Osteoarthritis: the importance of hormonal status in midlife women. Maturitas 2022;165:8–11.
67. de Klerk BM, Schiphof D, Groeneveld FPMJ, et al. No clear association between female hormonal aspects and osteoarthritis of the hand, hip and knee: a systematic review. Rheumatology 2009;48(9):1160–5.
68. Mei Y, Williams JS, Webb EK, et al. Roles of hormone replacement therapy and menopause on osteoarthritis and cardiovascular disease outcomes: a narrative review. Front Rehabil Sci 2022;3. https://doi.org/10.3389/fresc.2022.825147.

69. Stevens-Lapsley JE, Kohrt WM. Osteoarthritis in women: effects of estrogen, obesity and physical activity. Women's Health 2010;6(4):601–15.
70. Rahman A, Underwood M, Carnes D. Fibromyalgia. BMJ 2014;348:g1224.
71. Amris K, Wæhrens EE, Christensen R, et al, IMPROvE Study Group. Interdisciplinary rehabilitation of patients with chronic widespread pain: primary endpoint of the randomized, nonblinded, parallel-group IMPROvE trial. Pain 2014;155(7): 1356–64.
72. Li Y, Su Y, Chen S, et al. The effects of resistance exercise in patients with knee osteoarthritis: a systematic review and meta-analysis. Clin Rehabil 2016;30(10): 947–59.

Pelvic Pain and Pelvic Floor Disorders in Women

A Physiatrist's Approach to Epidemiology and Examination

Lisa Laurenzana, MD[a], Colleen Fitzgerald, MD[c],
Stacey Bennis, MD, CAQ-SM[b],*

KEYWORDS

- Chronic pelvic pain • Pelvic floor dysfunction • Pelvic floor history and examination

KEY POINTS

- Chronic pelvic pain has a significant impact on quality of life and disability in women across all ages.
- Chronic pelvic pain is complex and multifactorial; therefore, a holistic patient-centered approach is key in understanding and managing chronic pelvic pain.
- History taking of patients with chronic pelvic pain should not only focus on pain history, but also explore the gynecologic, urologic, gastrointestinal, psychological, and neurologic systems.
- The pelvic floor muscle examination is a specialized and sensitive examination and should be completed by those with specific training and understanding of pelvic floor anatomy and function.

DEFINING CHRONIC PELVIC PAIN
Definition and Prevalence

The American College of Obstetricians and Gynecologists defines chronic pelvic pain (CPP) as "pain symptoms perceived to originate from pelvic organs and structures typically lasting more than 6 months. It is often associated with negative cognitive behavioral, sexual, and emotional consequences as well as with symptoms suggestive of lower urinary tract, sexual, bowel, pelvic floor, myofascial, or gynecologic

[a] Department of Physical Medicine and Rehabilitation, McGaw Medical Center of Northwestern University, 420 East Superior Street Suite 9-900, Chicago, IL 60611, USA; [b] Department of Obstetrics and Gynecology, Loyola University Chicago, 2160 South First Avenue, Maywood, IL 60153, USA; [c] Department of Orthopedic Surgery and Rehabilitation/Obstetrics and Gynecology, Loyola University Chicago, 2160 South First Avenue, Maywood, IL 60153, USA
* Corresponding author.
E-mail address: Stacey.Bennis001@luhs.org

Phys Med Rehabil Clin N Am 36 (2025) 311–328
https://doi.org/10.1016/j.pmr.2024.11.008
pmr.theclinics.com
1047-9651/25/© 2024 Elsevier Inc. All rights are reserved, including those for text and data mining, AI training, and similar technologies.

dysfunction."[1,2] The prevalence of CPP in heterosexual women is estimated to be 5.7% to 26.6% as demonstrated by a 2014 systematic review of 7 CPP studies.[3] More recently, a 2022 study further characterized the prevalence of CPP in 6,150 US women of different sexual orientations and found an increased prevalence of lifetime CPP among women who identified as mostly heterosexual and lesbian when compared to completely heterosexual women.[4] In addition, CPP was found to be more common in women who reported to have both men and women as past sexual partners compared to women who reported only past male sexual partners.[4] Risk factors associated with CPP include psychological morbidity, history of sexual abuse, substance use disorders, low physical activity, and body mass index.[5,6]

CPP has a significant impact on quality of life and disability. CPP is associated with significant morbidity and contributes to long-term medical therapies. In a 1996 study, it was estimated that about $2.8 billion is spent annually on the management of CPP (about $5.5 billion in 2024).[7] Women with CPP account for 40% of laparoscopies and 12% of the hysterectomies in the United States, yet the origin of CPP is found to be not gynecologic in 80% of patients.[8,9]

Etiology of Chronic Pelvic Pain

CPP is multifactorial in nature and can be associated with visceral, neuropathic, musculoskeletal, and psychological symptoms. Additionally, there is significant overlap of these systems, making it difficult to target one system as the primary pain generator. For example, the visceral and somatic structures including the skin, muscles, and bones share neurologic pathways in the brain and spinal cord. The sharing of these pathways can lead to viscerosomatic convergence or viscero-viscero cross sensitization in which painful stimuli from one organ can result in painful stimulation in another organ or tissue.[10] Similarly, painful stimuli from muscle or tissue can lead to noxious stimuli in organs.[10] Due to the repeated stimulation into the central nervous system, responsiveness of the brain and spinal cord becomes enhanced leading to decreased pain inhibition. This can result in the phenomenon called central sensitization involving widespread hypersensitivity to pain in addition to associated sleep disturbances and poor mood and coping mechanisms.[11,12] There are several conditions which, when present with CPP, are strongly suggestive of central sensitization. These conditions include chronic low back pain, fibromyalgia, irritable bowel syndrome, temporomandibular joint disorder, endometriosis, interstitial cystitis, and chronic fatigue.[13] Organ-specific treatment is often insufficient to treat CPP in the setting of sensitization and myofascial dysfunction.[1,11] In fact, 50% to 90% of women who have a musculoskeletal examination of the pelvic floor, back, and hips have pain originating from these structures.[14–16] If the musculoskeletal examination is dismissed, patients may experience a delay in treatment, unnecessary surgical procedures, and prolonged pain.[12,17]

Overlapping Pain Diagnoses

Common comorbid contributors to pelvic pain include irritable bowel syndrome (IBS), interstitial cystitis or painful bladder syndrome, pelvic floor muscle myofascial pain, endometriosis, and depression. Prevalence of these conditions in women with CPP ranges from about 20% to 60%.[19–22] There are also several conditions in which the prevalence of CPP is higher including generalized hypermobility spectrum disorders such as Ehlers-Danlos[23] in addition to common chronic overlapping pain syndrome conditions including fibromyalgia, temporomandibular disorder, urologic syndrome, vulvodynia, chronic low back pain, chronic tension type headache, migraines, and chronic fatigue syndrome.[24] Additionally, patients with CPP have been found to often have comorbid endometriosis, vulvodynia, IBS, interstitial cystitis, hip or lumbar pain (**Table 1**).[25]

Mechanisms that may be involved in these overlapping disorders may include neurotransmitter or neuroendocrine dysfunction in the central nervous system, adverse childhood events, and psychological distress or psychiatric disorders.[1,13,26] Given the many overlapping conditions of numerous organ systems in addition to coordinating treatment for comorbid conditions, such as depression and anxiety, interdisciplinary care is critical for the treatment of CPP.[27,28]

ANATOMY OF THE PELVIC FLOOR

Women may be at an increased risk of developing pelvic floor disorders compared to men due to anatomic and biomechanical differences, namely the female pelvis is broader and shallower than the male pelvis. This broad shape puts greater strain on the muscles and ligaments of the pelvis which may predispose women to pelvic floor disorders.[29]

The pelvis is made up of bony and articular surfaces, including the ilium, ischium, and pubis, which act as the structural basis for the soft tissue of the pelvis. The coccyx is also a crucial point in the pelvis as it serves as a ligamentous and tendinous attachment for many pelvic floor muscles. The pelvic floor acts as a sling to support the internal organs including the bladder, reproductive organs, and rectum; it includes the muscles, ligaments, and fascia of the pelvis. The pelvic girdle maintains stability through force closure and form closure. Force closure refers to the stability created by tension from fascia and tendons. Form closure refers to stability formed by the bony congruency of joint surfaces.[29]

The Bony Pelvis

The posterior pelvic ring is made up of the 2 sacroiliac joints (SIJ) and the anterior and posterior sacroiliac ligaments. The anterior sacroiliac ligaments include the anterior longitudinal ligament, the anterior sacroiliac ligament, and the sacrospinous ligament. Their primary function is to resist upward movement of the sacrum and lateral movement of the ilium. The posterior sacroiliac ligaments include the supraspinous ligament, iliolumbar ligament, sacrotuberous ligament, and the short and long dorsal sacroiliac ligaments. They function to resist downward and upward movement of the sacrum and medial motion of the ilium. Importantly, the long dorsal sacroiliac ligament is thought to be a source of posterior pelvic pain as forces are transmitted from the SIJ and hip to the nociceptors in the ligament.[30] The anterior pelvic ring includes the pubic symphysis which is a cartilaginous joint between the 2 pubic bones. The 4 pubic ligaments, anterior, posterior, inferior, and superior pubic ligaments, help stabilize the pubic symphysis against tension or compression stresses.

The Pelvic Floor

The muscles of the pelvic floor function to maintain continence and allow micturition and defecation and assist in vaginal childbirth. When the muscles of the pelvic floor contract, they act to close the urethra, anal sphincters, and vagina, helping maintain

Table 1
Potential overlapping conditions associated with pelvic floor myofascial pain or dysfunction by system[18]

Gynectologic	Genitourinary	Gastrointestinal	Musculoskeletal	Neurologic	Psychological
Vulvdynia	Interstitial Cystitis/Painful Bladder Syndrome	Irritable Bowel Syndrome	Lumbar Spine Disorders	Radioculopathy	Anxiety
Dysmenorrhea	Urinary Urgency/Frequency Syndrome	Hemorrhoids	Pelvic Floor Myofascial Pain and Dysfunction	Plexopathy	Depression
Endometriosis	Urinary Incontinence (Stress, Urge or Mixed)	Dyssynergic Defecation	Pelvic Girdle Pain (Sacroiliac Joint/Pubic Symphysis Pain)	Peripheral Neuropathy (including pudendal neuropathy)	History of trauma (emotional, physical, sexual)
Fibroids	Pelvic Organ Prolapse	Fecal Incontinence	Coccydynia		
Ovarian Cyst			Hip Disorders		
Perineal Tear/Levator Avulsion			Hypermobility		

continence. When the muscles relax, they aid in micturition and defecation.[31] The muscles that make up the pelvic floor are organized into 3 categories: the superficial perineal layer, the deep urogenital diaphragm layer, and the pelvic diaphragm. In the superficial perineal layer are the bulbospongiosus, ischiocavernosus, and the superficial and deep transverse perineal muscles. The deep pelvic floor muscles include coccygeus and levator ani which is made up by the puborectalis, pubococcygeus, and iliococcygeus muscles (**Fig. 1**). The pelvic diaphragm is composed of levator ani, coccygeus, and the endopelvic fascia. The deep external rotators of the hip—piriformis and obturator internus muscles, while not directly a part of the pelvic floor, make up the lateral walls of the pelvis and can often contribute to pelvic pain.[18] A key structure in the pelvic floor is the perineal body, also called the central perineal tendon. The perineal body is the attachment for many pelvic muscles and sphincters and is located between the vagina and the anus. Of note, rupture of this entity, which can occur in childbirth, can lead to pelvic organ prolapse.[32]

Innervation of the Pelvic Floor

Innervation of the pelvic structures is through somatic, visceral, and central pathways (**Table 2**). The sacral plexus is responsible for the majority of innervation of the pelvic floor. The iliohypogastric, ilioinguinal, and genitofemoral nerves (L1 to L3 nerve roots) innervate the skin of the lower trunk, perineum, and proximal thigh. The lateral femoral cutaneous nerve innervates the lateral thigh and the obturator nerve innervates the skin of the medial thigh along with the adductor muscles in the medial thigh. The pudendal nerve originates from the ventral branches of S2 to S4 of the sacral plexus. The pudendal nerve takes a tortuous route in the pelvis, passing between the piriformis and coccygeal muscles, through the greater sciatic foramen, over the spine of ischium, and then reentering the pelvis through the lesser sciatic foramen. The pudendal nerve borders the lateral wall of the ischiorectal fossa where it is held in the sheath from the obturator fascia called Alock's canal.[18,29]

The pudendal nerve and its 3 branches, the inferior rectal/hemorrhoidal nerve, the perineal nerve, and the dorsal nerve of the clitoris, mainly innervate the superficial and anterior muscles in the pelvic floor. Namely, the pudendal nerve innervates the bulbospongiosus, ischiocavernosus, and anterior portions of levator ani muscles,

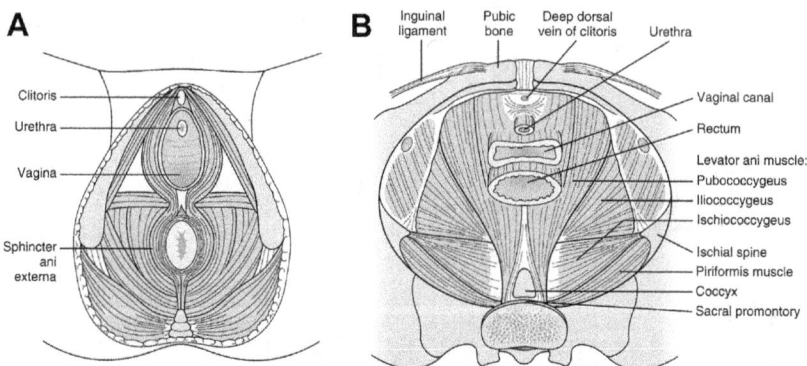

Fig. 1. Pelvic floor musculature. (*From Braddom's Physical Medicine and Rehabilitation, 774-788. Sixth edition. Copyright @ Elsevier, 2021. The muscles of the (A) superficial pelvic floor and (B) deep pelvic floor. Illustration by Elijah Leonard. Redrawn from Prather H, Dugan S, Fitzgerald C, Hunt D: Review of anatomy, evaluation, and treatment of musculoskeletal pelvic floor pain in women, PMR 2009;1:346–358.)*

Table 2
Pelvic floor muscles origin, insertion, action, and innervation

Muscle	Origin	Insertion	Action	Innervation
Ischiocavernosus	Ischiopubic rami & ischial tuberosities	Inferior & medial sides of the clitoris	Maintain erection of clitoris by compressing veins that drain it	Deep brain of perineal nerve (innervated by S2-S4 nerve roots)
Bulbospongiosus	Perineal body	Pubic arch	Assists in erection of clitoris, supports the perineal body	Deep branch of perineal nerve (innervated by S2-S4 nerve roots)
Superficial Transverse Perineal Muscles	Internal surface of ischiopubic rami and ischial tuberosities	Perineal body	Constricts urethra and vagina (maintains urinary continence)	Deep branch of perineal nerve (innervated by S2-S4 nerve roots)
Deep Transverse Perineal	Inner surface of inferior ischial rami	Sides of vagina	Stabilizes perineal body, supports the vagina	Perineal branches of pudendal nerve (S2, S3, S4)
Puborectalis	Pubic symphysis	None (wraps around rectum and re-inserts onto origin)	Inhibit defecation	Pudendal nerve
Pubococcygeus	Pubis and obturator fascia	Sacrum and coccyx	Controls urine flow and contracts during orgasm	Pudendal nerve
Iliococcygeus	Ischial spine and tendinous arch of pelvic fascia	Coccyx and anococcygeal raphe	Supports viscera in pelvic cavity	Pudendal nerve
Coccygeus	Sacrospinous ligament and ischial spine	Sacrum and coccyx	Pulls coccyx anteriorly post-defecation	Pudendal nerve and coccygeal nerve
Piriformis	Anterior surface of sacrum	Greater trochanter of femur	Thigh external rotation, thigh abduction	Nerve to piriformis (SI-S2)
Obturator Internus	Inferior margin of superior pubic ramus	Medial surface of greater trochanter of femur	External rotation of extended thigh, abduction of flexed thigh	Nerve to obturator internus (LS and SI)

the perineum, anus, external anal and urethral sphincters, and clitoris (**Fig. 2**). The pudendal nerve, therefore, is responsible for external genital sensation, continence, and orgasm. Of note, although the anterior portion of levator ani is innervated by the pudendal nerve, most of the levator ani is innervated directly from sacral nerves S3 to S5.[18,29] This innervation pattern is important when considering symptomatology for pudendal neuralgia which will be discussion in subsequent articles.

HISTORY TAKING

Gathering a thorough medical history during the evaluation of patients with CPP will include the history of present illness, medical and surgical history, social history, obstetric and gynecologic history, sexual history, psychiatric history (including history of trauma), relevant family history, and current and previous medications. It is also particularly important to obtain pregnancy history and, for women of child-bearing age, a menstrual history including birth control method if applicable. Pregnancy history includes number of pregnancies and children, delivery method and length, complications of past pregnancies, including use of instrumentation, and history of perineal tearing or episiotomy. For women of child-bearing age, it is important to ask if they are currently pregnant, trying to get pregnant, or are currently breastfeeding as this may impact the medical workup and treatment plans.

It is important to understand previously attempted treatments including past prescriptions, over the counter or supplemental medications, interventional procedures (ie, injections, cystoscopy, colonoscopy), surgeries (ie, exploratory laparoscopy, hysterectomy, or other surgical procedures), and modalities (ie, biofeedback, ultrasound, chiropractic, acupuncture, physical or occupational therapy, cold or heat).[17,33]

Regarding history taking, it is necessary to ascertain the onset of pain, including inciting events or injury, location, severity, and quality of pain, associated symptoms including radiation of pain, numbness or tingling, factors which improve and worsen pain, and temporal factors including timing of pain throughout the day.

There are certain features of the history, which should prompt an examiner to consider further evaluation for pelvic pain. For example, as discussed previously, history of trauma or premorbid mood disorder and generalized hypermobility spectrum

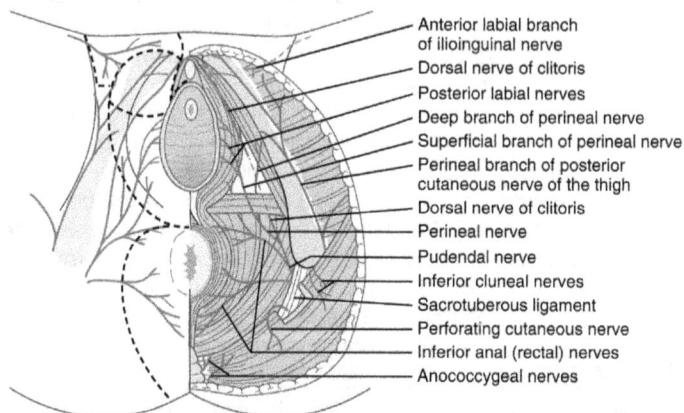

Fig. 2. Pelvic floor muscle innervation and nerve routes. (*From Braddom's Physical Medicine and Rehabilitation*, 774-788. Sixth edition. Copyright @ Elsevier, 2021. Redrawn from Prather H, Dugan S, Fitzgerald C, Hunt D: Review of anatomy, evaluation, and treatment of musculoskeletal pelvic floor pain in women. *PMR* 2009;1:346–358.)

disorders are associated with development of CPP.[23,28] Pain with intercourse, gynecologic speculum examination, or tampon use may be signs of pelvic floor myofascial pain or dysfunction. Urinary urgency, frequency, retention or incontinence, urinary tract infection symptoms in the absence of positive cultures, constipation or stool incontinence, and prior vaginal tearing during delivery may also be hints that the patient is experiencing pelvic floor myofascial pain or dysfunction.[31] Pelvic girdle pain, involving pain at the pubic symphysis or sacroiliac joints is suggestive of an SIJ or pubic symphysis disorder. Low back pain worse with coughing, sneezing, laughing, or bending may be suggestive of a discogenic process.[33]

A thorough history regarding back, hip, lower extremity, and pelvic symptoms is necessary in the assessment of patients with pelvic pain. **Table 3** below, adopted from a 2017 description of office evaluation of pelvic pain, outlines detailed questions organized by system, to guide differential diagnoses, physical examination, and diagnostic work up.[33]

THE CLINICAL PHYSICAL EXAMINATION

A thorough musculoskeletal physical examination is recommended for all patients presenting with pelvic or vaginal pain. A 2018 study reported about 50% to 90% of patients presenting for evaluation of pelvic pain were found to have musculoskeletal dysfunction.[17,34] The physical examination will include a thorough examination of the hips, lumbar spine, pelvic girdle, pelvic floor muscles, and lower limbs. Patients may present with symptoms more consistent with a primary condition involving the urologic, gastrointestinal, gynecologic, infectious, or oncologic systems. It is important to provide appropriate referrals when necessary, however, a physiatrist examination is still recommended, given the significant overlap of conditions contributing to pelvic pain.

The Pelvic Girdle Examination

The pelvic girdle is first assessed by inspection, evaluating for pelvic obliquity or shift when standing. The active straight leg raise test should be performed to assess for difficulty or heaviness when the patient is asked to raise 1 leg off the examination table in a supine position. If positive, the test should be repeated with manual compression or stabilization of the pelvis using an SIJ belt. If compression improves their symptoms with active straight leg testing, then it can be inferred the patient has SIJ dysfunction, hypermobility, and/or core instability.

There are several SIJ pain provocation tests which can help guide diagnosis of a symptomatic SIJ. The gold standard for diagnosing a symptomatic SIJ is with relief of pain from an intraarticular SIJ block. The following 6 tests can help predict who will benefit from an intraarticular SIJ block. The 6 tests include SIJ distraction, posterior pelvic pain provocation test (P4), Gaeslen's maneuver, compression test, sacral thrust, and drop test. When 3 out of all 6 are positive or 2 out the following 4 tests, distraction, compression, P4, or sacral thrust are positive, the patient is predicted to benefit from an intraarticular SIJ block (**Table 4**).[29,33,34]

The Pelvic Floor Examination

At a minimum, verbal consent from the patient should be obtained and the examination should be performed by a trained physician in a private room. Appropriate hand hygiene should be performed and gloves should be utilized for the examination. A chaperone should be always offered and is mandatory for treatment of opposite gender or for patients under the age of 18-years-old. A trauma-informed approach

Table 3
Review of systems questions for patients with pelvic pain

System	Questions
Neuromuscular	• Do you have low back or hip pain? • Do you have pain in your pelvis? • Do you have pain that radiates into your buttocks, legs, or feet? • Are there any positions that make your pain worse? • Is your pain worse with coughing, sneezing, or bending over? • Is your pain worse with transitional movements (getting in/out of chair, car, or bed) • Do you have weakness in your legs? Is it due to pain? • Do you have a history of tripping or falling? • Do you use an assistive device such as a cane or walker for ambulation? • Do you have numbness or tingling? • Can you feel the tissue paper when you wipe after urinating of having a bowel movement • Can you feel when you have a bowel movement or when you urinate?
Obstetric	• Gravida/para status: ○ How many times have you been pregnant? ○ How many children have you delivered? ○ Have you had any ectopic pregnancies, miscarriages, or abortions? Any procedures? • For each pregnancy: ○ Did you have pain during pregnancy? ○ Did you have a vaginal delivery or cesarean section? ○ What was the birth weight of your child? ○ How long were you in labor? ○ How long did you push/how long was your active labor? ○ Did your delivery require vacuum or forceps assistance? ○ Did you have any bowel or bladder changes after delivery?
Gynecologic	• Do you have a history of gynecologic surgery? Dilation & curettage? Biopsies? Loop electrosurgical excision procedures Tubal ligation? C-section? Hysterectomy? Salpingoopherectomy? Vaginal sling? Mesh? • Are gynecologic examinations painful for you? • Have you ever been diagnosed with endometriosis? How was it diagnosed? • Have you ever been diagnosed with chronic yeast infections? • For premenopausal women: ○ When was your last menstrual period? Are your periods regular? ○ Are you taking hormonal contraceptives? ○ Is there a chance you could be pregnant? ○ Do you wear tampons? Is it painful to wear tampons? • For menopausal/postmenopausal patients: ○ When was your last menstrual period? Do you ever have vaginal bleeding? ○ Did your pain start before or after menopause? ○ Have you been or are you currently on any hormonal replacement therapy? ○ Have you been diagnosed with vaginal atrophy, dryness, or lichen sclerosis or planus? ○ Have you ever been diagnosed with pelvic organ prolapse? Do you use a pessary?
Sexual History	• Are you sexually active? Do you have 1 partner or multiple? • Do you have pain with intercourse? What is painful? Initial penetration? Deep penetration? • Do you have pain after intercourse? How long does it last? • Is it painful when you orgasm?

(continued on next page)

System	Questions
Table 3 (*continued*)	
System	Questions
Gastrointestinal	• Do you have history of intraabdominal surgeries? • Do you ever have constipation or diarrhea? • Have you ever been diagnosed with irritable bowel syndrome? • How often do you have a bowel movement? • Do you have pain before, during, or after a bowel movement? • Do you have to strain to empty your bowels? • Do you ever have fecal urgency? • Do you ever have fecal incontinence or leakage? • Do you take any bowel medications?

Urologic	• Do you have a history of urologic disorders or surgeries?
	• General incontinence symptoms:
	  ○ Do you ever experience urinary incontinence or leaking? How often?
	  ○ Do you have to wear an incontinence pad? If so, how frequently do you have to change the pad?
	  ○ What do you drink throughout the day?
	• Stress urinary symptoms:
	  ○ Do you experience incontinence or leaking with coughing and sneezing? With standing from a chair or with exercise?
	• Urgency-frequency urinary symptoms:
	  ○ How often do you have to go to the bathroom to urinate?
	  ○ Do you ever have difficulty making it to the toilet?
	  ○ Do you ever have urinary incontinence or leaking when you have the urge to empty your bladder?
	• Nocturia symptoms:
	  ○ How many times per night do you wake up to use the bathroom?
	  ○ Do you ever have incontinence or leakage at night while sleeping?
	• Retention symptoms:
	  ○ Do you ever feel that you incompletely empty your bladder?
	  ○ Do you ever feel like you are straining to empty your bladder?
	• Urinary tract infection (UTI) symptoms:
	  ○ Do you have burning or pain with urination?
	  ○ Do you have blood in your urine?
	  ○ Do you have a history of UTIs? How frequently have you been treated for UTIs?
	• Urinary Symptoms associated with sexual intercourse:
	  ○ Do you have urinary incontinence or leakage with sexual intercourse?

Dermatologic	• Have you ever noticed rashes or lesions in the pelvic region? Any itchiness? • Have you noticed dryness of the skin in the pelvic region?
Infectious	• Have you had any recent fevers or chills? • Do you have vaginal discharge? • Have you ever been diagnosed with any sexually transmitted infections?
Oncologic	• Any recent unintentional weight loss? • Do you have any personal history of breast, ovarian, uterine or colon cancer? If so, any history of pelvic radiation? • Do you have any family history of breast, ovarian, uterine or colon cancer?
Psychiatric	• What are your hobbies? What do you enjoy doing in your spare time? • How many hours do you sleep on average? Do you have sleep aids? • Do you drink caffeinated beverages? How many per day? • Do you use tobacco? How many cigarettes per day and for how long? • Do you use alcohol? How many drinks per week and for how long? • Do you use any recreation drugs? Which drugs? How often and for how long?

(*continued on next page*)

Table 3
(continued)

System	Questions
	• Are you married, single, divorced or widowed?
	• Do you feel you have a strong support system?
	• Do you currently have any stressors in your life?
	• Do you feel safe at home and at work?
	• Have you ever been diagnosed with depression or anxiety?
	• Do you follow with a psychiatrist, psychologist, or social worker?
	• Have you ever been hospitalized for a psychiatric illness?
	• Have you ever had thoughts of harming yourself?
	• Have you ever been diagnosed with an eating disorder?
	• Have you ever been the victim of abuse? Physical? Verbal? Emotional? Sexual?

is recommended, and the patient should be given the autonomy to proceed with or stop the examination at any time.[35]

Examination of the pelvic floor muscles is essential due to its role in CPP.[34,36] Clinically, symptoms are improved through treatment of myofascial pain with pelvic floor physical therapy (PFPT); therefore, understanding the physical examination can help providers more effectively recommend, direct, and prescribe musculoskeletal rehabilitation treatment, including PFPT, and possibly avoid more invasive or risky treatment options.

The musculoskeletal pelvic floor examination is divided into 2 parts, the internal and external examination. The external examination begins with visual inspection of perineum, evaluating for possible lesions, scars, cysts, or swelling. The examiner should

Table 4
Sacroiliac joint pain tests

Test Name	Maneuver
SI Joint Distraction	Apply vertically oriented pressure to the bilateral anterior superior iliac spine, directed posteriorly
Posterior Pelvic Pain Provocation Test (P4)	Assesses ipsilateral SIJ by grounding the sacrum with one hand and applying a vertically oriented and posteriorly directed pressure with the other hand.
Gaenslen's Test	Tests ipsilateral SIJ in posterior rotation and contralateral SIJ in anterior rotation by applying a superior and posterior torsion force to the ipsilateral knee when the hip and knee are in flexion, and a posteriorly directed force to the contralateral knee which is flexed over the edge of the examination table.
Compression Test	Place the patient in side-lying and apply a vertically directed force through the iliac crest.
Sacral Thrust	Place the patient in prone and apply a vertically directed shearing force over the midline of the sacrum at its apex.
Drop Test	Assesses the ipsilateral SIJ by having the patient raise the ipsilateral heel off the floor to bear near full bodyweight then dropping the heel to the floor to create a force directed at the ipsilateral SIJ.
Patrick's or FABER Test (Flexion, Abduction, External Rotation)	With the patient supine, place the hip in flexion, abduction, and external rotation to assess pain provocation in the hip, groin, buttock, SIJ, or lumbar spine.

also take note of visible pelvic organ prolapse. The examiner will ask the patient to perform a voluntary Kegel contraction, and the examiner will attempt to visualize the lift of the perineal body. The examiner will then ask the patient to cough to create an involuntary contraction and a Valsalva maneuver to visualize involuntary relaxation. The examiner should take note of any inappropriate contraction or dyssynergia of the pelvic floor muscles with Valsalva.[33,36–38]

Next, the examiner can perform the Q-tip test to evaluate for vulvodynia. The cotton swab of a Q-tip is lightly brushed along the vulva and vestibule to evaluate if allodynia is elicited. An external sensory examination of the S2-S5 dermatomes is then performed to light touch and pinprick.[29] The anal wink reflex is tested near the anus and the bulbocavernosus reflex is tested near the labia minora lateral to the clitoris to visualize anal sphincter contraction. Both reflexes evaluate the sacral reflex arc. Lastly, the superficial pelvic floor muscles, including the bulbospongiosus, ischiocavernosus, and the transverse perineal muscle can be palpated externally.[33]

The internal examination can involve both digital vaginal and rectal examinations. The vaginal examination is best performed with the patient supine, knees bent, and ankles hip-width apart or in dorsal lithotomy using stirrups if available. The rectal examination is performed in the left lateral decubitus position. To palpate the pelvic floor musculature, a single lubricated, gloved finger is inserted into the vaginal introitus or anal canal.[38]

Internal palpation of musculature is guided by a clock face diagram to help correctly identify the positions of pelvic floor muscles. The pubic bone sits at the 12 o'clock position and the anus and coccyx at the 6 o'clock position. **Table 5**, adopted from a 2021 pelvic floor assessment guide, outline specific locations of muscles using clock face descriptions.[38] Tenderness with palpation at any of these sites may indicate muscle overactivity or trigger point sites. In an overactive muscle, the examiner may feel broad, thick fibers that are uncomfortable when palpated. In underactive muscles, the examiner may feel softer, less bulky muscles that are not typically tender. Of note, the obturator internus and levator ani are separated by the arcus tendinous, which feels like a guitar string on palpation (**Fig. 3**).

Muscle strength testing is evaluated with voluntary contraction, which is felt as a tightening or lifting of the examiners finger. Strength is graded using the modified Oxford scale which is a scale ranging from 0 to 5 out of 5 (**Table 6**).[39] Testing should be completed in 4 quadrants. Evaluation of strength and coordination of pelvic floor muscles can help guide providers toward diagnosis; for example, underactive pelvic floor muscles can lead to urinary incontinence or pelvic organ prolapse while overactive pelvic floor muscles can contribute to constipation or urinary retention. Initial baseline tone should be assessed on insertion prior to evaluating for muscle tenderness, strength, and coordination. Patients should also be asked to hold a voluntary contraction for 10 seconds (to test endurance) and to contract and relax sequentially and rapidly (to test coordination).

The Neurologic Examination

Strength, sensation to light touch, and pinprick particularly in the L2 to S2 nerve root distribution should be assessed in the evaluation of pelvic pain. Reflexes of the lower extremities should be tested in the patellar, medial hamstring, and Achilles tendons.

Gait should also be assessed, taking note of posture, stance, step and stride length, and any abnormal gait patterns such as antalgic gait, Trendelenburg gait, hip hiking, or steppage gait.

Table 5
Pelvic floor muscle

Examination 1	
Superficial Muscle Assessment	**Location Through Vaginal Examination**
Ischiocavernosus	11 o'clock and 1 o'clock
Bulbospongiosus	Immediately external to introitus
Superficial Transverse Perineal	3 o'clock and 9 o'clock
Levator Ani	7 o'clock and 5 o'clock
Anal Sphincter	Rectal: visual inspection and palpation at anus and surrounding tissue

Examination 2	
Deep Muscle Assessment	**Location Through Vaginal Examination**
Bulbocavernosus	At introitus
Levator Ani	1–2 knuckle depth: 5 o'clock and 7 o'clock
Rectum	Central 1–2 knuckle depth
Obturator Internus (place hand on outside of ipsilateral flexed and have patient push knee outward while resisting)	Vaginally: 2 knuckle depth: 3 o'clock and 9 o'clock Rectal: 4 o'clock and 8 o'clock beyond ischial spine
Puborectalis	Vaginally: 1 knuckle depth: 11 o'clock and 1 o'clock Rectally: just beyond internal/external sphincter
Bladder and Urethra	1–2 knuckle depth: 12 o'clock
Coccyx	Rectally: use external finger to guide internal examination to location of the coccyx
Coccygeus	Rectally: find the coccyx and palpate alone either side following the muscle laterally to the ischial spine

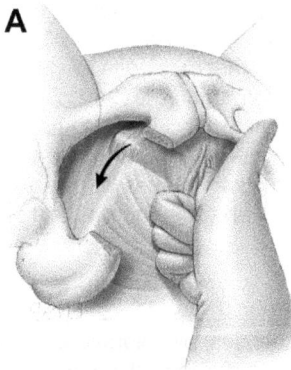

Obturator Internus   Levator Ani

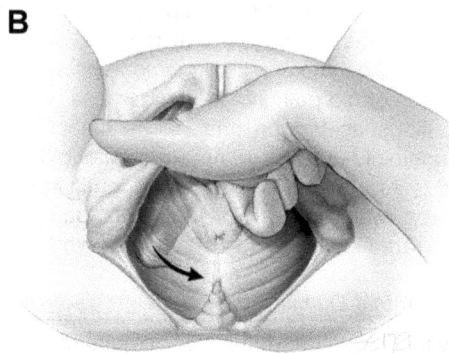

Fig. 3. Pelvic floor muscle internal exam. (Melanie R. Meister et al., Development of a standardized, reproducible screening examination for assessment of pelvic floor myofascial pain, American Journal of Obstetrics and Gynecology, 220 (3), 2019, 255.e1-255.e9, https://doi.org/10.1016/j.ajog.2018.11.1106.)

Table 6
Modified Oxford scale grading internal manual muscle testing of the pelvic floor muscles

Grading	Contraction?	Lift or Tightening?
0/5	No	No
1/5	Flicker	No
2/5	Weak	No
3/5	Moderate	Some lift and tightening, contraction is visible
4/5	Good	Holds for 5+ seconds
5/5	Strong	Holds for 10+ seconds

The Lumbosacral Spine Examination

Evaluation begins with inspection of the spine to assess alignment, shift, or presence of scoliosis. Palpation of the paraspinal muscles and spinous processes can help evaluate for tenderness, step-off deformities, and shifts. Range of motion evaluation should include assessment of restrictions or pain with forward flexion, extension, lateral side bending, and rotation.

Facet arthropathy and discogenic pain should routinely be assessed in patients with pelvic pain. The straight leg raise and seated slump test can be used to help assess discogenic pain while axial facet loading tests can help identify facet arthropathy.

The Hip Examination

Hip pain can be intraarticular, extraarticular, or it can be referred pain from the spine, SIJ, pelvic floor or the gastrointestinal or genitourinary systems. Hip pain can be experienced in the hip joint itself, but may also be felt in the groin, buttock, low back, and knee with or without pain in the hip joint.[40]

The hips should be assessed routinely in patients with pelvic pain. Passive and active range of motion can assess for asymmetry, restriction, or pain. Provocation tests such as the Stinchfield's test, also called the resisted hip flexion test, and the Scour test can be useful in helping to identify an intraarticular pathology.[33] Other hip examination maneuvers that may be helpful include FABER/Patrick's test and anterior and posterior hip impingement tests. Maneuvers that may point to extraarticular causes of hip pain include tenderness with palpation of the greater trochanteric region, iliopsoas tendon and iliacus muscles, adductor muscle origin, hamstring origin, conjoint tendon, inguinal ring/posterior inguinal canal, and pubic tubercle. Provocation tests that can be helpful in identifying extraarticular sources of pain are the Ober's test which may point to iliotibial band tightness and the Thomas test which may indicate hip contractures or psoas syndrome.[33]

The Abdominal Examination

Visually inspect the abdomen for obvious distension, hernias, discoloration, or scars. Auscultate the abdomen in all 4 quadrants to assess for bowel sound activity. Palpate with superficial and deep palpation in all 4 quadrants, also palpating the intraabdominal muscles and their insertions along with the iliacus and iliopsoas muscle. Pain with abdominal muscle activation can be assessed with Carnett's test. The test involves asking the patient to tense their abdominal muscles by raising their head off the table while the examiner holds pressure on the tender site. The test is positive if the pain becomes worse or is unchanged. A positive test suggests the pain is somatic in nature and originating from the abdominal wall rather than an intraabdominal origin.[41]

The examiner can test for diastasis rectus abdominis or "rectus diastasis" by asking the patient to do an abdominal crunch to the level of the shoulder blades raising from the examination table. If the space between the rectus abdominis is greater than 2 fingerbreadths, then rectus diastasis can be diagnosed. Mild rectus diastasis is characterized by 2 to 3 fingerbreadths, moderate is 3 to 4 fingerbreadths, and severe is >4 fingerbreadths.[33]

SUMMARY

Chronic pelvic pain presents a multifaceted challenge, affecting women across various stages of life with profound impacts on their daily functioning and well-being. When caring for women with chronic pelvic pain, practitioners should adopt a trauma-centered care approach and maintain a broad differential diagnosis. Symptoms often manifest across multiple organ systems and encompass diverse pain types such as visceral, neuropathic, musculoskeletal, and psychological, complicating both diagnosis and treatment. Effective management hinges upon a thorough understanding of specialized skills in history taking and physical examination tailored for the pelvic pain assessment. A thorough pain and medical history, encompassing gynecologic, obstetric, urologic, gastrointestinal, neurologic, musculoskeletal, and psychological aspects, is crucial. Physical examinations should include comprehensive neurologic and musculoskeletal assessments, along with external and internal pelvic examinations with patient consent. These examinations assess pelvic sensation, muscle tone, strength, coordination, and tenderness, providing valuable insights for accurate diagnosis and effective management strategies.

CLINICS CARE POINTS

- Practice a trauma-centered care approach when caring for women with chronic pelvic pain.
- Consider a broad differential diagnosis when evaluating pelvic pain.
- Often, organ-specific treatment alone is insufficient to treat chronic pelvic pain.
- Chronic overlapping pain conditions may complicate patient presentation, and it is important to gather a thorough pain and medical history.
- Key components of the pelvic pain history include pertinent gynecologic, obstetric, urologic, gastrointestinal, neurologic, musculoskeletal, and psychological history and complications.
- Physical examination should include a thorough neurologic and musculoskeletal examination of the back, hips, lower extremities, and pelvis, including an internal pelvic examination if the patient has consented.
- The external and internal pelvic examinations assess pelvic sensation, pelvic floor muscle tone, strength, coordination, and tenderness and can guide diagnosis and management.

DISCLOSURES

Dr S. Bennis is funded by NICHD and serves on the IPPS Advisory Board Member. Dr C. Fitzgerald serves as an UptoDate Editor, and is Funded by NIDDK, United States, NICHD, IPPS advisory board, speaker for UCSF, Kaiser, and the ShirleyRyan Ability Lab.

REFERENCES

1. Chronic Pelvic Pain: ACOG Practice Bulletin. Number 218. Obstet Gynecol 2020; 135(3):e98–109.
2. Gynecologists ACoOa. Gynecology data definitions (version 1.0). reVitalize. ACOG; 2018.
3. Ahangari A. Prevalence of chronic pelvic pain among women: an updated review. Pain Physician 2014;17(2):E141–7.
4. Tabaac AR, Chwa C, Sutter ME, et al. Prevalence of chronic pelvic pain by sexual orientation in a large cohort of young women in the United States. J Sex Med 2022;19(6):1012–23.
5. Latthe P, Mignini L, Gray R, et al. Factors predisposing women to chronic pelvic pain: systematic review. BMJ 2006;332(7544):749–55.
6. Stanford EJ, Koziol J, Feng A. The prevalence of interstitial cystitis, endometriosis, adhesions, and vulvar pain in women with chronic pelvic pain. J Minim Invasive Gynecol 2005;12(1):43–9.
7. Mathias SD, Kuppermann M, Liberman RF, et al. Chronic pelvic pain: prevalence, health-related quality of life, and economic correlates. Obstet Gynecol 1996; 87(3):321–7.
8. Allaire C, Williams C, Bodmer-Roy S, et al. Chronic pelvic pain in an interdisciplinary setting: 1-year prospective cohort. Am J Obstet Gynecol 2018;218(1): 114, e1-e12.
9. Lamvu G, Williams R, Zolnoun D, et al. Long-term outcomes after surgical and nonsurgical management of chronic pelvic pain: one year after evaluation in a pelvic pain specialty clinic. Am J Obstet Gynecol 2006;195(2):591–8, discussion 98-600.
10. Lamvu G, Carrillo J, Ouyang C, et al. Chronic pelvic pain in women: a review. JAMA 2021;325(23):2381–91.
11. Stratton P, Khachikyan I, Sinaii N, et al. Association of chronic pelvic pain and endometriosis with signs of sensitization and myofascial pain. Obstet Gynecol 2015;125(3):719–28.
12. Aredo JV, Heyrana KJ, Karp BI, et al. Relating chronic pelvic pain and endometriosis to signs of sensitization and myofascial pain and dysfunction. Semin Reprod Med 2017;35(1):88–97.
13. Maixner W, Fillingim RB, Williams DA, et al. Overlapping chronic pain conditions: implications for diagnosis and classification. J Pain 2016;17(9 Suppl):T93–107.
14. Bonder JH, Fitzpatrick L. Diagnosis of pelvic girdle pain. In: Fitzgerald CM, Segal NA, editors. Musculoskeletal health in pregnancy and postpartum : an evidence-based guide for clinicians. 1st 2015. Cham: Springer International Publishing; 2015. p. 69–80.
15. Mieritz RM, Thorhauge K, Forman A, et al. Musculoskeletal dysfunctions in patients with chronic pelvic pain: a preliminary descriptive survey. J Manip Physiol Ther 2016;39(9):616–22.
16. Sedighimehr N, Manshadi FD, Shokouhi N, et al. Pelvic musculoskeletal dysfunctions in women with and without chronic pelvic pain. J Bodyw Mov Ther 2018; 22(1):92–6.
17. Lamvu G, Carrillo J, Witzeman K, et al. Musculoskeletal considerations in female patients with chronic pelvic pain. Semin Reprod Med 2018;36(2):107–15.
18. Hwang S, Bennis S, Scott KM, et al. Pelvic floor disorders. In: Cifu DX, Eapen BC, editors. Braddom's physical medicine and rehabilitation. 6th edition. Philadelphia: Saunders/Elsevier; 2021. p. 774–8.

19. Learman LA, Gregorich SE, Schembri M, et al. Symptom resolution after hysterectomy and alternative treatments for chronic pelvic pain: does depression make a difference? Am J Obstet Gynecol 2011;204(3):269, e1-e9.

20. Williams RE, Hartmann KE, Sandler RS, et al. Recognition and treatment of irritable bowel syndrome among women with chronic pelvic pain. Am J Obstet Gynecol 2005;192(3):761–7.

21. Cheng C, Rosamilia A, Healey M. Diagnosis of interstitial cystitis/bladder pain syndrome in women with chronic pelvic pain: a prospective observational study. Int Urogynecol J 2012;23(10):1361–6.

22. Montenegro ML, Mateus-Vasconcelos EC, Rosa e Silva JC, et al. Importance of pelvic muscle tenderness evaluation in women with chronic pelvic pain. Pain Med 2010;11(2):224–8.

23. Hastings J, Forster JE, Witzeman K. Joint hypermobility among female patients presenting with chronic myofascial pelvic pain. PMR 2019;11(11):1193–9.

24. Till SR, Wahl HN, As-Sanie S. The role of nonpharmacologic therapies in management of chronic pelvic pain: what to do when surgery fails. Curr Opin Obstet Gynecol 2017;29(4):231–9.

25. Ye AL, Adams W, Westbay LC, et al. Evaluating disability-related quality of life in women with chronic pelvic pain. Female Pelvic Med Reconstr Surg 2020;26(8):508–13.

26. Turk DC, Fillingim RB, Ohrbach R, et al. Assessment of psychosocial and functional impact of chronic pain. J Pain 2016;17(9 Suppl):T21–49.

27. Miller-Matero LR, Saulino C, Clark S, et al. When treating the pain is not enough: a multidisciplinary approach for chronic pelvic pain. Arch Womens Ment Health 2016;19(2):349–54.

28. Yosef A, Allaire C, Williams C, et al. Multifactorial contributors to the severity of chronic pelvic pain in women. Am J Obstet Gynecol 2016;215(6):760, e1-e14.

29. Prather H, Dugan S, Fitzgerald C, et al. Review of anatomy, evaluation, and treatment of musculoskeletal pelvic floor pain in women. PMR 2009;1(4):346–58.

30. Vleeming A, Albert HB, Ostgaard HC, et al. European guidelines for the diagnosis and treatment of pelvic girdle pain. Eur Spine J 2008;17(6):794–819.

31. Messelink B, Benson T, Berghmans B, et al. Standardization of terminology of pelvic floor muscle function and dysfunction: report from the pelvic floor clinical assessment group of the International Continence Society. Neurourol Urodyn 2005;24(4):374–80.

32. DeLancey JO. The anatomy of the pelvic floor. Curr Opin Obstet Gynecol 1994;6(4):313–6.

33. Bennis S, Hwang S. Office evaluation of pelvic pain. Phys Med Rehabil Clin N Am 2017;28(3):461–76.

34. Laslett M. Evidence-based diagnosis and treatment of the painful sacroiliac joint. J Man Manip Ther 2008;16(3):142–52.

35. Gorfinkel I, Perlow E, Macdonald S. The trauma-informed genital and gynecologic examination. CMAJ (Can Med Assoc J) 2021;193(28):E1090.

36. Meister MR, Shivakumar N, Sutcliffe S, et al. Physical examination techniques for the assessment of pelvic floor myofascial pain: a systematic review. Am J Obstet Gynecol 2018;219(5):497, e1-e13.

37. Meister MR, Sutcliffe S, Ghetti C, et al. Development of a standardized, reproducible screening examination for assessment of pelvic floor myofascial pain. Am J Obstet Gynecol 2019;220(3):255, e1-e9.

38. Harm-Ernandes I, Boyle V, Hartmann D, et al. Assessment of the pelvic floor and associated musculoskeletal system: guide for medical practitioners. Female Pelvic Med Reconstr Surg 2021;27(12):711–8.
39. Ferreira CH, Barbosa PB, de Oliveira Souza F, et al. Inter-rater reliability study of the modified Oxford grading scale and the peritron manometer. Physiotherapy 2011;97(2):132–8 [published Online First: 20101022].
40. Prather H, Cheng A. Diagnosis and treatment of hip girdle pain in the athlete. PMR 2016;8(3 Suppl):S45–60.
41. Sun XX, Liu H, Qin XZ, et al. The diagnostic value of carnett's test with chronic abdominal pain: a narrative review. Curr Pain Headache Rep 2024;28(4):251–7.

Pelvic Pain and Pelvic Floor Disorders in Women

A Physiatrist's Approach to Diagnosis, Management, and Multidisciplinary Care

Lisa Laurenzana, MD[a], Colleen Fitzgerald, MD[b],
Stacey Bennis, MD, CAQ-SM[c,d],*

KEYWORDS

- Chronic pelvic pain • Pelvic floor dysfunction • Musculoskeletal causes of pelvic pain

KEY POINTS

- Many neuromusculoskeletal causes of pelvic pain can be identified through skillful history taking and physical examination.
- Pelvic floor physical therapy performed by certified, specialized therapists is often the first-line treatment of many musculoskeletal causes of pelvic pain.
- In conjunction with pelvic floor physical therapy, some patients with increased pelvic floor tone may benefit from the initiation of muscle relaxant vaginal suppositories, pelvic floor botulinum toxin, or trigger point injections to aid in therapy progression and quality of life improvement. It is important to understand the pelvic floor muscle examination and assessment prior to recommendation of these interventions.
- Physiatrists are a key member of the pelvic pain care team given the specialty's robust training in the management of chronic pain, bowel and bladder symptoms, and complex neuromusculoskeletal processes. Physiatrists can also help steer the focus of management to restoring function and improving quality of life, which is often the goal of many patients with chronic pelvic pain.

[a] Department of Physical Medicine and Rehabilitation, McGaw Medical Center of Northwestern University, 420 East Superior Street Suite 9-900, Chicago, IL 60611, USA; [b] Department of Obstetrics and Gynecology, Loyola University Chicago, 2160 South First Avenue, Maywood, IL 60153, USA; [c] Department of Orthopedic Surgery and Rehabilitation, Loyola University Chicago, 2160 South First Avenue, Maywood, IL 60153, USA; [d] Department of Obstetrics and Gynecology, Loyola University Chicago, 2160 South First Avenue, Maywood, IL 60153, USA
* Corresponding author. Department of Orthopedic Surgery and Rehabilitation, Loyola University Chicago, 2160 South First Avenue, Maywood, IL 60153.
E-mail address: Stacey.Bennis001@luhs.org

Phys Med Rehabil Clin N Am 36 (2025) 329–342
https://doi.org/10.1016/j.pmr.2024.11.014
1047-9651/25/© 2024 Elsevier Inc. All rights are reserved, including those for text and data mining, AI training, and similar technologies.

NEUROMUSCULOSKELETAL PELVIC PAIN ETIOLOGIES AND MANAGEMENT

Although there are several etiologies of musculoskeletal pelvic pain, we will focus our discussion on common diagnoses, including presentation, evaluation, and management.

Pelvic Floor Myofascial Pain

Myofascial pelvic pain (MFPP), also known as pelvic floor myofascial pain and dysfunction, is defined by pain in the pelvic floor muscles (PFMs), connective tissue, and nearby fascia causing painful trigger points or taut bands in the PFMs.[1] MFPP may also be known under other terminology including levator ani syndrome or tension myalgia. MFPP often develops from overuse, weakness, repetitive strain, or dysfunctional posturing. MFPP can either be secondary to several abdominopelvic pain disorders or be its own syndrome. MFPP can contribute to symptoms of dyspareunia, dyschezia, constipation, and bladder pain. Prevalence of MFPP on vaginal physical examination was found to be about 13% in a recent study.[2] Another study demonstrated MFPP was the second most common cause of pelvic pain behind endometriosis.[3] A simple screen for myofascial pain by light palpation of the levator ani, obturator internus, bulbospongiosus, ischiocavernosus, and transverse perineal muscles was recently shown to have good reliability in screening for myofascial pain.[4]

History

As discussed in the prior article, "Pelvic Pain and Pelvic Floor Disorders in Women: A Physiatrist's Approach to Epidemiology and Examination", it is important to obtain obstetric and gynecologic history including labor complications, lacerations, instrumentation, and menstrual history. It is also important to take note of comorbid pain conditions or comorbid mood disorders. Key descriptors that may suggest MFPP include descriptors such as "deep" or "internal" pain worse with sitting or associated with dyspareunia, dyschezia, or dysuria.[1]

Examination

As described in the previous article, "Pelvic Pain and Pelvic Floor Disorders in Women: A Physiatrist's Approach to Epidemiology and Examination", a detailed musculoskeletal physical examination of the lumbar spine, hips, pelvic girdle, lower limbs, and PFMs should be performed. The characteristic examination findings of MFPP are found on the internal examination. Internally, the examiner will likely find referring trigger points, taut bands and tenderness, often in the levator ani or obturator internus, although these findings can be in any of the PFMs.[1] During the examination, patients may experience muscle spasms, referred pain to the lumbar spine, gluteal region or hips, or neuropathic pain.

Patients with MFPP may have pain with the active straight leg raise test, which is typically associated with pelvic girdle pain (PGP), because the test also causes a contraction of the PFMs. Additionally, patients may have weakness, poor ability to relax, or poor coordination. Findings of improper contraction or weakness may suggest a possible nerve injury, especially in patients with a history of childbirth or pelvic floor surgery.

Diagnostic testing

MFPP is a clinical diagnosis that can be made with adequate history taking and the examination findings of painful trigger points and taut bands as described earlier. However, PFM physical examination is subjective and may change among providers. A recent 2024 systematic review, demonstrated electromyography, ultrasonography, and manometry are the most common, objective measures of pelvic floor dysfunction and may provide objective data to aid in the diagnosis of MFPP.[5] Imaging, such as pelvic, hip, or lumbar radiographs, may be useful to help rule out other musculoskeletal causes of lumbopelvic pain. If there is concern for more serious causes of pelvic pain such as fracture, malignancy, lumbosacral disc herniation or infection, magnetic resonance imaging (MRI) of the spine, pelvis, or hip may be indicated.

Myofascial trigger points have been evaluated with ultrasound and magnetic resonance elasticity, by some groups, but none have been specifically studied in PFMs.[6–8] On ultrasound, myofascial trigger points appear as focal, hypoechoic regions with reduced vibration amplitude.[6] On MRI, the taut muscle bands have increased stiffness compared to normal tissue.[7,8] A recent systematic review highlights the lack of diagnostic tests currently available in myofascial pain assessment.[9]

Treatment

MFPP is treated conservatively through several different approaches with the goal being to return the pelvic floor musculature back to normal function and coordination through pelvic floor therapy, behavioral modifications, and bowel and bladder management. Pain management medications such as nonsteroidal anti-inflammatory drugs (NSAIDs), antidepressants, muscle relaxants, and neuromodulators can also be considered after obtaining adequate history, though there is little evidence to support their use. Given the knowledge that MFPP can occur both independently and secondary to other medical conditions, it is important to address multiple systems and tailor treatment to each patient.

Pelvic floor physical therapy (PFPT) is the mainstay treatment of most pelvic floor disorders, including MFPP.[10] A highly trained, specialized pelvic floor therapist will complete a history and examination including external and internal pelvic examination and rectal examination if indicated. PFPT may include neuromuscular re-education, PFM strengthening, soft tissue mobilization, relaxation techniques, biofeedback, behavioral modifications, education, bowel and bladder training, and creation of a home exercise program.[1,10] As the muscle groups release and stretch, pelvic floor strengthening techniques can be incorporated. Home exercise programs may include the use of a mirror so the patient may visualize the lifting and relaxation of the pelvic floor with contractions. Pelvic floor therapists may also recommend the use of vaginal dilators or pelvic wands. Typically, patients are advised to avoid activities such as Kegel exercises, prolonged sitting, or wearing tight clothing.[10]

Vaginal baclofen or diazepam suppositories can be prescribed for use before PFPT, prior to intercourse, or before sleep in an effort to reduce pelvic floor muscular tone and pain.[1] Vaginal diazepam has, in the past, shown to be effective in women with high-tone pelvic floor dysfunction,[11,12] but in more recent studies it has demonstrated no benefit in terms of vaginal muscle tone or pain.[13,14] Given there is systemic uptake of vaginal valium, there can be a sedating effect similar to oral dosing, as well as risk for tolerance and dependence.[14]

Myofascial trigger point injections with anesthetic agents or botulinum toxin can be considered if therapy and medication treatment does not provide adequate pain relief.[15,16] A recent 2021 systematic review evaluating 9 studies demonstrated significant improvement in pain scores among patients with chronic pelvic pain (CPP) at 6 and 12 weeks after botulin toxin injections.[17] It is important to note that injections should not be used alone, but rather as a part of rehabilitation plan to improve progress in therapy and overall function. An ultrasound-guided trigger point injection to the piriformis or obturator internus may also be considered if the patient has posterior pelvic myofascial pain.

Medications commonly used as first-line treatments for MFPP include acetaminophen and for acute pain, NSAIDs.[18] NSAIDs should not be taken long term due to the risk of bleeding as well as gastrointestinal, renal, and cardiovascular side effects. Opioids are not recommended in the treatment of CPP. Oral muscle relaxants can be effective when combined with therapies, though to date there is little supportive evidence. Neuromodulating medication such as gabapentin, pregabalin, antiepileptics, or serotonin norepinephrine reuptake inhibitors (SNRIs) may be useful particularly for patients with overlapping neurologic diagnoses such as radiculopathy, peripheral neuropathy, central sensitization, or fibromyalgia.[1] A recent randomized control trial showed no benefit of gabapentin compared to placebo in the treatment of women aged between 18 and 50 years with CPP.[19] Given the side effects and potential harm of these medications, it may be helpful to explore other treatment options prior to initiation of off-label neuromodulating medications such as gabapentin.

Vulvodynia

Vulvodynia refers to vulvar pain that has been present for at least 3 months without an identifiable cause. Recently, a consensus statement was released, which divides vulvar pain into 2 categories: vulvar pain secondary to another disorder (such as infection, malignancy, neurologic, inflammatory, hormonal, or iatrogenic causes) and vulvodynia.[20] Vulvodynia is a causative diagnosis in chronic pelvic pain, estimated to affect between 8% and 15% of women; this prevalence is stable throughout reproductive years and begins to decline gradually in women aged over 70 years.[21,22] The etiology of vulvodynia is not well understood. Several factors associated with vulvodynia include genetics, hormonal factors, inflammation, musculoskeletal issues, structural defects, neuroproliferation, comorbid pain syndromes, and psychosocial factors.[20] Additionally, vulvodynia often overlaps with or may be secondary to other diagnoses such as MFPP or pudendal neuralgia.

History

It is critical to understand the patient's description of pain to adequately characterize vulvodynia. Vulvodynia can be provoked or unprovoked, referring to pain exacerbated by contact or pain that is spontaneous. Provoked vulvodynia is initiated or provoked by contact, such as inserting a tampon or sexual activity. Unprovoked vulvodynia is spontaneous pain and is present regardless of contact. This distinction is important as it can help guide treatment.[23] Vulvodynia is also characterized by location, for example, if pain is localized to one part of the vulva such as the vestibule versus generalized or mixed. Onset and temporal pattern can also help further describe vulvodynia.[20,24]

Examination

Although not always positive, the characteristic physical examination finding in vulvodynia is the Q-tip test.[25] The test involves applying mild pressure with a cotton swab to various areas of the vulva and asking the patient to rate their pain levels on a Likert scale of 0 to 10. The tested positions typically move laterally to medially and include the labia majora and minora and vulvar vestibule. During the Q-tip test, the examiner may also visually inspect the vulva, which is typically normal in patients with vulvodynia.

Patients with vulvodynia often have accompanying sexual and pelvic floor dysfunction. Specifically, it is common to see high tone in the PFMs, weakness with voluntary and involuntary contractions, and muscle tenderness on examination.[25] In 2015, the Evidence-Based Vulvodynia Assessment Project demonstrated that 90% of women with vulvodynia had muscular abnormalities in the pelvic floor.[24] Therefore, it is important to do a complete external and internal pelvic floor examination in patients presenting with vulvodynia.

Treatment

PFPT is recommended as the first-line treatment of vulvodynia[26,27] in conjunction with multidisciplinary approaches including psychotherapy, sex therapy, and pharmacotherapy.[28] Physical therapy modalities often used include manual techniques, desensitization, PFMs exercises, stretching, and insertional techniques using dilators or pelvic wands.[29,30] A recent large, randomized control trial demonstrated that physical therapy is effective and superior in reducing vulvodynia symptoms when compared to overnight topical lidocaine.[31]

Although there is currently a lack of literature to support pharmacotherapy, in practice, often oral or topical neuromodulators are used in the treatment of vulvodynia. Oral neuromodulators such as gabapentin or pregabalin are often used in the management of unprovoked or generalized vulvodynia while topical compound creams are used for provoked vulvodynia.[23] In women with vulvovaginal atrophy, commonly seen in postmenopausal women, topical estrogen therapy should be the first-line therapy.[28] In some cases, symptoms may be refractory to multidisciplinary management, and it may be beneficial to consider the use of baclofen suppositories or botulinum toxin injections, which may help relax the PFMs and relieve pain. Often, patients with vulvodynia have associated high tone and shortening of the PFMs that may inhibit progress in PFPT, and the clinician may consider pharmacotherapy to aid in relaxation of the PFMs. Although botulinum toxin remains off label for use in the pelvic floor, a recent 2019 study demonstrated localized botulinum toxin injections were helpful in reducing dyspareunia and improving quality of life in treatment refractory, localized, provoked vulvodynia.[32] Therefore, injections may be considered for specific, refractory cases of vulvodynia.

Nerve Injuries

Nerve injuries can contribute to pelvic pain and dysfunction. The iliohypogastric, ilioinguinal, genitofemoral, and pudendal nerves provide innervation to the PFMs and overlying skin and, therefore, can cause pelvic floor dysfunction if injured. Specifically, pudendal nerve damage can lead to urinary and fecal incontinence as well as sexual dysfunction due to its motor innervation of many of the PFMs. Nerves of the pelvis can be damaged in pelvic surgeries, inguinal hernia repair, or trauma.[33,34] More superficial nerves that provide sensation to the perineum can be damaged if a Pfannenstiel or low transverse incision is dissected beyond the edge of the rectus abdominus muscles.[35] The genitofemoral nerve can be damaged by compression from self-retaining retractors during gynecologic or pelvic surgeries.[35]

Pudendal neuralgia refers to damage of the pudendal nerve itself. The incidence of pudendal neuralgia ranges from 1% to 4%.[34] The pudendal nerve can be injured in vaginal delivery, which may contribute to postpartum urinary and fecal incontinence.[36] Bicycle riding, repetitive squatting, and chronic straining during defecation can also lead to pudendal neuralgia.[34]

History

Obtaining a thorough history, paying close attention to pain descriptions and location of pain can be most helpful in making a diagnosis, especially because motor, sensory, and reflex examination may often be normal.[34] Pain described as burning or numbness should raise suspicion for neuropathic pain. Patients may describe a foreign body sensation in the perineum or rectum. Patients with neuropathic pain may also have associated pelvic floor dysfunction, and it can be difficult to determine whether the muscle or nerve is the primary source of the pain as hypertonic PFMs may be the cause or the consequence of a pudendal neuroalgia.[34]

Examination

Neuropathic pelvic pain can be difficult to assess on physical examination due to overlapping borders of the pelvic nerves. The Nantes criteria are a validated set of clinical conditions that are sensitive, but not specific for pudendal neuralgia.[37] The criteria involve pain in the anatomic territory of the pudendal nerve, worse with sitting, not awakened from sleep by pain, no sensory loss on examination, and positive anesthetic nerve block.[37] The criteria may be helpful in characterizing pain; however, several components of the criteria are often present with overactive pelvic floor dysfunction and, therefore, are not specific for pudendal neuralgia.[38]

Diagnostic testing

To confirm a diagnosis of neuropathic pelvic pain, diagnostic nerve blocks are performed. Nerve blocks are considered reliable for the iliohypogastric, ilioinguinal, and genitofemoral nerves, but are less clear for the pudendal nerve.[39] It has been proposed that patients with primary pelvic floor dysfunction may also respond well to a pudendal nerve block because the pudendal nerve innervates the sphincters and PFMs. Therefore, the block may not be helpful in determining if the pudendal nerve is the primary source of pain, despite possible improvements in symptoms following the block.[37,40] Magnetic resonance (MR) neurography technology has recently began to be recognized as one of the most effective tools for diagnosing nerve injury as it is thought to be superior to MRI for nerve visualization.[41] The lumbosacral plexus, specifically, is demonstrated well on MR neurography and can be useful in visualizing injury to the iliohypogastric, ilioinguinal, genitofemoral, and pudendal nerves.[42]

Treatment

PFPT, often in conjunction with medications, is the first-line treatment of neuropathic pelvic pain. Neuromodulating medications typically used include gabapentin, pregabalin, SNRIs, or tricyclic antidepressants (TCAs). These medications may also be compounded into creams or vaginal/rectal suppositories[23]; data are minimal to support their effectiveness. Image-guided corticosteroid injections mixed with local anesthetic have also been reported as helpful for neuropathies of the pelvic floor.[34,39,40] In some severe cases, surgery, typically a neurectomy or nerve resection, may be recommended for the iliohypogastric, ilioinguinal, and genitofemoral nerves. For severe groin pain, a triple neurectomy where all 3 nerves are resected or transected may be performed.[43,44] Pain relief after neurectomy of the iliohypogastric, ilioinguinal, and genitofemoral nerves has been reported in 66% to 100% of patients.[43,44] However, surgical outcomes for pudendal neuralgia have not been consistent.[45,46]

Pelvic Girdle Pain

Pelvic girdle pain (PGP) refers to musculoskeletal pain between the posterior iliac crest and the gluteal fold.[47] The etiology is multifactorial but can be from instability, biomechanical dysfunction, abnormal motor control, or ligamental laxity in the pelvic joints. Persistent malalignment and instability of the sacroiliac joint (SIJ) may lead to spams and tension in the PFMs, which can further contribute to pelvic pain. PGP can be characterized by the location of painful joints. The most common pain pattern is double-sided SIJ, followed by double-sided SIJ and pubic symphysis pain, then single-sided SIJ pain followed by isolated pubic symphysis pain.[48]

Although, PGP can occur in patients of any age, it is particularly important to discuss in the context of pregnancy as the prevalence in this population has been noted to be 20% to 65%.[47–50] PGP is also reported to be the second most common reason for sick leave among pregnant women.[51] Onset of pain typically occurs between 18 and 36 weeks' gestation.[52]

History

Patients often experience pain in the SIJ or pubic symphysis described as pain in their low back, buttock, or hip. Pain often worsens with transitional movements and impact ability to stand, sit, and walk. Patients may describe a feeling of giveaway weakness on the effected side, pain in the groin with legs crossed, or pain with increases in speed when walking or stair climbing.[53] Patients may describe difficulty finding comfortable positions to sleep or pain when rolling in bed. Pain may radiate down the posterior thigh, sometimes with associated numbness and tingling, and therefore, etiologies such as lumbosacral plexopathy, herniated disc, and radiculopathy should be ruled out before a diagnosis of PGP is given. Other etiologies that should be included in the differential diagnosis include inflammatory disorders, hip disorders, collagen abnormalities, infections, sacral fractures, and tumors.

Examination

The examination should include evaluation of gait, posture, strength, sensation, and reflexes. Evaluation of the lumbar spine and hips should also be performed. Pain provocation tests for PGP include Patrick's/FABER, posterior pelvic pain provocation test (P4), Gaenslen's test, Modified Trendelenburg, and assisted straight leg raise test (for detail, see the previous article, "Pelvic Pain and Pelvic Floor Disorders in Women: A Physiatrist's Approach to Epidemiology and Examination"). Examination maneuvers specific to PGP include a positive Patrick's/FABER, active straight leg raise, and P4. FABER and P4 are the most sensitive tests for pregnancy-related PGP.[47] Pain originating from the pubic symphysis should be suspected when there is tenderness to palpation of the pubic symphysis that lasts more than 5 seconds after the examiner removes their finger. Modified Trendelenburg may also be present with pubic symphysis pain.[53]

Treatment

First-line treatment of PGP is physical therapy, which may focus on posture, stabilizing exercises, motor control, and strengthening. Strengthening of the entire spine is recommended in addition to pelvic stabilization due to conflicting evidence with the use of pelvic stabilization techniques alone.[54] Pelvic stabilizing belts may also be used to provide passive force closure of the pelvis and relieve pain. A recent study demonstrated significant pain reduction and function improvement with the use of stabilizing belts in pregnancy-related PGP.[55] There is also evidence to support the use of stabilizing belts in non–pregnancy-related PGP.[54,56–58] The addition of PFPT may be helpful if patients have PFM pain or dysfunction on physical examination.

Medications such as NSAIDs or acetaminophen can be taken for pain relief. However, NSAIDs should be avoided in the pregnant population. Recent studies have found benefit in osteopathic manipulations and acupuncture in this population, when other medications or injections may be less desirable.[59,60] Other medications that may be used in the pregnant or nonpregnant population include topical lidocaine patches, antispasmodic, or muscle relaxant medication (pregnancy category B). Oral steroids can also be considered. Steroid injections into the SIJ or pubic symphysis can be helpful for severe pain refractory to conservative management. Steroid injections should only be considered in the pregnant population on a case-by-case basis as steroids are pregnancy category C medications.[23]

Coccydynia

Coccydynia refers to pain in the coccyx region, the terminal segment of the spine. The coccyx is a triangular bone with 3 to 5 fused segments. It is anteriorly bordered by the levator ani muscles and the sacrococcygeal ligament. The coccyx serves as the insertion site for the coccygeal and gluteus maximus muscles, the sacrotuberous and sacrospinous ligaments on the lateral edges and the iliococcygeus muscle tendon on the inferior edge.[61] The coccyx is, therefore, a key structure for function of the PFMs.

Coccydynia commonly occurs due to direct trauma to the coccyx such as a fall on the buttock or trauma from cycling or parturition.[62] The exact prevalence in the general population is not well documented; however, it has been estimated that about 7% of women have postpartum coccydynia, with even higher reports up to 50% in women who required instrumentation during delivery.[63] Other studies have estimated postpartum coccydynia with instrumentation to be lower at 12% to 17%.[64] Nontraumatic coccydynia etiologies, which should be ruled out, include infection, degenerative joint or disc disease, masses or tumors, hypermobility or hypomobility, and variant coccygeal morphology.[61]

History

Patients with coccydynia typically report worsened pain when sitting or standing up from a seated position. They may report frequent urge to defecate or pain with defecation. They may also have pain with intercourse. History should be taken with note of recent trauma and onset of pain.

Examination

Examination will reveal tenderness to palpation over the coccyx. Rectal examination will allow the examiner to palpate the coccyx internally. The coccyx is grasped between the forefinger and thumb to allow for manipulation and evaluation of pain and hypermobility or hypomobility of the sacrococcygeal joint. Normal range of motion is 13°.[65] The muscles of the pelvic floor may also be tender on palpation with the internal or external examination as the PFMs often tighten and shorten in response to coccyx pain, which can further contribute to pelvic pain.

Diagnostic testing

Coccydynia itself can be diagnosed through history and physical examination. However, radiographic images can help further evaluate for anterior angulation, subluxation/dislocation, fractures, degenerative changes, or masses that may be causing or contributing to coccyx pain. Dynamic radiographs, taken when standing and sitting, and MRI can help evaluate for sacrococcygeal joint mobility.

Treatment

Conservative treatment is successful in 90% of cases, and many cases resolve without any medical management.[66,67] Early participation in physical therapy can be helpful as reports have shown benefit of physical therapy over placebo, with further benefit demonstrated when therapy was started within 1 year of onset of symptoms.[68] Activity modification such as adopting proper sitting posture and using circular-shaped or wedge-shaped pillows can help relieve pressure on the coccyx. Often NSAIDs may be recommended, especially in acute injury, but opioids should be avoided.

Patients who are not improving with conservative measures may be evaluated for fluoroscopy-guided injections around the coccyx, sacrococcygeal joint, or sacrococcygeal ligaments. Studies have shown that injection alone has a 60% success rate, while the combination of injection with coccygeal manipulation, as done in physical therapy, has an 85% success rate over a 3 month period.[69] Epidural steroid injections have been used to treat coccyx pain secondary to Tarlov cysts causing lower radicular pain.[70] Ganglion impar blocks can also be performed in treatment refractory cases. Surgical treatment involving coccygectomy is not recommended as the procedure has high major complication rates.[71,72] Additionally, coccygectomy can negatively impact the PFMs as several muscles insert onto the coccyx.

MULTIDISCIPLINARY CARE FOR CHRONIC PELVIC PAIN

A common theme throughout this chapter is the complexity of pelvic pain, often involving overlapping diagnoses within several organ systems. It is critical for management to be coordinated succinctly for optimal patient care.[73,74] Patients often see multiple specialties and receive numerous diagnoses that put patients at risk for overmedication or inadequate treatment. Due to possible fatigue and frustration, patients are also at risk for missing routine preventative screenings or being overlooked if new, red flag pain features develop in the setting of chronic pain.

Physiatrists are uniquely equipped to lead a large multidisciplinary team as is required for treating pelvic pain given the specialty's knowledge of management of chronic pain, bowel, and bladder symptoms and complex neuromusculoskeletal processes. Additionally, physiatrists can help steer the focus of management to restoring function and improving quality of life, which is often the goal of many patients with chronic pelvic pain.

SUMMARY

Pelvic pain encompasses a spectrum of conditions stemming from various sources, making diagnosis and management complex across multiple medical disciplines. Many neuromusculoskeletal causes of pelvic pain, including pelvic floor myofascial pain, vulvodynia, nerve injuries, pelvic girdle pain, and coccydynia, can be effectively evaluated through comprehensive history taking and skillful physical examination. PFPT stands as primary treatment of many musculoskeletal pelvic pain conditions. Depending on examination findings, specific diagnoses, and response to therapy, additional medical interventions may include neuromodulation via oral or topical medications, vaginal muscle relaxants, or injections of botulinum toxin or trigger points in the PFMs. A multidisciplinary approach is crucial for comprehensive care, integrating expertise from physiatry, gynecology, urology, gastroenterology, pain management, and physical and occupational therapy to address the multifaceted nature of pelvic pain effectively.

CLINICS CARE POINTS

- PGP (ie, musculoskeletal pain) is common in women presenting with pelvic pain.

- Pelvic floor myofascial pain is a component of PGP.

- Examination techniques specific to the SIJ and pubic symphysis are critical in evaluating musculoskeletal causes of pelvic pain.

- Examination maneuvers include Patrick's/FABER, active straight leg raise, P4, SIJ distraction, Gaenslen's maneuver, compression test, sacral thrust, and drop test.

- Workup may include plain radiographs and MRI of the low back, hips, and pelvis to evaluate a broad differential.

- Treatment is multifactorial with the mainstay of treatment being pelvic floor focused physical therapy.

- Additional diagnosis-specific management may include oral or topical analgesia or neuromodulation, pelvic floor trigger point or botulinum toxin injections.

- Utilizing the multidisciplinary team approach is key for holistic care of women with chronic pelvic pain.

DISCLOSURE

Dr S. Bennis is funded by NICHD and serves on the IPPS Advisory Board Member. Dr C. Fitzgerald serves as an UptoDate Editor and is funded by NIDDK, United States, NICHD, IPPS advisory board, speaker for UCSF, Kaiser, and the ShirleyRyan Ability Lab.

REFERENCES

1. Bonder JH, Chi M, Rispoli L. Myofascial pelvic pain and related disorders. Phys Med Rehabil Clin 2017;28(3):501–15.
2. Bedaiwy MA, Patterson B, Mahajan S. Prevalence of myofascial chronic pelvic pain and the effectiveness of pelvic floor physical therapy. J Reprod Med 2013;58(11–12):504–10.
3. Montenegro ML, Mateus-Vasconcelos EC, Rosa e Silva JC, et al. Importance of pelvic muscle tenderness evaluation in women with chronic pelvic pain. Pain Med 2010;11(2):224–8 [published Online First: 20091209].
4. Bhide AA, Puccini F, Bray R, et al. The pelvic floor muscle hyperalgesia (PFMH) scoring system: a new classification tool to assess women with chronic pelvic pain: multicentre pilot study of validity and reliability. Eur J Obstet Gynecol Reprod Biol 2015;193:111–3 [published Online First: 20150731].
5. Michalik D, Herman U, Stangel-Wojcikiewicz K. Quantitative tools to assess pelvic floor muscle function - systematic review. Ginekol Pol 2024. https://doi.org/10.5603/gpl.90873 [published Online First: 20240320].
6. Sikdar S, Shah JP, Gebreab T, et al. Novel applications of ultrasound technology to visualize and characterize myofascial trigger points and surrounding soft tissue. Arch Phys Med Rehabil 2009;90(11):1829–38.
7. Chen Q, Basford J, An KN. Ability of magnetic resonance elastography to assess taut bands. Clin Biomech 2008;23(5):623–9 [published Online First: 20080221].
8. Chen Q, Wang HJ, Gay RE, et al. Quantification of myofascial taut bands. Arch Phys Med Rehabil 2016;97(1):67–73 [published Online First: 20151014].
9. Kapurubandara SC, Lowes B, Sansom-Daly UM, et al. A systematic review of diagnostic tests to detect pelvic floor myofascial pain. Int Urogynecol J 2022; 33(9):2379–89 [published Online First: 20220707].
10. FitzGerald MP, Kotarinos R. Rehabilitation of the short pelvic floor. II: treatment of the patient with the short pelvic floor. Int UrogynEcol J Pelvic Floor Dysfunct 2003; 14(4):269–75 [discussion 75].
11. Rogalski MJ, Kellogg-Spadt S, Hoffmann AR, et al. Retrospective chart review of vaginal diazepam suppository use in high-tone pelvic floor dysfunction. Int Urogynecol J 2010;21(7):895–9 [published Online First: 20100112].
12. Holland MA, Joyce JS, Brennaman LM, et al. Sr. Intravaginal diazepam for the treatment of pelvic floor hypertonic disorder: a double-blind, randomized, placebo-controlled trial. Female Pelvic Med Reconstr Surg 2019;25(1):76–81.
13. Crisp CC, Vaccaro CM, Estanol MV, et al. Intra-vaginal diazepam for high-tone pelvic floor dysfunction: a randomized placebo-controlled trial. Int Urogynecol J 2013;24(11):1915–23 [published Online First: 20130517].
14. Carrico DJ, Peters KM. Vaginal diazepam use with urogenital pain/pelvic floor dysfunction: serum diazepam levels and efficacy data. Urol Nurs 2011;31(5): 279–84, 99.
15. Till SR, Wahl HN, As-Sanie S. The role of nonpharmacologic therapies in management of chronic pelvic pain: what to do when surgery fails. Curr Opin Obstet Gynecol 2017;29(4):231–9.

16. Moldwin RM, Fariello JY. Myofascial trigger points of the pelvic floor: associations with urological pain syndromes and treatment strategies including injection therapy. Curr Urol Rep 2013;14(5):409–17.

17. Meister MR, Brubaker A, Sutcliffe S, et al. Effectiveness of botulinum toxin for treatment of symptomatic pelvic floor myofascial pain in women: a systematic review and meta-analysis. Female Pelvic Med Reconstr Surg 2021;27(1):e152–60.

18. Srinivasan AK, Kaye JD, Moldwin R. Myofascial dysfunction associated with chronic pelvic floor pain: management strategies. Curr Pain Headache Rep 2007;11(5):359–64.

19. Horne AW, Vincent K, Hewitt CA, et al. Gabapentin for chronic pelvic pain in women (GaPP2): a multicentre, randomised, double-blind, placebo-controlled trial. Lancet 2020;396(10255):909–17.

20. Bornstein J, Goldstein AT, Stockdale CK, et al. 2015 ISSVD, ISSWSH and IPPS consensus terminology and classification of persistent vulvar pain and vulvodynia. Obstet Gynecol 2016;127(4):745–51.

21. Harlow BL, Stewart EG. A population-based assessment of chronic unexplained vulvar pain: have we underestimated the prevalence of vulvodynia? J Am Med Women's Assoc (1972) 2003;58(2):82–8.

22. Arnold LD, Bachmann GA, Rosen R, et al. Assessment of vulvodynia symptoms in a sample of US women: a prevalence survey with a nested case control study. Am J Obstet Gynecol 2007;196(2):128.e1–6.

23. Hwang S, Bennis S, Scott KM, et al. Pelvic floor disorders. In: Cifu DX, Eapen BC, editors. Braddom's physical medicine and rehabilitation. 6th edition. Philadelphia: Saunders/Elsevier; 2021.

24. Lamvu G, Nguyen RH, Burrows LJ, et al. The evidence-based vulvodynia assessment project. a national registry for the study of vulvodynia. J Reprod Med 2015; 60(5–6):223–35.

25. Edwards L. Vulvodynia. Clin Obstet Gynecol 2015;58(1):143–52.

26. Goldstein AT, Pukall CF, Brown C, et al. Vulvodynia: assessment and treatment. J Sex Med 2016;13(4):572–90 [published Online First: 20160325].

27. Nunns D, Mandal D, Byrne M, et al. Guidelines for the management of vulvodynia. Br J Dermatol 2010;162(6):1180–5 [published Online First: 20100316].

28. Stenson AL. Vulvodynia: diagnosis and management. Obstet Gynecol Clin N Am 2017;44(3):493–508.

29. Hartmann D, Strauhal MJ, Nelson CA. Treatment of women in the United States with localized, provoked vulvodynia: practice survey of women's health physical therapists. J Reprod Med 2007;52(1):48–52.

30. Morin M, Carroll MS, Bergeron S. Systematic review of the effectiveness of physical therapy modalities in women with provoked vestibulodynia. Sex Med Rev 2017;5(3):295–322 [published Online First: 20170328].

31. Morin M, Dumoulin C, Bergeron S, et al. Multimodal physical therapy versus topical lidocaine for provoked vestibulodynia: a multicenter, randomized trial. Am J Obstet Gynecol 2021;224(2). 189.e1-89.e12.

32. Hedebo Hansen T, Guldberg R, Meinert M. Botulinum toxin-treatment of localized provoked vulvodynia refractory to conventional treatment. Eur J Obstet Gynecol Reprod Biol 2019;234:6–9 [published Online First: 20181215].

33. Hakeem A, Shanmugam V. Inguinodynia following Lichtenstein tension-free hernia repair: a review. World J Gastroenterol 2011;17(14):1791–6.

34. Hibner M, Desai N, Robertson LJ, et al. Pudendal neuralgia. J Minim Invasive Gynecol 2010;17(2):148–53 [published Online First: 20100112].

35. Bradshaw AD, Advincula AP. Postoperative neuropathy in gynecologic surgery. Obstet Gynecol Clin N Am 2010;37(3):451–9.
36. Connolly AM, Thorp JM Jr. Childbirth-related perineal trauma: clinical significance and prevention. Clin Obstet Gynecol 1999;42(4):820–35.
37. Labat JJ, Riant T, Robert R, et al. Diagnostic criteria for pudendal neuralgia by pudendal nerve entrapment (Nantes criteria). Neurourol Urodyn 2008;27(4): 306–10.
38. Elkins N, Hunt J, Scott KM. Neurogenic pelvic pain. Phys Med Rehabil Clin 2017; 28(3):551–69 [published Online First: 20170512].
39. Starling JR, Harms BA. Diagnosis and treatment of genitofemoral and ilioinguinal neuralgia. World J Surg 1989;13(5):586–91.
40. Vancaillie T, Eggermont J, Armstrong G, et al. Response to pudendal nerve block in women with pudendal neuralgia. Pain Med 2012;13(4):596–603 [published Online First: 20120305].
41. Petchprapa CN, Rosenberg ZS, Sconfienza LM, et al. MR imaging of entrapment neuropathies of the lower extremity. Part 1. The pelvis and hip. Radiographics 2010;30(4):983–1000.
42. Soldatos T, Andreisek G, Thawait GK, et al. High-resolution 3-T MR neurography of the lumbosacral plexus. Radiographics 2013;33(4):967–87.
43. Chen DC, Hiatt JR, Amid PK. Operative management of refractory neuropathic inguinodynia by a laparoscopic retroperitoneal approach. JAMA Surg 2013; 148(10):962–7.
44. Loos MJ, Scheltinga MR, Roumen RM. Surgical management of inguinal neuralgia after a low transverse Pfannenstiel incision. Ann Surg 2008;248(5):880–5.
45. Mauillon J, Thoumas D, Leroi AM, et al. Results of pudendal nerve neurolysis-transposition in twelve patients suffering from pudendal neuralgia. Dis Colon Rectum 1999;42(2):186–92.
46. Robert R, Labat JJ, Bensignor M, et al. Decompression and transposition of the pudendal nerve in pudendal neuralgia: a randomized controlled trial and long-term evaluation. Eur Urol 2005;47(3):403–8.
47. Vleeming A, Albert HB, Ostgaard HC, et al. European guidelines for the diagnosis and treatment of pelvic girdle pain. Eur Spine J 2008;17(6):794–819 [published Online First: 20080208].
48. Albert HB, Godskesen M, Westergaard JG. Incidence of four syndromes of pregnancy-related pelvic joint pain. Spine 2002;27(24):2831–4.
49. Larsen EC, Wilken-Jensen C, Hansen A, et al. Symptom-giving pelvic girdle relaxation in pregnancy. I: prevalence and risk factors. Acta Obstet Gynecol Scand 1999;78(2):105–10.
50. FitzGerald MP, Kotarinos R. Rehabilitation of the short pelvic floor. I: background and patient evaluation. Int UrogynEcol J Pelvic Floor Dysfunct 2003;14(4):261–8 [published Online First: 20030802].
51. Dørheim SK, Bjorvatn B, Eberhard-Gran M. Sick leave during pregnancy: a longitudinal study of rates and risk factors in a Norwegian population. Bjog 2013; 120(5):521–30 [published Online First: 20121107].
52. Ostgaard HC, Andersson GB, Karlsson K. Prevalence of back pain in pregnancy. Spine 1991;16(5):549–52.
53. Bonder JH, Fitzpatrick L. Diagnosis of pelvic girdle pain. In: Fitzgerald CM, Segal NA, editors. Musculoskeletal health in pregnancy and postpartum : an evidence-based guide for clinicians. 1st 2015. Cham: Springer International Publishing; 2015.

54. Elden H, Hagberg H, Olsen MF, et al. Regression of pelvic girdle pain after delivery: follow-up of a randomised single blind controlled trial with different treatment modalities. Acta Obstet Gynecol Scand 2008;87(2):201–8.

55. Fitzgerald CM, Bennis S, Marcotte ML, et al. The impact of a sacroiliac joint belt on function and pain using the active straight leg raise in pregnancy-related pelvic girdle pain. Pm r 2022;14(1):19–29 [published Online First: 20210520].

56. Elden H, Ostgaard HC, Fagevik-Olsen M, et al. Treatments of pelvic girdle pain in pregnant women: adverse effects of standard treatment, acupuncture and stabilising exercises on the pregnancy, mother, delivery and the fetus/neonate. BMC Compl Alternative Med 2008;8:34 [published Online First: 20080626].

57. Pool-Goudzwaard AL, Slieker ten Hove MC, Vierhout ME, et al. Relations between pregnancy-related low back pain, pelvic floor activity and pelvic floor dysfunction. Int UrogynEcol J Pelvic Floor Dysfunct 2005;16(6):468–74 [published Online First: 20050401].

58. Verstraete EH, Vanderstraeten G, Parewijck W. Pelvic girdle pain during or after pregnancy: a review of recent evidence and a clinical care path proposal. Facts Views Vis Obgyn 2013;5(1):33–43.

59. Franke H, Franke JD, Belz S, et al. Osteopathic manipulative treatment for low back and pelvic girdle pain during and after pregnancy: a systematic review and meta-analysis. J Bodyw Mov Ther 2017;21(4):752–62 [published Online First: 20170531].

60. Foster NE, Bishop A, Bartlam B, et al. Evaluating acupuncture and standard carE for pregnant women with Back pain (EASE Back): a feasibility study and pilot randomised trial. Health Technol Assess 2016;20(33):1–236.

61. Lirette LS, Chaiban G, Tolba R, et al. Coccydynia: an overview of the anatomy, etiology, and treatment of coccyx pain. Ochsner J 2014;14(1):84–7.

62. Patijn J, Janssen M, Hayek S, et al. 14. Coccygodynia. Pain Pract 2010;10(6):554–9 [published Online First: 20100906].

63. Maigne JY, Rusakiewicz F, Diouf M. Postpartum coccydynia: a case series study of 57 women. Eur J Phys Rehabil Med 2012;48(3):387–92 [published Online First: 20120723].

64. Revicky V, Mukhopadhyay S, Morris EP, et al. Induction of labour and the mode of delivery at term. J Obstet Gynaecol 2011;31(4):304–6.

65. Maigne JY, Doursounian L, Chatellier G. Causes and mechanisms of common coccydynia: role of body mass index and coccygeal trauma. Spine 2000;25(23):3072–9.

66. Trollegaard AM, Aarby NS, Hellberg S. Coccygectomy: an effective treatment option for chronic coccydynia: retrospective results in 41 consecutive patients. J Bone Joint Surg Br 2010;92(2):242–5.

67. Capar B, Akpinar N, Kutluay E, et al. [Coccygectomy in patients with coccydynia]. Acta Orthop Traumatol Turcica 2007;41(4):277–80.

68. Maigne JY, Chatellier G, Faou ML, et al. The treatment of chronic coccydynia with intrarectal manipulation: a randomized controlled study. Spine 2006;31(18):E621–7.

69. Wray CC, Easom S, Hoskinson J. Coccydynia. Aetiology and treatment. J Bone Joint Surg Br 1991;73(2):335–8.

70. Foye PM, Buttaci CJ, Stitik TP, et al. Successful injection for coccyx pain. Am J Phys Med Rehabil 2006;85(9):783–4.

71. De Andrés J, Chaves S. Coccygodynia: a proposal for an algorithm for treatment. J Pain 2003;4(5):257–66.

72. Khan SA, Kumar A, Varshney MK, et al. Dextrose prolotherapy for recalcitrant coccygodynia. J Orthop Surg 2008;16(1):27–9.
73. Hwang SK. Advances in the treatment of chronic pelvic pain: a multidisciplinary approach to treatment. Mo Med 2017;114(1):47–51.
74. Miller-Matero LR, Saulino C, Clark S, et al. When treating the pain is not enough: a multidisciplinary approach for chronic pelvic pain. Arch Womens Ment Health 2016;19(2):349–54 [published Online First: 20150505].

Rheumatologic Issues in Women and Rehabilitation

Seema Malkana, DO[a], Jaclyn Joki, MD[b,c,d,*], Vivien Hsu, MD[e]

KEYWORDS

- Rheumatologic conditions • Rheumatoid arthritis • Lupus • Sjogren's syndrome
- Inflammatory myopathy • Systemic sclerosis • Women

KEY POINTS

- Rheumatologic conditions frequently affect women more commonly than men, including most connective tissue diseases such as rheumatoid arthritis and lupus.
- Rheumatoid arthritis presents with symmetric joint inflammation leading to joint damage and deformities if not treated early. Ankle and foot involvement is commonly overlooked.
- Systemic lupus erythematosus primarily affects young women and can involve various organ systems, leading to significant morbidity and mortality.
- Inflammatory myopathies are more common in women and can present with progressive proximal muscle weakness and extramuscular manifestations, requiring immunosuppressive therapy and rehabilitation.
- Systemic sclerosis predominantly affects women and can lead to skin and visceral organ fibrosis, with significant impacts on quality of life and survival.

INTRODUCTION

Rheumatologic conditions affect the joints, muscles, and connective tissues, frequently impairing musculoskeletal function and impacting functional mobility and activities of daily living (ADLs). Beyond the local effects causing muscle weakness, joint pain, stiffness, swelling, and instability, many of these conditions may have more systemic involvement with negative effects on the central nervous system and cardiopulmonary system, which increases risk for further reduced overall function and quality of life.

[a] Division of Rheumatology, Department of Medicine, Rutgers Robert Wood Johnson Medical School, 125 Paterson Street, MEB 496, New Brunswick, NJ 08873, USA; [b] Department of Physical Medicine and Rehabilitation, Hackensack Meridian School of Medicine; [c] Department of Physical Medicine and Rehabilitation, Rutgers Robert Wood Johnson Medical School; [d] Director, PM&R Consult Service at RWJUH, HMH JFK Johnson Rehabilitation Institute, 65 James Street, Edison, NJ 08820, USA; [e] Director, Rutgers-Robert Wood Johnson Scleroderma Program, Division of Rheumatology, Department of Medicine, Rutgers Robert Wood Johnson Medical School, 125 Paterson Street, MEB 458, New Brunswick, NJ 08903, USA
* Corresponding author.
E-mail address: Jaclyn.joki@hmhn.org

Phys Med Rehabil Clin N Am 36 (2025) 343–360
https://doi.org/10.1016/j.pmr.2024.11.010
1047-9651/25/© 2024 Elsevier Inc. All rights reserved, including those for text and data mining, AI training, and similar technologies.

Abbreviations	
ADLs	activities of daily living
ANA	antinuclear antibody
CTDs	connective tissue disorders
DM	dermatomyositis
DMARDs	disease-modifying antirheumatic drugs
EMG	electromyography
HRQoL	health-related quality of life
IgG	immunoglobulin G
IL	interleukin
ILD	interstitial lung disease
JIA	juvenile idiopathic arthritis
lcSSc	limited cutaneous systemic sclerosis
MCP	metacarpophalangeal
OA	osteoarthritis
OT	occupational therapy
PIP	proximal interphalangeal
PM	polymyositis
PMR	polymyalgia rheumatica
PR	pulmonary rehabilitation
pSS	primary Sjogren's syndrome
PT	physical therapy
RA	rheumatoid arthritis
RF	rheumatoid factor
ROM	range of motion
SLE	systemic lupus erythematosus
SSc	systemic sclerosis

These conditions can affect individuals of any gender; however, certain conditions tend to be more prevalent in female individuals or present differently in women. Appropriate diagnosis and treatment plans in conjunction with effective rehabilitation management with an emphasis on understanding the unique challenges faced by women with rheumatologic conditions are important to promote optimal health.

BACKGROUND

Rheumatic disorders, including rheumatoid arthritis (RA) and other connective tissue disorders (CTDs), affect women more commonly than men.[1] Younger women are at 3 times higher risk of developing more severe and deforming RA than men.[2] Up to 80% of patients who develop CTDs such as scleroderma are women in their prime adult years and beyond.[3] Another similar CTD is dermatomyositis (DM), where the prevalence is twice as high in women of childbearing age.[4] Patients with these disorders have higher risk of developing lung disease, including interstitial lung disease (ILD).[5,6]

Many patients with rheumatism have systemic inflammation, as well as other clinical features including fatigue, stiffness, muscle weakness, joint changes causing pain, instability, loss of range of motion (ROM) leading to contracture development, and emotional issues that may negatively influence their general wellness and cause disability. These patients benefit from early intervention and management, including rehabilitation and exercise. These have demonstrated improved muscle and joint function, bone strength, aerobic and cardiopulmonary function, and improved health-related quality of life (HRQoL) measures, all of which improve self-esteem.[7] There is evidence to support the beneficial effects of exercise through myogenic and vascular mechanisms on sleep, pain, fatigue, and bowel flora.[8,9]

DISCUSSION

We will review rheumatologic conditions that have a greater incidence or more unique presentation in women. We will discuss features of the disease conditions that may include presentation, diagnosis, management, and rehabilitation to reduce disease burden or progression of disease, improve pain, maintain function, and optimize quality of life.

Rheumatoid Arthritis

RA most commonly affects the small joints but can also affect intermediate and large joints, particularly in juvenile idiopathic arthritis (JIA). RA affects women more commonly than men in adult onset (3:1 female:male) and in all juvenile onset forms except for enthesitis-related JIA (1.5:1 male:female) and systemic JIA (1:1 male:female).[10] Population studies in Minnesota show a rising trend in the incidence of RA in women more recently (**Fig. 1**).[11] Autoantibody production may predate clinical arthritis by up to 5 years or more, but the transition from this preclinical stage to early and then chronic arthritis, in terms of synovial inflammation and joint damage, can be rapid. Beginning treatment within 12 weeks of clinical onset has significant benefit in achieving remission.[10] Later time to diagnosis, later start of disease-modifying antirheumatic drugs (DMARDs) and seropositivity (positive rheumatoid factor [RF] and anticyclic citrullinated peptide antibodies) are associated with more difficult to treat disease and increased risk of joint damage, deformity, and extra-articular manifestations.

The hallmark of RA is symmetric joint inflammation (pain, stiffness, swelling, and redness) that is frequently worse in the morning and improves after greater than 1 hour of activity. Periarticular erosions at the wrists, metacarpophalangeal (MCP) joints, proximal interphalangeal (PIP) joints, and metatarsal heads can aid in diagnosis as compared to sites more prevalent in gout or erosive osteoarthritis but are not pathognomonic. Carpal tunnel syndrome is common at diagnosis or with active disease, due to inflammation in the wrist. Classic RA hand deformities include radial deviation at the wrist, volar subluxation and ulnar deviation at MCP joints, and swan neck and boutonniere deformities of fingers. Wrist hand orthoses and finger orthoses and splints (**Fig. 2**) can be used to relieve pain, stabilize joints, and improve function. The swan neck ring splint prevents PIP joint hyperextension, and the boutonniere

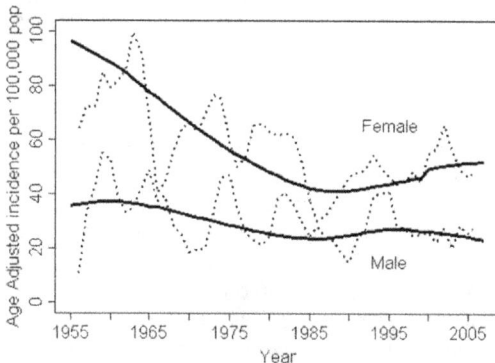

Fig. 1. Rising incidence of RA in women from 1996 to 2007. (*From* Firestein GS, Budd RC, Gabriel SE, McInnes IB, O'Dell JR, Koretzky G. Kelley and Firestein's Textbook of Rheumatology. 11th ed. Elsevier, Philadelphia, 2020.)

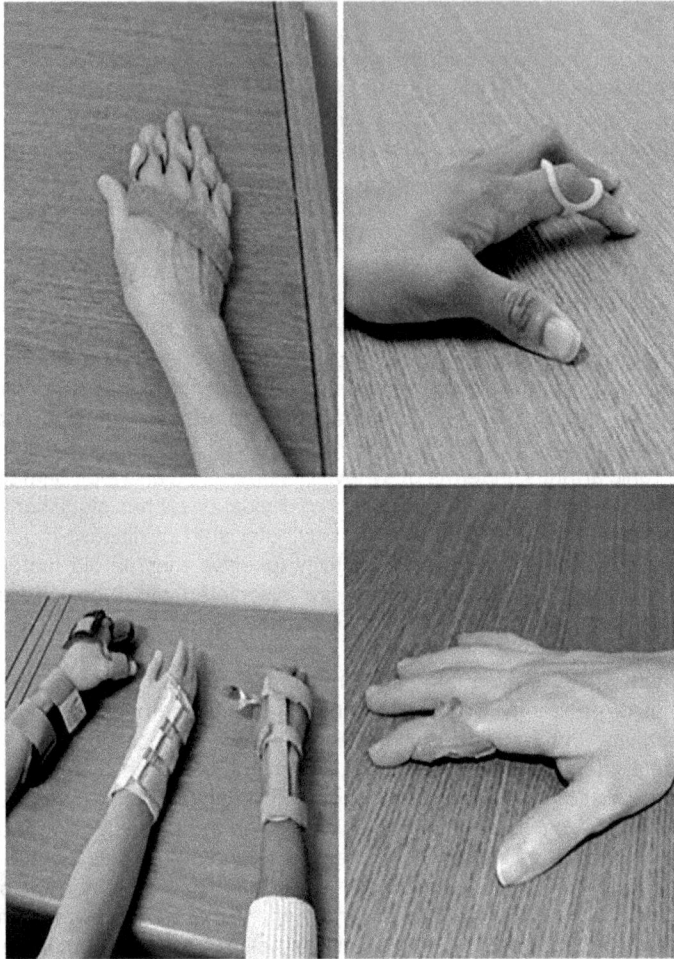

Fig. 2. Wrist, hand and finger orthoses. Left Top: ulnar deviation correction splint, Left Bottom: from left to right; resting wrist and hand orthosis, functional wrist splint, ADL splint with utensil holder/universal cuff. Right Top: Swan neck splint. Right Bottom: Boutonnière splint. (*From* Firestein GS, Budd RC, Gabriel SE, McInnes IB, O'Dell JR, Koretzky G. Kelley and Firestein's Textbook of Rheumatology. 11th ed. Elsevier, Philadelphia, 2020.)

ring splint prevents PIP joint flexion.[11] Some women with RA may prefer ring splints that resemble jewelry where they are made of metal (silver or gold) and may have a decorative pattern or include gemstones.

Up to 89% of patients with RA will experience ankle or foot symptoms.[12] Despite the importance of the feet in patient-reported outcomes and observed joint damage and disability, disease-specific measures such as the Disease Activity Score (of 28 joints) and Clinical Disease Activity Index do not include the foot joints! Metatarsophalangeal joints are often affected early. Tenosynovitis, rheumatoid nodules, and inflamed bursae are common, and atrophy of fat pads can occur.[13] Cartilage loss and changes in weight-bearing joints in the foot ultimately leads to valgus and hindfoot deformity posteriorly, and fibular deviation anteriorly. Tarsometatarsal joint subluxation can result in a "rocker-bottom" foot deformity similar to Charcot joint.[12] Observation for characteristic deformities such as metatarsal head subluxation, hallux valgus deformity, hammertoes and toe clawing, metatarsal squeeze testing, and assessment for rheumatoid nodules or Morton's neuroma along the plantar aspect, should be included in physician evaluation of women with RA, especially those that report foot pain or issues.

Insoles, foot orthoses, and shoe modifications including additional depth (to accommodate custom-molded foot orthotics), high toe box (for hammer toes), and wide toe box (for bunion/hallux valgus) can make a dramatic difference for quality of life by reducing pain, improving gait mechanics, and avoiding the need for corticosteroid injections, which carry a risk of tendon rupture and fat pad necrosis.[11,13] Shoe modifications include inner sole excavation relief (usually under metatarsal heads), metatarsal pads (placed proximal to the metatarsal heads and transfers load to the metatarsal shaft and relieves stress/pressure at metatarsal heads); **Fig. 3**, toe crests (relieves pressure at distal end and plantar surface for hammertoes), and foot orthoses.[13] A rocker bottom shoe may also be beneficial to reduce pain and improve gait mechanics (**Fig. 4**).

Systemic or intra-articular glucocorticoids may be helpful with acute inflammation but due to their toxicity profile, chronic use should be avoided. Therapeutic treatment options continue to expand for RA and include conventional synthetic DMARDs such

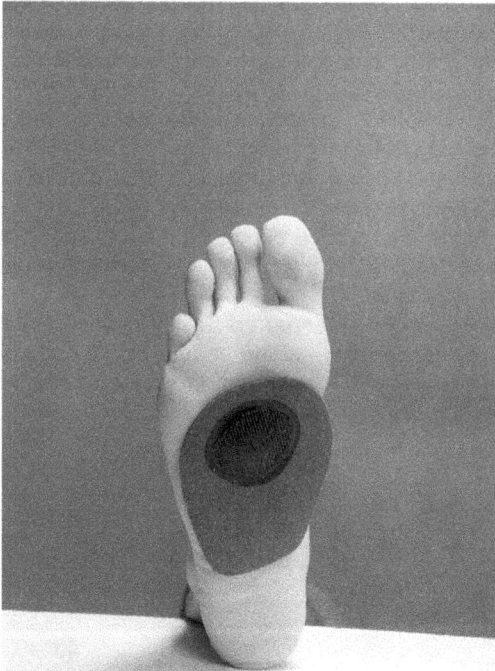

Fig. 3. Metatarsal pad. (*From* Braddom, RL. Physical Medicine and Rehabilitation. 4th Edition; Elsevier, Philadelphia, PA, 2011.)

as methotrexate, oral small molecules such as janus kinase inhibitor (JAK) inhibitors, and biologic medications targeting tumor necrosis factor, interleukin (IL)-6r, IL-1r, and B cell marker (CD20).

Acutely inflamed joints should be rested with relative rest. Nighttime splints and immobilizers, allowing for local rest of an inflamed joint, can be helpful in the short term; however, complete immobilization as was popular prior to the introduction of DMARDs is counterproductive and causes decline in muscle strength. Twice daily full and slow passive ROM should be done to prevent soft tissue contracture. Isometric strengthening is recommended as this causes the least amount of periarticular bone destruction, pain, and joint inflammation especially during an acute flare; additionally, it helps to maintain and restore strength by generating muscle tension with minimal work, fatigue, and stress. Isotonic strengthening exercises are recommended after achieving remission. Aquatic therapy can improve pain while providing joint and muscle support due to buoyancy of water.[11]

Physical modalities for inflamed joints include therapeutic cold or cryotherapy to reduce pain and swelling (but avoid in patients with Raynaud phenomenon). Therapeutic heat should be avoided in acutely inflamed joints as it increases collagenase enzyme activity that causes increased joint destruction; however, after acute inflammation improves, superficial heat including moist heat, paraffin wax (**Fig. 5**), and fluidotherapy can decrease pain and increase collagen extensibility for symptom management. Orthoses for distal upper and lower extremity joints can also be helpful to provide pain relief, decrease joint motion (joint stabilization), reduce weight through joint, facilitate relative rest, decrease inflammation, and support improved biomechanics to allow for better mobility and ADLs (see **Fig. 2**). Assistive and adaptive devices can be recommended and utilized to improve function and compensate for impairments allowing for increased independence (**Fig. 6**).[11]

As with most CTDs, pregnancy outcomes in RA are improved with better disease control. Contraception and the care of pregnant women with RA and other rheumatic disease must be discussed and tailored to the individual patient with an emphasis on safety and efficacy.[14] Best pregnancy outcomes will result if the pregnancy is planned so that safer medications can be used during the preconception period, during pregnancy, and while breastfeeding. Poorly controlled rheumatic diseases are associated with poor pregnancy outcomes.[15–18]

Postpartum, patients with RA self-report disability in physical domains of parenting such as carrying, hygiene, feeding, getting up and down, and household shopping. Difficulty with ADLs in the first trimester and presence of erosive disease increase the risk of high parenting disability postpartum.[19]

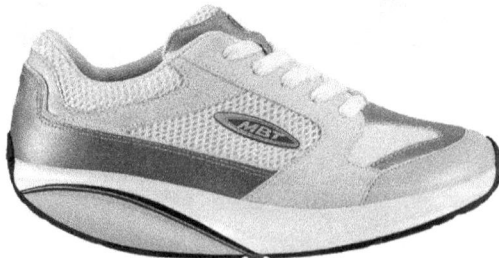

Fig. 4. Rocker bottom shoe. (*From* Braddom, RL. Physical Medicine and Rehabilitation. 4th Edition; Elsevier, Philadelphia, PA, 2011.)

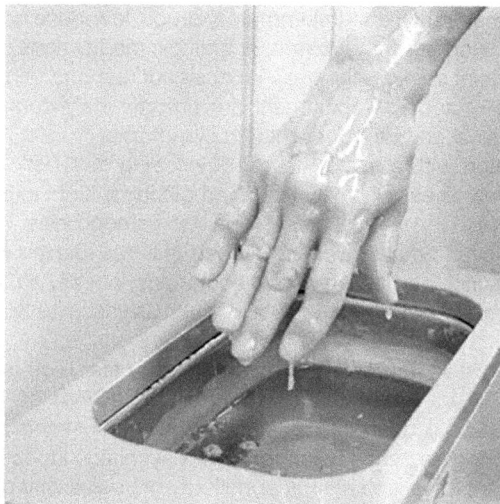

Fig. 5. Paraffin wax.

Systemic Lupus Erythematosus

Systemic lupus erythematosus (SLE [lupus]) is a pleomorphic autoimmune disease that primarily affects young women of reproductive age. In the United States, an estimated 200,000 persons are affected, with a female:male ratio of at least 9:1, and it is more common in persons of African origin than Northern European origin.[20] In addition to the classic malar rash, patients may experience constitutional, hematologic, mucocutaneous, musculoskeletal, renal, and central nervous system manifestations. Classification criteria require a positive antinuclear antibody (ANA) of at least 1:80, in addition to clinical and immunologic criteria.

Jaccoud's arthropathy is a nonerosive, fully reducible arthropathy that mimics RA in appearance (MCP dorsal subluxation and ulnar deviation, swan neck and boutonniere deformities, and thumb interphalangeal joint hyperextension), but does not cause joint destruction as it involves ligamentous and capsular laxity with periarticular inflammation.[11] Persons with Jaccoud's changes do not typically experience limitations in ADLs

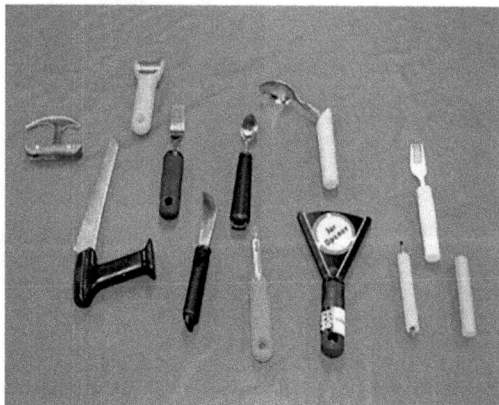

Fig. 6. Utensils with adaptive or built-up handles.

or ROM (**Fig. 7**). Nonsteroidal anti-inflammatory drugs, low-dose corticosteroids, conventional DMARDs such as methotrexate, or biologic medications such as belimumab may be needed for joint pain or stiffness that does not respond to hydroxychloroquine alone. Work disability and unemployment are unfortunately common, though influenced by both physical and neuropsychiatric symptoms.[20]

Lupus is associated with a higher risk of developing metabolic bone disease and osteonecrosis. Lupus disease activity itself and glucocorticoid exposure for its treatment both contribute to the risks of osteopenia and osteoporosis. The femoral head is the most common joint to develop osteonecrosis in lupus and it is frequently bilateral. Contributing factors include the use of corticosteroids, obesity, lupus disease activity itself, and immune microenvironmental factors such as vasculitis and antiphospholipid antibody syndrome.[11]

Patients with a positive lupus anticoagulant, or high titer (>40 units) anticardiolipin immunoglobulin G (IgG) or anti-beta 2 glycoprotein 1 (B2GP 1) IgG or immunoglobulin M, are at an increased risk of arterial or venous thrombotic events and obstetric complications.[11] A high degree of suspicion for neuropsychiatric lupus is necessary in patients with established lupus and antiphospholipid antibodies who present with altered mental status along with stroke, seizure, posterior reversible encephalopathy syndrome, or retinal vasculitis. Lumbar puncture and brain MRI and magnetic resonance angiography (MRA) or digital subtraction angiography can assist with diagnosis and with ruling out mimics including infection.[21] Events may be recurrent despite therapeutic anticoagulation and immunosuppressive treatment.

Peak disease incidence of lupus occurs during reproductive years and pregnancies in these patients are considered high risk for maternal and fetal mortality. Reproductive failure and obstetric complications such as pre-eclampsia, preterm birth, and intrauterine growth restriction are more common with a history of lupus nephritis or positive antiphospholipid antibodies, and in the setting of uncontrolled disease.[11] Pregnancy itself may increase disease activity in previously well-controlled patients.[21] High-grade cervical dysplasia and cervical cancer are also increased by 1.5 times in women with lupus.[21] The effects and limitations of difficult to control disease on women's reproductive health outcomes are an area of ongoing research.

Patients with lupus can experience debilitating effects on overall energy, mood, and quality of life as a result of their diagnosis and from medication side effects. Studies of women with lupus have found that as many as 40% felt distressed or unable to cope as a result of their diagnosis. In symptom surveys, fatigue is rated worse than pain,

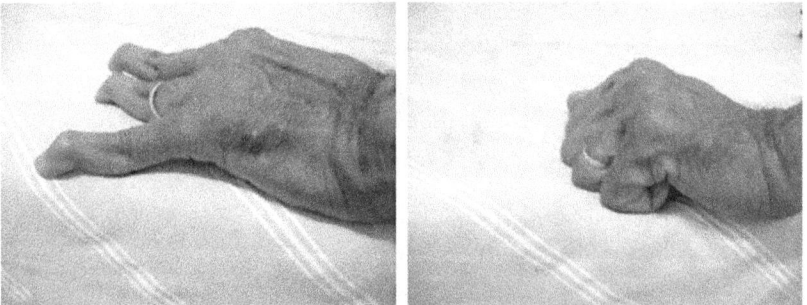

Fig. 7. Jaccoud's arthropathy with reversible swan neck deformities. (*From* Fontera, WR., Rizzo, TD., Silver, JK. Essentials of Physical Medicine and Rehabilitation, Fourth Edition. Elsevier, Philadelphia, 2019.)

depression, or anxiety.[22] Cognitive dysfunction may occur in as many as 80% of patients, manifested by trouble with thinking, memory, or concentration.

Given the wide spectrum of disease features a multidisciplinary team of specialists would be best to optimize overall outcomes for patients with SLE as they may benefit from physiatry, physical therapy (PT), occupational therapy (OT), speech and cognitive therapy, recreational therapy, psychology and psychiatry services, vocational rehabilitation, and social work with continued education and supportive resources.

Sjogren's Syndrome

Patients with Sjogren's syndrome experience the sicca complex of keratoconjunctivitis sicca and xerostomia. This may manifest as a secondary Sjogren's syndrome in association with other CTDs (most commonly RA or SLE), or primary Sjogren's syndrome (pSS) with sicca and extraglandular features (fatigue, Raynaud phenomenon, xerosis, polyarthritis, ILD, neuropathy, and vasculitis). A female prevalence in pSS stands out even among related CTDs—as much as 10:1 female:male prevalence—with peak incidence after middle age.[11] In addition to symptoms and specific antibodies (anti-Ro/SS-A or anti-La/SS-B), diagnosis can be confirmed with objective measures of dry eyes or dry mouth, and histopathology of a minor salivary gland (lip biopsy) showing focal lymphocytic sialadenitis. Biopsy is encouraged for patients who are seronegative for SSA/SSB, and to help rule out keratoconjunctivitis sicca or xerostomia due to aging, hormonal changes, meibomian gland dysfunction, and anticholinergic medications.

Polyarthralgia presents in nearly half of patients with Sjogren's syndrome.[11] Patients who present with a positive ANA or RF and joint pains may initially be classified with lupus or RA, until or unless screened for sicca and extraglandular symptoms, or evaluated for specific antibodies. Peripheral neuropathy (sensory, motor, or sensorimotor axonal polyneuropathies; mononeuritis multiplex; autonomic neuropathy; cranial nerve neuropathy; or demyelinating polyradiculoneuropathy) and small fiber neuropathy are both found in patients with pSS due to type II (mixed) cryoglobulinemia.[11] These patients will be treated with neuropathic pain medications and immunosuppressive medications and respond well to OT and PT when combined with drug therapy.

Sicca complex is primarily treated with topical agents and preventive care, while additional glandular symptoms like arthritis, rashes, and ILD may respond to antimalarials and other common conventional immunosuppressive medications.[23]

Fatigue is challenging to treat in Sjogren's and does not respond to immunosuppressive medications, including biologic therapies, in trials to date. Fatigue may manifest as tiredness, functional impairment, pain, or depression.[24] Physical exercise, including a supervised walking program, provides measurable benefits in aerobic capacity, fatigue, and ratings of perceived exertion and depression as compared to controls.[24] Combination OT and PT have also shown benefits in small cohort studies. Mimics or comorbid conditions including chronic fatigue syndrome, fibromyalgia, and certain vitamin deficiencies, should also be addressed.[11]

Inflammatory Myopathies

The idiopathic inflammatory myopathies, including polymyositis (PM), DM, and immune-mediated necrotizing myositis, are almost twice as common in women as in men. Although rare, occurring in 8 in 1,000,000 persons, all races and ethnicities are affected.[11] Inflammatory myopathy may also manifest as an overlap syndrome in other autoimmune diseases such as scleroderma, SLE, Sjogren's syndrome, mixed connective tissue disease, and sarcoidosis.

Muscle pain and weakness may worsen insidiously until patients present with diminishing quality of life. Patients present with objective, symmetric, progressive, or insidious weakness of proximal upper and lower extremities; in the neck, flexor muscles are weaker than extensors. In addition to muscle strength testing, patients should be assessed for fatigue with repetitive movements. Extramuscular manifestations include dysphagia, cardiomyopathy, ILD, arthritis, Raynaud phenomenon, and rash.[25] Lung involvement contributes to major morbidity and mortality and can be caused by respiratory muscle weakness or ILD.[11] Pulmonary function testing should, therefore, also include measurement of the negative inspiratory force.

On examination, patients have proximal more than distal weakness. Early atrophy points to inclusion body myositis or another cause, rather than PM or DM. Sensory deficits are also less likely to be present in myositis. Classic skin manifestations in DM include the heliotrope rash, shawl and V signs, Gottron's papules (**Fig. 8**), and sleeve and holster signs; hyperkeratotic mechanic's hands and hiker's feet may also be seen. A careful search for malignancy is indicated in the first 1 and 5 years after diagnosis. In adult women, this should include a mammogram and pelvic ultrasound regardless of age.[11]

Elevations of CK (5–100 times the upper limit of normal), and/or other laboratories such as lactate dehydrogenase (LDH), aspartate aminotransferase (AST), alanine aminotransferase (ALT), and aldolase support the inflammatory myositis diagnosis.[26] For example, consider muscle disease when AST, ALT, or LDH are elevated in the setting of normal gamma-glutamyl transferase (GGT) and alkaline phosphatase (ALP). Obtain exercise fasted laboratories for mildly elevated creatine kinase (CK) without symptoms, or test over the weekend for patients who have physically demanding jobs. Myositis specific antibodies including the anti-a myositis specific auto-antibody (Jo-1) (antisynthetase syndrome with myositis, fever, Raynaud, ILD, and arthritis), anti-an autoantibody that targets the signal recognition particle (SRP) (African-American women with refractory necrotizing myositis), and anti-autoantibody that targets the Mi-2 nuclear antigen (Mi-2) (older women with classic shawl sign and other rashes) antibodies, represent specific phenotypic presentations and have prognostic value.[27]

Electromyography (EMG) is sensitive but not specific for inflammatory myopathies; it can be useful to exclude neuromuscular mimics including motor neuron disease, muscular dystrophy, motor neuropathies, and neuromuscular junction disorders. EMG abnormalities in myositis may include the presence of increased insertional activity, abnormal spontaneous fibrillations, positive sharp waves, and low-amplitude short-duration polyphasic motor unit potentials.[28] Early recruitment represents the use of more motor units being required to generate a certain level of force due to the diminished number of functioning muscle fibers. Muscle biopsy is the "gold standard" for inflammatory myopathy and should be done on affected, nonend-stage muscle on the contralateral side as the EMG due to the risks of needle necrosis from the procedure. MRI with short tau inversion recovery (STIR) imaging can provide visual quantification of inflammation and help guide location for biopsy, which is typically in the rectus femoris for PM and DM (**Fig. 9**).

Treatment involves moderate-to-high dose glucocorticoids followed by steroid-sparing immunosuppressive medications. Patients with dysphagia may respond better to intravenous immunoglobulin (IVIG) than steroids. PT and OT should begin alongside immunosuppressive therapy and can themselves decrease systemic inflammation in addition to improving muscle strength, functional mobility, and ADLs. The Functional Index in Myositis-2 can be administered by a physical therapist in 20 minutes and is more sensitive for fatigability or endurance in proximal muscle groups than manual muscle testing to assess response to therapy.[11]

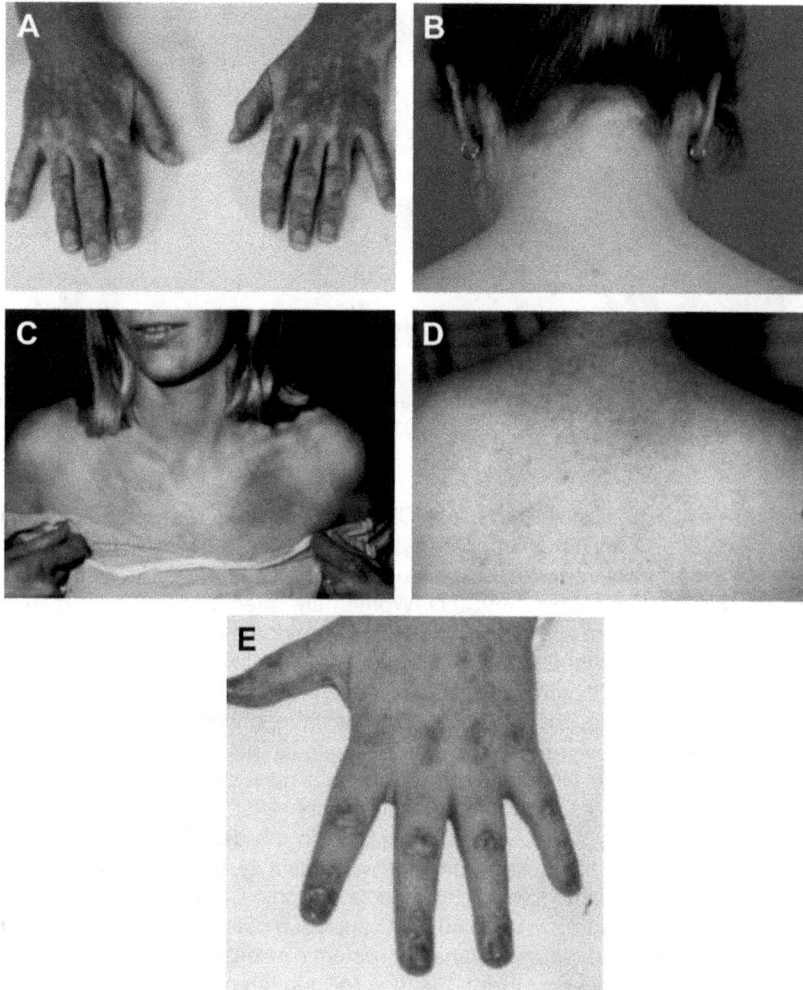

Fig. 8. Dermatomyositis rashes. (*A*) Linear erythema (*B*) Scalp Rash (*C*) V-like sign (*D*) Shawl sign (*E*) Gottron's sign. (*From* Firestein GS, Gabriel SE, McInnes IB, O'Dell JR. Kelley and Firestein's Textbook of Rheumatology. 10th ed. Elsevier, Philadelphia, 2017.)

In patients who were previously responding to therapy and then develop new weakness or reduced CK levels, consider steroid myopathy. These patients will have weak proximal muscles except for preserved strength in the neck flexors.

Systemic Sclerosis/Scleroderma

Systemic sclerosis (SSc) or scleroderma, is a complex CTD involving an occlusive microangiopathy that leads to fibrosis of the skin (hallmark of this disease), joints, and visceral organs.[29] Skin and organ involvement are progressive and result in increased disability and mortality. Limited cutaneous systemic sclerosis (lcSSc) and diffuse cutaneous systemic sclerosis are used to describe characteristic patterns of skin involvement and are each associated with specific autoantibodies. The limited form, previously known as (Calcinosis, Raynaud, Esophageal, Sclerodactyly,

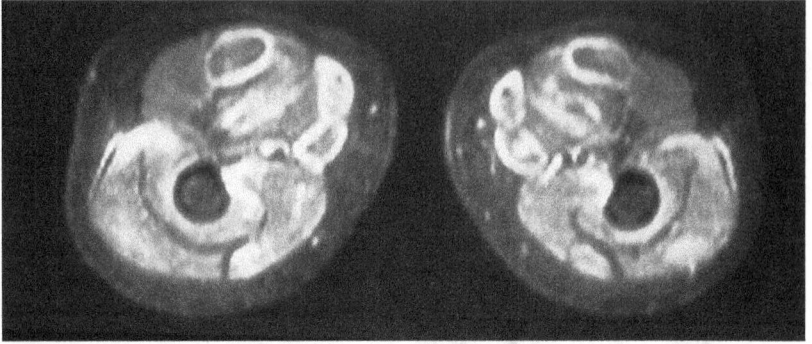

Fig. 9. MRI of symmetric thigh inflammation in myositis—Fig 85-11 from Kelley's 10th ed. (*From* Firestein GS, Gabriel SE, McInnes IB, et al. Kelley and Firestein's Textbook of Rheumatology. 10th edition. Philadelphia: Elsevier. 2017.)

Telangiectasia (a subset of scleroderma) [CREST]) syndrome, is associated with anti-centromere B antibodies and pulmonary hypertension, and the diffuse form is associated with anti-antiscleroderma-associated autoantigen of 70-kDa (Scl-70) or antitopoisomerase I antibodies and ILD. Women are affected more than men (4:1), and onset is typically from age 40 to 50 years.[11] Vasculopathy and tissue fibrosis affect not just the skin but lungs, GI tract, heart, kidneys, and skeletal muscle. Mortality is high, especially related to cardiac or lung disease. Overlap features with other CTDs include arthritis, myositis, and sicca. Similarly to lupus, a worse disease course and higher mortality have been reported in African American patients with scleroderma.[30]

An early phase of acute inflammation that predates classic skin thickening in scleroderma can be described as "puffy hands" or fingers. After this edematous phase, a fibrotic phase develops with collagen deposition in the dermis and deeper layers, causing the classic skin thickening alongside sclerodactyly, tendon friction rubs, contractures of small and large joints, and muscle atrophy. Contractures are the most prevalent of these, occurring in up to 30% of patients, mostly those with the antitopoisomerase I antibody and diffuse cutaneous systemic sclerosis (dcSSc) phenotype.[11] Patients may have reduced mobility, function, or grip strength that will benefit from occupational therapy modalities including splinting or from paraffin wax (see **Fig. 5**) followed by passive ROM exercises. Even a short 4 week supervised rehabilitation protocol was associated with improvements in disability, hand function, and handgrip and pinch for up to 6 months afterward.[31] However, a large international cohort found that fewer than one-quarter of patients with SSc used PT or OT interventions despite having more severe musculoskeletal manifestations and higher pain and disability.[32]

Muscle atrophy and weakness is compounded by gastrointestinal manifestations of the disease (dysmotility, chronic esophageal reflux, and small bowel bacterial overgrowth) due to abnormally slow bowel motility may lead to malabsorption and malnutrition.[11] Psychosocial impacts of these cutaneous and visceral organ complications include anxiety, depression, and body image dissatisfaction, which are common in men across all age groups and in younger women.

Raynaud phenomenon, a characteristic triphasic color change (white, blue, then red) of the fingers or toes due to cold or stress, is caused by vasospasm of the distal arterioles and capillaries and begins at mean 1.2 years prior to systemic disease onset.[11] Progressive endothelial dysfunction and structural vessel damage occurs, and digital pits and ulcerations can occur. Keeping core temperature warm or wearing

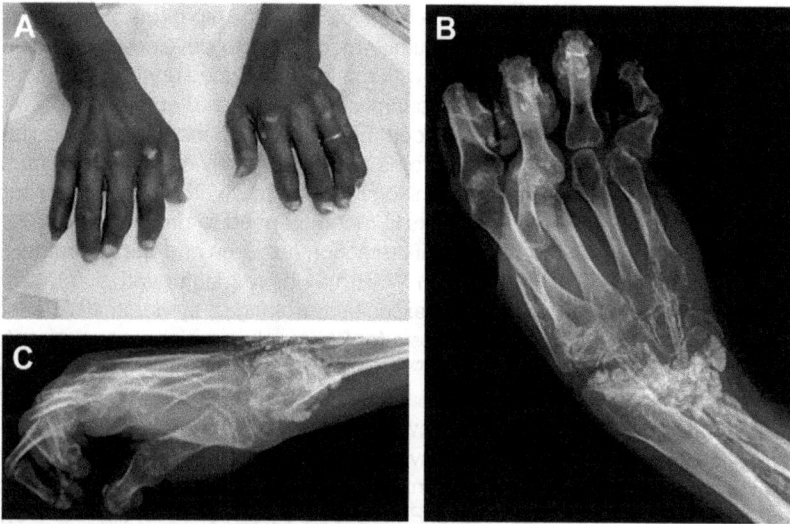

Fig. 10. Hands of patient with scleroderma and radiographs showing acro-osteolysis, calcinosis, and joint erosions. (*A*) Pigmented Gottron's rash over metacarpal joints of a patient with Dermatomyositis. (*B*) Posterior-Anterior xray view of a hand with severe finger contracture associated with tumorous calcinosis deposits in the wrist, metacarpal and proximal interphalageal joints. (*C*) Lateral xray view of the same hand showing tumorous calcinosis at the wrist with bony erosions of the carpal bones. (*From* Firestein GS, Budd RC, Gabriel SE, McInnes IB, O'Dell JR, Koretzky G. Kelley and Firestein's Textbook of Rheumatology. 11th ed. Elsevier, Philadelphia, 2020.)

warming gloves, as well as smoking cessation, biofeedback, low-dose calcium channel blockers, and phosphodiesterase-5 inhibitors can mediate these symptoms. In the case of severe vasospasm, if overt digital ischemia occurs, treatment can include topical nitroglycerin, hyperbaric oxygen, intravenous prostacyclin, endothelin receptor antagonists, and sympathectomy. Peripheral vascular disease can also contribute to acro-osteolysis (**Fig. 10**).[11]

Treatments including DMARDs such as methotrexate and mycophenolate mofetil have been used in SSc but have not yet shown statistically significant impact on onset of skin progression or forced vital capacity decline.[11] Other immunosuppressive therapies including cyclophosphamide and biologic DMARDs, as well as antifibrotic therapies, can be tried in patients with ILD. SSc has the highest mortality rate of any autoimmune rheumatologic disease, most commonly from cardiac involvement or lung disease, up to 6.6% at 3 years of follow-up from diagnosis.[11]

ILD is the leading cause of death in those with scleroderma spectrum disorders.[33] Although there is no cure, survival has improved over the years with earlier intervention, including the use of appropriate immunosuppression and antifibrotic therapy; however, 30% to 40% develop ILD and the 10 year mortality is still 40%. African Americans with SSc and those with antitopoisomerase 1 antibodies are at higher risk for morbidity and mortality from lung complications.[30]

Polymyalgia Rheumatica

Patients aged 60 years or older who experience acute onset of severe pain and stiffness of the shoulder and/or hip girdles should be evaluated for polymyalgia rheumatica (PMR). Pain and stiffness may begin unilaterally but will shortly become bilateral and may extend from the shoulder to the neck and from the hip girdle and buttocks to the proximal thighs. Women are 2 to 3 times more likely to develop the condition.[11] Ninety percent of cases of PMR present with markedly elevated erythrocyte sedimentation rates and a moderate degree of anemia; fever, malaise, anorexia, and weight loss are also common. The majority of community-dwelling independent adults can recall the date of abrupt onset of symptoms and will similarly experience a dramatic and complete clinical response to prednisone 15 mg daily within 2 days, although a slow steroid taper of 1 mg every 5 weeks is recommended to prevent relapse.[34,35]

Imaging in PMR shows periarticular inflammation (tendons and bursae) rather than synovitis such as in RA.[36] Patients with PMR may have painful active and passive ROM, but they should not be truly weak unless prolonged symptoms have led to disuse atrophy.[37] The differential diagnosis for PMR includes malignancy, neurologic disease, thyroid disease, depression, PM (which should display elevated muscle enzyme and proximal weakness more than pain), elderly onset RA, adhesive capsulitis, and fibromyalgia (though there is a low incidence of de novo onset fibromyalgia in older adults unless a physiologic or psychological trauma has occurred).[37] Due to epidemiologic, pathophysiologic, and clinical features overlapping between the 2 conditions, patients with a new diagnosis of PMR should be screened for signs and symptoms of giant cell arteritis.

Crystal-Induced Arthropathy

Both gout and pseudogout are more common in male individuals, so we will not discuss them further; however, Milwaukee shoulder syndrome or cuff-tear arthropathy is a crystal deposition disease most commonly found in elderly women. This is a destructive arthritis caused by periarticular or intra-articular deposition of calcium hydroxyapatite crystals.[38] Patients present with sudden joint effusion with limited ROM of one or both shoulders. Despite the name, it can also occur in the knees in 50% of cases. Synovial fluid is typically hemorrhagic but noninflammatory, and hydroxyapatite crystals are seen with the alizarin red S stain.[39] With recurrent episodes, rotator cuff tears develop, and there is a rapid decline in joint function. Radiographs will show calcific tendinitis and loss of the normal glenohumeral and subacromial spaces, sometimes with erosion of the articular surfaces, allowing for proximal migration of the humeral head.[11] Rotator cuff repair can be tried but patients with cuff-tear arthropathy will need reverse total shoulder arthroplasty for a stabilized, functional joint. Chronic joint overuse and repetitive arm elevation may contribute to failure of conservative therapy.

Osteoarthritis

Osteoarthritis (OA) is the most common type of arthritis, occurring most frequently in the knee joint. After the age of 50 years, there is a marked increase in prevalence among women, and additionally, obesity is also associated with knee OA.[11] Conservative treatment includes PT and OT for ROM and strengthening exercises (quadriceps strengthening), weight loss, assistive devices, braces, joint protection, and energy conservation education. Hot and cold modalities, medication management, and injection treatments to decrease pain and reduce inflammation.[11]

Spondyloarthropathies

Ankylosing spondylitis is more common in male individuals, therefore not discussed here; however, it is important to note patients can develop restrictive lung disease due to impaired chest wall excursion. Additionally, because it is more common in men, diagnosis in women may be missed or delayed.

Pulmonary Rehabilitation

Chronic respiratory diseases, including but not limited to chronic obstructive pulmonary disease, asthma, cystic fibrosis, pulmonary fibrosis, and pulmonary hypertension, may lead to disabling shortness of breath, fatigue, weakness, increased hospitalization, anxiety, depression, and reduced quality of life, all of which contribute to increased morbidity and mortality.[40] Many rheumatologic patients as discussed earlier develop chronic respiratory disease including pulmonary hypertension and restrictive lung disease secondary to chest wall excursion limitations and/or ILD including pulmonary fibrosis.

The American Thoracic Society recommends pulmonary rehabilitation (PR) as an integral component of the management for all stable respiratory diseases.[40] PR programs generally include both aerobic and resistance training conducted in a supervised rehabilitation facility lasting 1 to 2 months or longer, followed by a maintenance program. Education in breathing retraining and self-management exercises is often included in the training program. Those who participate report improvement in their physical function and sense of well-being, decline in dyspnea sensation, and increased exercise capacity[41] as measured by HRQoL[42] compared to those who do not participate. In patients with fibrotic ILD, improved performance after PR was associated with improved survival.[43] In another randomized study of patients with fibrotic ILD from various causes, twice-weekly supervised outpatient exercise training program consisting of 30 minutes aerobics, cycling, walking, upper and lower resistance training, significantly improved the 6 minute walk distance and dyspnea symptoms, as well as HRQoL measures. Sustained benefit was found in those with milder lung disease who adhered to their exercise program.[44] For best results, PR training should include both aerobic and resistance training.[45]

SUMMARY

Rheumatological conditions that predominantly affect women, including RA, SLE, Sjogren's syndrome, inflammatory myopathies, SSc, and PMR, were reviewed. These conditions impact more than one organ system and often have significant implications on day-to-day life for women living with these diseases. They can cause physical limitations and disability by reducing independence with functional mobility and ADLs. Weakness and fatigue, in addition to reduced overall general health with cardiopulmonary impairment, make these challenging conditions to address without multidisciplinary teams working together to maximize outcomes. Women already typically juggle caring for themselves while caring for others. These chronic and debilitating diseases need close monitoring, medical management, rehabilitation care with continued patient education, and guidance to prevent, minimize, and delay the potentially rapid progressive functional decline and morbidity and mortality that can be associated with these conditions.

CLINICS CARE POINTS

- SLE: Jaccoud's is a nonerosive arthropathy involving pericapsular inflammation and does not cause fixed deformities. Splinting can help with pain, but it does not require increased immunosuppression.
- RA: Foot and ankle arthritis can lead to significant deformities and gait abnormalities. Early evaluation and intervention with orthoses can improve pain and gait mechanics and defer need for surgical interventions.

- Myositis: In patients who previously responded to therapy but present with weakness and normal or lower CK than at diagnosis, consider steroid myopathy or disuse atrophy.
- Scleroderma: Progressive SSc can cause contractures of small and large joints. Early and frequent occupational therapy interventions can improve pain, strength, and function.

DISCLOSURE

The authors have nothing to disclose.

REFERENCES

1. Crowson CS, Matteson EL, Myasoedova E, et al. The lifetime risk of adult-onset rheumatoid arthritis and other inflammatory autoimmune rheumatic diseases. Arthritis Rheum 2011;63(3):633–9.
2. Shin S, Park EH, Kang EH, et al. Sex differences in clinical characteristics and their influence on clinical outcomes in an observational cohort of patients with rheumatoid arthritis. Joint Bone Spine 2021;88(3):105124.
3. Mayes MD, Lacey JV, Beebe-Dimmer J, et al. Prevalence, incidence, survival and disease characteristics of systemic sclerosis in a large US population. Arthritis Rheum 2003;48(8):2246–55.
4. Kronzer VL, Kimbrough BA, Crowson CS, et al. Incidence, prevalence, and mortality of dermatomyositis: a population-based cohort study. Arthritis Care Res 2023;75(2):348–55.
5. Sun KY, Fan Y, Wang YX, et al. Prevalence of interstitial lung disease in polymyositis and dermatomyositis: a meta-analysis from 2000 to 2020. Semin Arthritis Rheum 2021;51(1):175–91.
6. Joy GM, Arbiv OA, Wong CK, et al. Prevalence, imaging patterns and risk factors of interstitial lung disease in connective tissue disease: a systematic review and meta-analysis. Eur Respir Rev 2023;32(167):220210.
7. Benatti FB, Pedersen BK. Exercise as an anti-inflammatory therapy for rheumatic diseases- myokine regulation. Nat Rev Rheumatol 2015;11(2):86–97.
8. Monda V, Villano I, Messina A, et al. Exercise modifies the gut microbiota with positive health effects. Oxid Med Cell Longev 2017;2017. https://doi.org/10.1155/2017/3831972.
9. Natalello G, Bosello SL, Sterbini PF, et al. Gut microbiota analysis in systemic sclerosis according to disease characteristics and nutritional status. Clin Exp Rheumatol 2020;38(3):73–84.
10. Guo Q, Wang Y, Xu D, et al. Rheumatoid arthritis: pathological mechanisms and modern pharmacologic therapies. Bone Res 2018;6:15.
11. Firestein GS, Budd RC, Gabriel SE, et al. Kelley and Firestein's Textbook of Rheumatology. 11th ed. Philadelphia: Elsevier; 2020.
12. Borman P, Ayhan F, Tuncay F, et al. Foot problems in a group of patients with rheumatoid arthritis: an unmet need for foot care. Open Rheumatol J 2012;6: 290–5. Epub 2012 Oct 4. PMID: 23066434; PMCID: PMC3468872.
13. Uustal H, Baerga E, Joki J, et al. Prosthetics and orthotics. In: Cuccurullo S, editor. Physical medicine and rehabilitation board review. Fourth Edition. New York, NY: Demos Medical; 2020.
14. Sammaritano LR, Bermas BL, Chakravarty EE, et al. American college of Rheumatology guideline for the management of reproductive health in rheumatic and musculoskeletal diseases. Arthritis Care Res 2020;72(4):461–88.

15. Langen ES, Chakravarty EF, Liaquat M, et al. High rate of preterm birth in pregnancies complicated by rheumatoid arthritis. Am J Perinatol 2014;31:9–13.
16. Chakravarty EF, Nelson L, Krishnan E. Obstetric hospitalizations in the United States for women with systemic lupus erythematosus and rheumatoid arthritis. Arthritis Rheum 2006;54:899–907.
17. Ruiz-Irastorza G, Lima F, Alves J, et al. Increased rate of lupus flare during pregnancy and the puerperium: a prospective study of 78 pregnancies. Br J Rheumatol 1996;35:133–8.
18. Eisfeld H, Glimm AM, Burmester GR, et al. Pregnancy outcome in women with different rheumatic diseases: a retrospective analysis. Scand J Rheumatol 2021;50(4):299–306.
19. Smeele HTW, de Man YA, Röder E, et al. Parenting problems postpartum can be detected early in pregnancy in patients with rheumatoid arthritis. RMD Open 2020;6:e001276. https://doi.org/10.1136/rmdopen-2020-001276.
20. Kaul A, Gordon C, Crow M, et al. Systemic lupus erythematosus. Nat Rev Dis Prim 2016;2:16039.
21. Fanouriakis A, Tziolos N, Bertsias G, et al. Update on the diagnosis and management of systemic lupus erythematosus. Ann Rheum Dis 2021;80:14–25.
22. Schmeding A, Schneider M. Fatigue, health-related quality of life and other patient-reported outcomes in systemic lupus erythematosus. Best Pract Res Clin Rheumatol 2013;27(3):363–75.
23. Ramos-Casals M, Brito-Zerón P, Bombardieri S, et al, On behalf of the EULAR-Sjögren Syndrome Task Force Group. EULAR recommendations for the management of Sjögren's syndrome with topical and systemic therapies. Ann Rheum Dis 2020;79:3–18.
24. Mæland E, Miyamoto ST, Hammenfors D, et al. Understanding fatigue in sjögren's syndrome: outcome measures, biomarkers and possible interventions. Front Immunol 2021;12:703079. https://doi.org/10.3389/fimmu.2021.703079. PMID: 34249008; PMCID: PMC8267792.
25. Lundberg IE, Tjärnlund A, Bottai M, et al. European League against Rheumatism/American College of Rheumatology classification criteria for adult and juvenile idiopathic inflammatory myopathies and their major subgroups. Ann Rheum Dis 2017;76(12):1955–64. https://doi.org/10.1136/annrheumdis-2017-211468 [published correction appears in Ann Rheum Dis. 2018 Sep;77(9):e64].
26. Volochayev R, Csako G, Wesley R, et al. Laboratory test abnormalities are common in polymyositis and dermatomyositis and differ among clinical and demographic groups. Open Rheumatol J 2012;6:54–63. https://doi.org/10.2174/1874312901206010054.
27. Love LA, Leff RL, Fraser DD, et al. A new approach to the classification of idiopathic inflammatory myopathy: myositis-specific autoantibodies define useful homogeneous patient groups. Medicine (Baltim) 1991;70(6):360–74. PMID: 1659647.
28. Paganoni S, Amato A. Electrodiagnostic evaluation of myopathies. Phys Med Rehabil Clin N Am 2013;24(1):193–207. https://doi.org/10.1016/j.pmr.2012.08.017.
29. Jaafar S, Lescoat A, Huang S, et al. Clinical characteristics, visceral involvement, and mortality in at-risk or early diffuse systemic sclerosis: a longitudinal analysis of an observational prospective multicenter US cohort. Arthritis Res Ther 2021;23(1):170. PMID: 34127049; PMCID: PMC8201684.
30. Moore DF, Kramer E, Eltaraboulsi R, et al. Increased morbidity and mortality of scleroderma in African Americans compared to non-African Americans. Arthritis Care Res 2019;71(9):1154–63.

31. Waszczykowski M, Dziankowska-Bartkowiak B, Podgórski M, et al. Role and effectiveness of 28complex and supervised rehabilitation on overall and hand function in systemic sclerosis patients—one-year follow-up study. Sci Rep 2021;11:15174.

32. Becetti K, Kwakkenbos L, Carrier ME, et al. Physical or occupational therapy use in systemic sclerosis: a scleroderma patient-centered intervention network cohort study. J Rheumatol 2019;46(12):1605–13. Epub 2019 May 1. PMID: 31043542.

33. Perelas A, Silver RM, Arrossi AV, et al. Systemic sclerosis-associated interstitial lung disease. Lancet Respir Med 2020;8(3):304–20.

34. Dejaco C, Singh YP, Perel P, et al. Recommendations for the management of polymyalgiarheumatica: a European League against rheumatism/American College of Rheumatology collaborative initiative. Ann Rheum Dis 2015;74:1799–807.

35. Weyand CM,GJ. Clinical practice: giant-cell arteritis and polymyalgia rheumatica. N Engl J Med 2014;371(1):50–7.

36. Fruth M,SA. Diagnostic capability of contrast-enhanced pelvic girdle magnetic resonance imaging in polymyalgia rheumatica. Rheumatology 2020. https://doi.org/10.1093/rheumatology/keaa0.

37. Pipitone N,SC. Update on polymyalgia rheumatica. Eur J Intern Med 2013;24:583–9.

38. Halverson P, Carrera G. Milwaukee shoulder syndrome: fifteen additional cases and a description of contributing factors. JAMA Intern Med 1990;150(3):677–82.

39. Ea H,LF. Calcium pyrophosphate dihydrate and basic calcium phosphate crystal induced arthropathies: update on pathogenesis, clinical features, and therapy. Curr Rheumatol Rep 2004;6:221–7.

40. Rochester CL, Alison JA, Carlin B, et al. Pulmonary rehabilitation for adults with chronic respiratory disease: an official American thoracic society for clinical practice guideline. Am J Respir Crit Care Med 2023;208(4):e7–26.

41. McCarthy B, Casey D, Devane D, et al. Pulmonary rehabilitation for chronic obstructive pulmonary disease. Cochrane Database Syst Rev 2015;2015:CD003793.

42. Jaeschke R, Singer J, Guyatt GH. Measurement of health status. Ascertaining the minimal clinically important difference. Contr Clin Trials 1989;10:407–15.

43. Guler SA, Hur SA, Stickland MK, et al. Survival after inpatient or outpatient pulmonary rehabilitation in patients with fibrotic interstitial lung disease: a multicentre retrospective cohort study. Thorax 2022;77(6):589–95.

44. Dowman LM, McDOnald CF, Hill CJ, et al. The evidence of benefits of exercise training in interstitial lung disease: a randomized controlled trial. Thorax 2017;72:610–9.

45. Ortega F, Toral J, Cejudo P, et al. Comparison of effects of strength and endurance training in patients with chronic obstructive pulmonary disease. Am J Respir Crit Care Med 2002;166:669–77.

Osteoporosis Issues Regarding Rehabilitation in Women

Casey Schoenlank, MD*, Alphonsa Thomas, DO, Raisa Bakshiyev, MD, SuAnn Chen, MD

KEYWORDS

- Osteoporosis • Vertebral and hip fractures • DXA scan • Postmenopausal
- Bone mineral density • Osteopenia

KEY POINTS

- Osteoporosis is the result of reduced structural bone integrity and remains a serious health concern impacting women over the age of 50 worldwide.
- Dual X-ray absorptiometry is the gold standard for bone mineral density testing and is a component of the diagnostic workup for osteoporosis.
- A multifactorial approach to treatment includes pharmacologic and nonpharmacologic recommendations, specifically lifestyle changes centered around nutrition and exercise.
- Skeletal fractures are often the first clinical indication of this disease with the most common being vertebral fractures.
- Osteoporosis is a preventable and treatable condition in women that can result in significant morbidity and mortality if left unattended.

INTRODUCTION AND EPIDEMIOLOGY

The World Health Organization (WHO) defines osteoporosis as a condition of a change in bone microarchitecture, such as reduced bone mass and density, decreased cortical bone thickness, and a decrease in the trabeculae of cancellous bone, resulting in bone fragility and increased fracture incidence. It is the most common metabolic bone disease, affecting 1 in 3 women over the age of 50 across the world.[1] In the United States, an estimated 10 million adults (80% female) have osteoporosis and another 44 million have low bone mass, placing them at higher risk for fracture.[2] Osteoporosis accounts for 2 million fractures annually, and this is projected to reach 3 million fractures annually by 2025.[3] One in 2 women will break a bone because of

Department of Physical Medicine and Rehabilitation, Hackensack Meridian Johnson Rehabilitation Institute at Ocean University Medical Center (OUMC), 425 Jack Martin Boulevard, Brick, NJ 08724, USA
* Corresponding author.
E-mail address: casey.schoenlank@hmhn.org

Phys Med Rehabil Clin N Am 36 (2025) 361–370
https://doi.org/10.1016/j.pmr.2024.11.004
1047-9651/25/© 2024 Elsevier Inc. All rights reserved, including those for text and data mining, AI training, and similar technologies.

osteoporosis, and the incidence of osteoporotic fracture is greater than that of heart attack, stroke, and breast cancer combined.[4] Osteoporosis is a disease of increasing age, as bone tissue loss is known to progress over time. The loss of gonadal function, especially after menopause, precipitates rapid bone loss—up to 20% in the first 5 to 7 years.[3] By age 80, Caucasian women will lose about 20% of their hip bone density.[3]

Hip fractures play a large role in morbidity and mortality, loss of independence and financial burden, especially in women over the age of 50. Six months after a hip fracture, only 15% of patients can walk across a room unaided.[3] About 24% of patients die within 1 year of hip fracture.[3] The annual economic burden of osteoporosis in the United States is $19 billion and is anticipated to rise to $25 billion by 2025.[3] Despite these exponential costs, less than 1 in 4 women over the age of 67 years with an osteoporosis related fracture gets bone mineral density (BMD) testing or initiates treatment.[5] Increased fear of falls along with anxiety and depression due to loss of independence can impact emotional health in a woman diagnosed with osteoporosis. She may develop poor body image due to a decrease in stature, kyphotic curvature of the spine and wounds that can develop on pressure points, or as a result of a more sedentary lifestyle.

RISK OF FACTORS OF OSTEOPOROSIS

Risk factors for osteoporosis can be classified as Nonmodifiable and Modifiable. Nonmodifiable factors include: older age, female gender, Caucasian or Asian ethnicity, early menopause, fracture in adulthood, inflammatory diseases, and family history of osteoporosis. Modifiable factors include: nutrition with relation to calcium, vitamin D, and protein intake, low body mass index (BMI) or anorexia, smoking and alcohol use, hormone deficiency, inactivity or lack of weight-bearing, and medication side effects (ie, Steroids, PPI). It should be noted that obesity, in fact, decreases the risk of this disease.[5,6]

PATHOPHYSIOLOGY

Bone is live tissue that grows and evolves over the course of one's life. The natural process of bone metabolism is maintained by a continuous balance between bone formation and bone resorption. At the cellular level, osteoblasts are cells that build bone and osteoclasts are cells that resorb bone. Cortical bone makes up the most the human skeleton and is found at the shaft of long bones, accounting for the primary mechanical strength. Trabecular bone is found in vertebrae, flat bones, and the ends of long bones.

The chemical composition of bone involves vitamin D, which impacts calcium and phosphorus absorption in the kidneys and intestine. Vitamin D deficiency is the most common cause of osteomalacia or impaired bone mineralization resulting in soft bones. Calcitonin is manufactured in the thyroid gland's C-cells and it decreases osteoclast activity thus aiding in calcium incorporation into bone. Parathyroid Hormone (PTH) stimulates both resorption and formation of bone to maintain calcium homeostasis. Ninety nine percent of the body's calcium is found in bone, and its levels in the body are regulated by Vitamin D, Calcitonin, and PTH.[7] Any discrepancies in the above processes will manifest as either increased rate of bone loss or decreased production of trabecular bone. The rate of bone loss is most rapid after menopause due to hormonal changes and may also be expedited by initially low peak bone mass—that is, anorexia and immobility.

SCREENING AND DIAGNOSIS

All postmenopausal women 50 years and older should be assessed for osteoporosis risk.[5] A history of fractures (proximal femur, distal forearm, hip, or vertebral body), usually associated with minimal trauma, often is the first indicator of a heightened risk for osteoporosis. There are clinical fracture risk assessment tools available and should be included in the initial evaluation for osteoporosis, such as the Fracture Risk Assessment Tool (FRAX®). FRAX® is a web-based algorithm that was designed to predict the 10-year probability of major osteoporosis-related fractures based on clinical risk factors and BMD. Included in this assessment are other risk factors (ie, alcohol/smoking, medications, and inflammatory disease) to better identify those individuals who are at risk of future fractures, but perhaps who do not have low BMD.[5,8]

Further investigation can be initiated with laboratory testing, especially to evaluate for secondary causes of osteoporosis. Testing may include complete blood count, comprehensive metabolic panel, ionized calcium level, vitamin D level, PTH, sedimentation rate, thyroid function tests, hormone tests (estradiol, testosterone, and follicle stimulating hormone). Markers for bone resorption/breakdown include urine studies (elevated levels of calcium/creatinine ratio) and tartrate resistant acid phosphatase. Bone formation markers would include total and bone specific alkaline phosphatase.

Imaging studies include the gold standard test for BMD, Dual X-ray Absorptiometry (DXA, formerly DEXA). This is an accurate, precise, and fast examination, with low-radiation exposure. Evaluation uses comparison of one's BMD to that of a young adult reference population. Results are reported as T-scores (number of standard deviations away from the mean of a reference population, such as a young adult population) and Z-scores (number of standard deviations away from mean compared with adults of the same age and gender). Other imaging tests remain available but may overall have less impact on diagnosing the disease. X-ray, though useful in diagnosing acute fractures, is not as sensitive as DXA for detecting bone demineralization. Single photon absorptiometry and dual photon absorptiometry both require the use of radioactive isotopes. Quantitative Computed Tomography (CT) is expensive with the use of high-dose radiation, and ultrasound does not offer a precise measure of BMD.[9]

WORLD HEALTH ORGANIZATION DEFINITIONS

The WHO classifies osteopenia and osteoporosis within a range of T-scores. Normal bone density is noted as a T-score between −1 and +1 standard deviations. Osteopenia range is a T-score between −1 and −2.5 standard deviations, whereas osteoporosis has a T-score less than −2.5. Diagnosis of osteoporosis can be made, per 2020 AACE (American Association of Clinical Endocrinologists) Guidelines, if any of the following criteria are met. First, a fragility fracture (usually at a vertebrae or hip) results from minimal trauma and qualifies one regardless of BMD. Similarly, a T-score less than −2.5 in the lumbar spine, femoral neck, total proximal femur, and distal $\frac{1}{3}$ radius, would meet the criteria for osteoporosis. A T-score between −1.0 and −2.5 and either a fragility fracture of proximal humerus, pelvis or distal forearm, or a high risk of fracture on assessment tools (ie, FRAX score) also qualifies.[5,8]

Classification of Osteoporosis

Osteoporosis can be broken down to primary, which is the most common, and secondary. Primary osteoporosis includes postmenopausal or type 1, which usually occurs during the 15 to 20 years after menopause (50–65-years-old women). Type 1 osteoporosis results from a rapid decline in bone mass during a time when the protective effect of estrogen on the skeletal system is reduced. Trabecular bone loss is greater than cortical bone loss in this scenario. Type 2 or age-associated (senile) oste-oporosis affects females more than males in a 2:1 ratio and those over the age of 70 year old. In type 2 osteoporosis, loss of trabecular and cortical bone is about equal. Some cases would be classified as idiopathic in those less commonly affected individuals, such as juveniles, premenopausal women. Secondary osteoporosis (or type 3) results from another medical condition namely acquired or inherited diseases (**Table 1**).

TREATMENT RECOMMENDATIONS

In 2016, the AACE and the American College of Endocrinology created "Clinical Practice Guidelines for the Diagnosis and Treatment of Postmenopausal Osteoporosis", updated in 2020, and endorsed by the American Academy of Orthopedic Surgeons in December 2023 based on meta-analysis and reviews of prior clinical evidence.[5] Postmenopausal women with osteoporosis can be stratified according to high-risk and very high-risk features, including prior fractures. This stratification drives the choice of initial treatment agents and duration of therapies.[5]

Pharmacologic Management

Pharmacologic therapy is strongly recommended for patients with osteopenia or low bone mass and a history of fragility fracture of the hip or spine.[5] Clinicians in a variety of fields, including primary care, physical medicine, and rehabilitation, orthopedics, and rheumatology, may initiate treatment. Most osteoporotic patients with high fracture risk should be treated with oral bisphosphonates, such as Alendronate or Risedronate, as an appropriate initial therapy.[5] For those patients who are unable to tolerate oral therapy, infusion therapy with Abaloparatide, Denosumab, Romosozumab, Teriparatide, or Zoledronate should be considered as initial treatment.[5] Vitamin and mineral supplementation with Calcium and Vitamin D are additional recommendations.[5] Calcium is the mainstay for prevention and treatment, whereas Vitamin D works on osteoblasts to increase calcium absorption in the gut.

Bisphosphonates, as mentioned above, were first introduced in the 1990s and are the most widely used osteoporosis treatment medications.[5] The mechanism of action is that it binds to hydroxyapatite in the bone and reduces the activity of bony osteoclasts, or bone breakdown. The recommendation is oral administration after fasting overnight and then at least 30 min before eating breakfast.[5] Caution should be taken in patients with active esophageal disease; this group of medication is contraindicated in patients with drug hypersensitivity or hypocalcemia and should be used with caution in those with reduced renal function.[5]

Monoclonal Antibody Treatment, including denosumab (Prolia), romosozumab (Evenity), as mentioned above, work by decreasing both the differentiation of precursor cells into mature osteoclasts and the function and survival of activated osteoclasts. This class of medication offers broad-spectrum antifracture efficacy as early as 12 months after starting therapy.[5] Other recommendations include calcitonin nasal spray (Miacalcin, Fortical), which works by directly inhibiting osteoclast activity and has been shown to decrease pain in acute compression fractures, by stimulating beta endorphins.[5]

Selective estrogen-receptor modulators (SERMs), for example raloxifene (Evista), are approved by the Federal Drug Administration (FDA) for prevention and treatment of osteoporosis.[5] This class has been found to have an added benefit of reducing the risk of breast cancer in postmenopausal women. bazedoxifene (Duavee) is a SERM that has been studied for use in combination with conjugated equine estrogen.

Table 1
Classification of osteoporosis

Primary osteoporosis

Postmenopausal (type 1)   Age-associated or senile (type 2)

Secondary osteoporosis (type 3)

Endocrine/Metabolic	Nutritional/GI Conditions	Drug Side Effects	Collagen Disorders
• Acromegaly	• Alcoholism	• Antiepileptic drugs	• Ehlers-Danlos syndrome
• Diabetes mellitus	• Anorexia nervosa	• Aromatase inhibitors	• Homocystinuria
• Growth hormone deficiency	• Calcium deficiency	• Chemotherapy/immunosuppressants	• Marfan Syndrome
• Hypercortisolism	• Chronic liver disease	• Medroxyprogesterone acetate	• Osteogenesis imperfecta
• Hyperparathyroidism	• Malabsorption syndromes	• Glucocorticoids	Chronic Illness
• Hyperthyroidism	• Malnutrition	• Gonadotropin-releasing hormone agents	• AIDS/HIV
• Hypogonadism	• Vitamin D deficiency	• Heparin	• COPD
• Pregnancy	• Total parenteral nutrition	• Lithium	• Renal failure
• Porphyria		• Proton pump inhibitors	• Rheumatoid arthritis
		• Selective serotonin reuptake inhibitors	• Myeloma
		• SGLT2-inhibitors	
		• Thiazolidinediones	
		• Thyroid hormone.	

This pair is indicated for use in women with a uterus with moderate-to-severe vaso-motor symptoms associated with menopause.[5] Estrogen and other menopausal hormone therapies work on inhibiting osteoclasts by interleukin-6 suppression to decrease bone resorption and increase calcium absorption in the gut. Other anabolic agents include abaloparatide (Tymlos) and teriparatide (Forteo), which are injectable forms of recombinant human PTH.[5]

So how would one evaluate for successful treatment of osteoporosis? Clinicians will look for stable or increasing BMD, with no evidence of new fractures. Bone turnover markers can be a target for response to therapy for patients taking antiresorptive agents, and these markers should appear at or below the median value for premenopausal women. There may also be a significant increase in bone formation markers.[5]

Nonpharmacologic Treatment

Lifestyle changes are the main nonpharmacologic option for treatment. Weight-bearing activities and exercises are encouraged, as well as alcohol and smoking cessation. Multiple studies have shown that women who smoke cigarettes are at higher risk for osteoporotic fracture than nonsmokers, though the exact mechanism is unknown.[5] Excessive alcohol use dysregulates calcium and hormone signaling.

Nutritional considerations factor into osteoporosis treatment. Patients should be recommended calcium and Vitamin D3, especially those that are deficient in Vitamin D on bloodwork. A negative calcium balance will increase PTH and thus increase bone resorption. Postmenopausal women, between the ages of 51 and 70 years are recommended to have at least 1,200 mg of calcium per day from all sources.[5] Calcium supplementation remains a controversial topic; however, as various studies have suggested, there may be an increased risk of cardiovascular disease, stroke, and kidney stones associated with daily intake greater than 1,500-2,100 mg/day.[5] Individuals with a low body mass are at increased risk for rapid bone loss and low bone mass.

Physical exercise and activity remains a recommendation for treatment of osteoporosis. A history of fracture may lead an individual to develop avoidance and fear of physical activities and exercise. Avoidance can lead to further bone and muscle loss and risk for further disability and immobility. A physical therapy regimen should be tailored to each individual, and activities can be modified to mitigate risk and allow for safe participation. For example, rapid, weighted, repetitive or sustained exercises may be avoided, along with far end-range twisting or flexion of the spine and axial loading.[10] Exercise programs should target balance, gait and muscle strength, as these are the most effective way to prevent falls in older adults.

COMPLICATIONS OF OSTEOPOROSIS

Fracture risk increases with age, osteopenia, osteoporosis, falls, prior osteoporotic fractures, and certain medical comorbidities, such as chronic steroid use.[11] The first clinical indication of osteoporosis is usually a fracture due to minor trauma. Fractures can result in chronic pain, disfigurement, temporary disability but can also lead to a large decline in function resulting in a loss of independence for patients.

Vertebral Fractures

The most common of osteoporotic fractures are vertebral compression fractures. They are frequently seen in the lower thoracic and upper lumbar regions. More than two-thirds of patients with vertebral fractures are asymptomatic or found incidentally.[11] Evaluation of these patients include a thorough history and physical and

Table 2
Acute versus chronic vertebral fractures management

	Acute Vertebral Fractures	Chronic Vertebral Fractures
Symptoms	Severe pain at the fracture site	Less pain or asymptomatic
Treatment	Analgesics for pain relief Restrict flexion based activities Spinal bracing (see below). Physical therapy: Targeted to optimizing core strength, balance, flexibility, and body mechanics. Spinal augmentation procedures (see below)	Relative rest Analgesics for pain relief as needed Avoid flexion based activities Soft spinal brace for comfort Physical therapy

imaging (plain radiographs, CT scan, MRI, bone scan). The classic radiographic finding is an anterior wedge-shaped fracture (**Table 2**).

Spinal augmentation procedures
Spinal augmentation procedures are an option for those patients with inadequate pain relief with conservative measures. Balloon kyphoplasty is a minimally invasive procedure aimed at restoring vertebral body height and reducing pain. A needle is inserted into the site of the fracture and then a balloon is inflated thus restoring the height and shape of the vertebra. The balloon is later deflated and the remaining cavity is filled with cement.[11] A vertebroplasty is similar to kyphoplasty, but no balloon is used, rather cement is injected directly into the vertebral body. Common complications of these procedures include extravasation of cement, infection, embolism, and neurologic injury.[11]

Spinal bracing
Bracing of vertebral fractures is indicated for pain relief (spinal immobilization leading to decreased paraspinal muscle spasms), spinal stabilization, decrease flexion, and to compensate for weak erector spinae muscles (**Table 3**). Bracing is not typically used for patients with hiatal and inguinal hernias, orthopnea secondary to chronic obstructive pulmonary disease (COPD) and kyphoscoliosis. Long term use is not indicated due to atrophy of the core musculature with prolonged use.

Hip Fractures

Hip fractures often occur due to weakness in the lower extremities and disequilibrium from individuals with kyphotic postures. They are the most serious complication of osteoarthritis (OA) and the most severe of osteoporotic fractures.[12] They are a significant cause of morbidity and mortality. The incidence of hip fractures increases largely between the ages of 60 to 85.[12] The typical presentation is that of an externally rotated and shortened limb. Patients should be evaluated with a thorough history and physical and radiographic imaging (X-rays, CT scan, MRI).

Treatment of hip fractures includes analgesics for pain relief as needed and surgical fixation depending on the site of the fracture. Types of fractures include intracapsular (ie: femoral neck) and extracapsular (ie: trochanteric) fractures. Intracapsular fractures require surgical fixation with internal fixation, hemiarthroplasty, or total hip arthroplasty, whereas extracapsular fractures can be managed with internal fixation. All surgical patients will require therapy postoperatively. Of note, other low trauma fractures

Table 3
Types of available spinal orthoses

	Type	Example	Benefits
Non-Rigid Bracing	Abdominal binder	Elastic type	Increases intraabdominal pressure and reduced axial load Used in stable fractures
Rigid Bracing	Thoracolumbar brace	Jewett brace, cruciform anterior spinal hypertension CASH brace	Increases intraabdominal pressure Assists in spine extension and limits flexion
	TLSO	Taylor brace, Knight-Taylor brace	Most restrictive

Abbreviations: CASH, cruciform anterior spinal hypertension; TLSO, Thoracolumbosacral orthosis.

that are also commonly seen in those with osteoporosis are fractures at the proximal humerus, pelvis, and distal forearm.

Prevention of Fractures

Prevention begins with managing medical conditions that predispose one to falls and/or osteoporosis, including, but not limited to, obesity, insulin resistance, celiac disease, rheumatologic disorders, hormonal imbalances, vision correction, cautious use of medications that cause dizziness, or chronic glucocorticoid use in chronic illness. Similarly, exercise programs that target balance, gait and muscle strength are the most effective way to prevent falls in older adults.[13] Particularly effective are exercises that improve leg strength through resistance and strength training, including balance, gait, coordination, and functional exercises for activities of daily living.[14] One study found that back extensor strengthening exercises helped prevent refracture rates in patients with prior vertebral fractures.[15]

DISCUSSION
Future Considerations

Osteoporosis prevalence and burden of care are forecasted to increase over the following years given the aging population.[16] Current researchers are looking into new ways to help detect and treat osteoporosis. Biomarkers such as microRNA and long-noncoding RNA control gene expression and are promising in the development of future therapeutic agents to manage osteoporosis.[16] Research into novel biomarkers that will help with the early detection of osteoporosis is also being done. The modulation of osteocyte activity is also a potential target in optimizing bone mass.[17] It has been noted that one of the biggest challenges is optimizing the use of the treatments that already exist, making room for changes and/or ways to optimize existing treatment models and for newer treatments to come.[17]

Current Controversies

Menopausal Hormone Therapy (MHT) has become a controversial topic in women's health care. A benefit–risk evaluation does support the use of MHT in women less than 10 years from onset of menopause, less than 60 year old, and those at low risk for adverse events—that is, cardiovascular events, thromboembolic disease, stroke-, and breast cancer.[18] The risks of these hormone therapies differ depending on the type, dose, duration of use, route of administration, timing of initiation, and whether a progestogen is used. Frequent reevaluation is necessary to ensure continued benefit outweighs risk. MHT has shown significant antifracture efficacy while in use but without lasting skeletal benefits after being stopped.[18]

Overall, despite the wide availability of screening tools and FDA approved medications for the diagnosis and treatment of osteoporosis, many patients remain undiagnosed and untreated. Medication compliance has been impacted by societal concerns about the safety of these drugs in the setting of rare but serious side effects being discussed in the news - that is, atypical femoral fractures and osteonecrosis of the jaw. Early detection and education are key to treating this patient population.

SUMMARY

Osteoporosis prevalence and burden of care are a rising concern worldwide due to an aging female population. Broad screening can assist with early detection of low BMD and associated risk factors that could help reduce fracture rates and thus morbidity and mortality. Fracture rates can be further reduced by making lifestyle changes, including exercise, nutritional supplementation, smoking and alcohol cessation. Those who have had fractures and are at higher osteoporotic risk should be initiated on pharmacologic therapy. Furthermore, it is important to use a multidisciplinary approach in caring for woman with osteoporosis, and this should include, primary care monitoring, rehabilitative efforts, including pain management and bracing, as well as psychosocial support.

CLINICS CARE POINTS

- Screening: DXA scan for women over the age of 50 and inclusion of other fracture-risk assessment tools.
- Diagnosis, one of the following criteria:
  - Low trauma fragility fracture
  - T score less than -2.5 at the lumbar spine, femoral neck, total hip or distal $\frac{1}{3}$ radius on dual X-ray absorptiometry scan
  - T score between -1.0 and -2.5 with elevated fracture risk on risk assessment tools
- Treatment: Risk assessment drives pharmacologic choice and duration.
- Evaluate: For secondary causes of osteoporosis.
- Prevention: Exercise, nutrition, and lifestyle modification.
- Complications: Fractures due to minimal trauma are most commonly seen as vertebral compression fractures, but also include hip, proximal humerus, pelvis and distal radius fractures.

DISCLOSURES

The authors have nothing to disclose.

REFERENCES

1. Lorentzon M, Johansson H, Harvey NC, et al. Osteoporosis and fractures in women: the burden of disease. Climacteric 2022;25(1):4–10.

2. Clynes MA, Harvey NC, Curtis EM, et al. The epidemiology of osteoporosis. Br Med Bull 2020;133(1):105–17.

3. Osteoporosis fast facts, *Bone Health and Osteoporosis Foundation*, 2024, Available at: https://www.bonehealthandosteoporosis.org/patients/what-is-osteoporosis (Accessed 18 April 2024).

4. Epidemiology of osteoporosis and fragility fractures, *International Osteoporosis Foundation*, 2024, Available at: https://www.osteoporosis.foundation/facts-statistics/epidemiology-of-osteoporosis-and-fragility-fractures#ref_17 (Accessed 18 April 2024).

5. Camacho PM, Petak SM, Binkley N, et al. AMERICAN association of clinical endocrinologists/AMERICAN college of endocrinology clinical practice guidelines for the diagnosis and treatment of postmenopausal OSTEOPOROSIS-2020 update. Endocr Pract 2020;26(Suppl 1):1–46.

6. "Osteoporosis", NIH: National Institute of arthritis and Musculoskeletal and Skin disease, Available at: https://www.niams.nih.gov/health-topics/osteoporosis/basics/symptoms-causes, (Accessed 18 April 2024), 2024.

7. Renkema KY, Alexander RT, Bindels RJ, et al. Calcium and phosphate homeostasis: concerted interplay of new regulators. Ann Med 2008;40(2):82–91.

8. Silverman SL, Calderon AD. The utility and limitations of FRAX: a US perspective. Curr Osteoporos Rep 2010;8(4):192–7.

9. Sabri SA, Chavarria JC, Ackert-Bicknell C, et al. Osteoporosis: an update on screening, diagnosis, evaluation, and treatment. Orthopedics 2023;46(1):e20–6.

10. Giangregorio L, Katzman WB. Exercise and other physical therapy interventions in the management of osteoporosis, Chapter 69, . Marcus and Feldman's Osteoporosis. p. 1649–63.

11. McCarthy J, Davis A. Diagnosis and management of vertebral compression fractures. Am Fam Physician 2016;94(1):44–50.

12. Ip TP, Leung J, Kung AW. Management of osteoporosis in patients hospitalized for hip fractures. Osteoporos Int 2010;21(Suppl 4):S605–14.

13. Khandelwal S, Lane NE. Osteoporosis: review of etiology, mechanisms, and approach to management in the aging population. Endocrinol Metab Clin N Am 2023;52(2):259–75.

14. Poulton G, Matney BF, Williams T, et al. Exercise to reduce falls in older adults. Am Fam Physician 2020;101(1):42–3.

15. Huntoon E, Schmidt CK, Sinaki M. Significantly fewer refractures after vertebroplasty in patients who engage in back-extensor-strengthening exercises. Mayo Clin Proc 2008;83(1):54–7.

16. Adami G, Fassio A, Gatti D, et al. Osteoporosis in 10 years time: a glimpse into the future of osteoporosis. Ther Adv Musculoskelet Dis 2022;14. 1759720X221083541.

17. Bone H. Future directions in osteoporosis therapeutics. Endocrinol Metab Clin North Am 2012;41(3):655–61.

18. Rozenberg S, Al-Daghri N, Aubertin-Leheudre M, et al. Is there a role for menopausal hormone therapy in the management of postmenopausal osteoporosis? Osteoporos Int 2020;31(12):2271–86.

Considerations for Long COVID Rehabilitation in Women

Monica Verduzco-Gutierrez, MD[a],*, Talya K. Fleming, MD[b,1],
Alba M. Azola, MD[c,2]

KEYWORDS

- Long coronavirus disease
- Post-acute sequelae of severe acute respiratory syndrome coronavirus 2
- Postural orthostatic tachycardia syndrome • Myalgic encephalomyelitis • Women
- Female • Gender differences

KEY POINTS

- Long coronavirus disease 2019 (COVID), or post-acute sequelae of severe acute respiratory syndrome coronavirus 2, presents a complex and prolonged disease course that extends beyond the acute phase of COVID-19 infection.
- Women are disproportionately affected by long COVID, with higher prevalence rates compared to men, despite traditional risk factors not fully explaining this disparity.
- Rehabilitation efforts for long COVID in women must address health equity concerns and consider the historic context of stigmatized infection-associated chronic conditions.

INTRODUCTION

In the wake of the coronavirus disease 2019 (COVID-19) pandemic, the world faces a new challenge beyond the acute phase of infection: long COVID. Emerging as a consequence of severe acute respiratory syndrome coronavirus 2 (SARS-CoV-2) infection, Long COVID or post-acute sequelae of SARS-CoV-2 (PASC) presents a complex and prolonged disease course that extends far beyond the initial acute illness

[a] Department of Rehabilitation Medicine, University of Texas Health Science Center at San Antonio, 7703 Floyd Curl Drive, MC7798, San Antonio, TX 78229, USA; [b] Department of Physical Medicine and Rehabilitation, JFK Johnson Rehabilitation Institute at Hackensack Meridian Health, 65 James Street, Edison, NJ, USA; [c] Pediatrics Division of Adolescent Medicine, Department of Physical Medicine and Rehabilitation, Johns Hopkins University School of Medicine
[1] Present address: 1346 Bradford Street, Plainfield, NJ 07063.
[2] Present address: 10116 Falls Road, Lutherville, MD 21093.
* Corresponding author.
E-mail address: Gutierrezm19@uthscsa.edu

Phys Med Rehabil Clin N Am 36 (2025) 371–387
https://doi.org/10.1016/j.pmr.2024.11.009
1047-9651/25/© 2024 Elsevier Inc. All rights reserved, including those for text and data mining, AI training, and similar technologies.

pmr.theclinics.com

Abbreviations	
AAPM&R	American Academy of Physical Medicine and Rehabilitation
CFS	chronic fatigue syndrome
COVID-19	coronavirus disease 2019
GET	graded exercise therapy
ICU	intensive care unit
ME	myalgic encephalomyelitis
PASC	post-acute sequelae of severe acute respiratory syndrome coronavirus 2
PEM	post-exertional malaise
POTS	Postural orthostatic tachycardia syndrome
SARS-CoV-2	severe acute respiratory syndrome coronavirus 2

with different definitions putting a time course of anywhere from symptoms at 4 weeks to 3 months and lasting years. Defined by a myriad of new, recurring, or ongoing fluctuating and unpredictable signs and symptoms persisting after an acute COVID-19 infection, long COVID can impact many organ systems including respiratory, vascular, cardiac, neurologic, autonomic, gastrointestinal, immunologic, endocrinologic, and musculoskeletal. Other terms have been used to refer to this disease state including the aforementioned PASC, post-COVID syndrome, and post-COVID conditions. This article will use long COVID, a term created by the patient community and now given a standardized definition by the National Academy of Science, Engineering, and Medicine.[1]

Delving into the history and background of long COVID unveils a landscape rife with unanswered questions and evolving understanding as often occurs with infection-associated chronic conditions. Initially characterized by its association with acute COVID-19 infection, long COVID has since emerged as a distinct entity, marked by its persistence and variability in symptomatology. Despite concerted efforts to unravel its pathophysiological mechanisms and identify risk factors, diagnostic and treatment modalities for long COVID remain inadequate.

An intriguing aspect of long COVID lies in its disproportionate impact on women. While mortality and acute morbidity from COVID-19 infection tend to be lower in females compared to males, females find themselves overrepresented among patients grappling with long COVID.[1-7] Women are more likely than men to ever have long COVID, and women are also more likely than men to currently have long COVID.[7] Notably, factors traditionally associated with a heightened risk of severe acute COVID-19, such as advanced age or male sex, fail to align with the increased prevalence of long COVID among women. The reasons underlying disparities in sex and gender distribution between acute and chronic COVID-19 manifestations continue to elude definitive explanation but are being researched.

This article explores considerations specific to the rehabilitation of women affected by long COVID. Identifying that there have always been well-known health disparities for females—who are also more impacted by other infection-associated chronic conditions like myalgic encephalomyelitis/chronic fatigue syndrome (ME/CFS) or dysautonomia[8] coronavirus disease 2019—it is essential to recognize the health equity concerns and provide the best rehabilitation care for these individuals. Multidisciplinary collaborative consensus guidance statements have been developed that address multiple symptoms related to long COVID (eg, fatigue,[9] cognitive deficits,[10] cardiovascular sequelae,[11] respiratory sequelae,[12] autonomic dysfunction,[8] neurologic disorders,[13] mental health conditions,[14] and pediatric impacts[15]). These statements specifically also address issues related to health equity inclusive of assessments and solutions to address biologic sex differences. By considering the historic context of stigmatized infection-associated chronic conditions and understanding the background of long COVID's multiple signs, symptoms, and related conditions, we aim to shed light on the unique challenges and opportunities in addressing long COVID in this demographic. Through a comprehensive understanding of the intersection between sex, gender, and long COVID, we hope to pave the way for more effective rehabilitation strategies tailored to the needs of women enduring the lingering effects of this novel coronavirus.

EPIDEMIOLOGY

The estimated prevalence of long COVID varies depending on how studies define long COVID, the population studied, and the methodology. A global metanalysis systematic review reported the prevalence to be 54% for hospitalized patients and 34% for non-hospitalized, with a wide range contributing to this estimate (9%–81%).[16] Albeit wide ranges in overall prevalence, they all consistently reported higher prevalence in females (49%) versus males (37%).[16] The Centers for Disease Control estimates that 6.9% of all US adults have experienced long COVID.[7] Women are predominantly affected (8.5%) compared to males (5.2%), with over 14 million American women living with long COVID. A large cross-sectional US study identified middle age, female sex, lack of a college degree, and severity of acute COVID-19 infection as risk factors for long COVID.[17] UK data on non-hospitalized patients with Long COVID noted risk factors including female sex, belonging to an ethnic minority, socioeconomic deprivation, smoking, and obesity, with an increased risk along a gradient of decreasing age.[18]

Several theoretic explanations are proposed to explain the female preponderance in Long COVID, including hormonal differences that perpetuate a hyperinflammatory status, stronger immunoglobulin G production, and the hypothesis that women are generally more attentive to their body and related distress.[19] Long COVID shares similar features with post-acute infectious syndromes, such as ME/CFS and post-treatment Lyme disease, which also disproportionately affect female patients. In 1970, 2 psychiatrists in the United Kingdom (UK) reviewed reports of 15 outbreaks of benign ME. They concluded that these outbreaks *were psychosocial phenomena caused by one of two mechanisms, either mass hysteria on the part of the patients or altered medical perception of the community.*[20] They based their conclusions on the higher prevalence of the disease in females and the lack of physical signs in these patients. The historic perception that the etiology of these clinical entities is non-organic has pervaded through modern medicine, which as a community, generally questions the existence or seriousness of this disease in females. Scientific advancement and a growing interest in understanding sex differences promise to advance the biologic underpinnings of the factors playing a role in the high female prevalence.

CLINICAL PRESENTATION
Overview of Long Coronavirus Disease in Women

Understanding the basic tenets of long COVID is critical in understanding how its influence may affect women differently. Symptom presentation of long COVID is heterogeneous, varies depending on the time course after infection, and is largely underreported. Current research postulates potentially overlapping etiologies with systemic consequences (eg, organ injury, immune dysregulation, autoimmunity, tissue and organ injury, pathogen persistence/reactivation, hypoperfusion, fibrin amyloid microclots, neuroinflammation and autonomic dysfunction, and gut microbiome dysbiosis).[21,22] Research suggests that the most frequent symptoms are fatigue, post-exertional malaise, and cognitive dysfunction.[21,23] A larger study revealed that the frequencies of new-onset symptoms were post-exertional malaise (PEM) (28%), fatigue (37%), dizziness (21%), brain fog (20%), and gastrointestinal symptoms (20%).[21] There have been documented over 203 symptoms of long COVID, with symptoms recognized in over 10 organ systems.[23] PEM refers to the aggravation of symptoms after engaging in even minor physical or mental activity. This phenomenon is characterized by a gradual worsening of symptoms that can last for days or even weeks, with the symptoms often peaking between 12 and 48 hours after the activity.[9] The severity of the symptoms may vary depending on the individual and the nature of the activity. It is important to note that PEM is a significant challenge for individuals with long COVID, as it can severely limit their ability to engage in daily activities and have a negative impact on their quality-of-life. PEM and post-exertional symptom exacerbation may trigger relapses in symptoms after physical, cognitive, emotional, or psychological stress.[23]

According to the Centers for Disease Control and Prevention, in the United States, women (8.5%) were more likely than men (5.2%) to ever have long COVID, and women (4.4%) were also more likely than men (2.3%) to currently have long COVID.[24–26] Factors contributing to poorer long-term outcomes included younger age, female sex, less education,[25] and higher severity of acute disease.[22] Females under age 50 and those with more severe in-hospital acute disease had the worst long-term outcomes.[22] Compared to men, females under the age of 50 years were twice as likely to feel worsened fatigue (adjusted odds ratio [OR] 2.06, 95% confidence interval [CI] 0.81–3.31), 7 times more likely to become more breathless (adjusted OR 7.15, 95% CI 2.24–22.83), 5 times less likely to report feeling recovered (adjusted OR 5.09, 95% CI 1.64–15.74), and more likely to have a greater disability (adjusted OR 4.22, 95% CI 1.12–15.94).[22] Moreover, the female sex was significantly associated with increased problems in the usual activity, pain/discomfort, and anxiety/depression domains, leading to a diminished quality-of-life.[22] Females are more likely to survive severe acute COVID-19 disease than men, possibly resulting in worse long-term outcomes.[22,27] Beyond the hormonal impact of estrogen, more research is needed to elucidate the biopsychosocial determinants that may explain differences between the sexes.[22,26 28]

Select Neuropsychiatric Disparities

Evidence supports that females are disproportionately affected by post-acute neurologic sequelae of SARS-CoV-2.[29] In a large sample of hospitalized adults, approximately 70% of patients had multiple neurologic symptoms at the first follow-up (median = 102 days).[29] Notable gender differences were documented as women experienced more headaches, compared to paresthesias, anosmia, disorientation, confusion, and sleep disorders noted in both genders.[30] Compared to males, females (OR = 1.34, CI = 1.237, 1.451) are more likely to have cognitive deficits with difficulty remembering.[31] The most prevalent reported psychiatric symptoms were anxiety, depression, post-traumatic stress disorder, poor sleep qualities, somatic symptoms, and cognitive deficits.[32] Being female and having a previous psychiatric diagnosis were risk factors for the development of the reported psychiatric long COVID symptoms.[32,33] At 12 months, anosmia and dysgeusia were resolved in most patients, although fatigue, altered consciousness, and myalgia remained unresolved in greater than 10% of the cohort.[29] In females, neurologic symptom prevalence was higher and had a longer time to the resolution (5.2 vs 3.4 months) at follow-up for those with more than 1 neurologic symptom.[29]

Select Cardiovascular Disparities

Several cardiovascular derangements exist after long COVID, which are more prevalent in women. Postural orthostatic tachycardia syndrome (POTS) is a common form of autonomic dysregulation characterized as excessive tachycardia upon standing in the presence of orthostatic intolerance.[34] POTS is a common representation of the cardiovascular dysfunction that can occur after long COVID. The prevalence of POTS in the general US population varies, with estimates between 0.1 and 1%, and a higher incidence among females.[35,36] Despite its prevalence, POTS in the general population is likely significantly underdiagnosed.[37] POTS occurs most frequently in females ages 12 to 50, and is uncommon in young children.[38] Patients may report clinical symptoms of palpitations and tachycardia, worsened with positional changes from seated to standing or lying to seated positions. Of the patients who reported tachycardia, 72.8% reported being able to measure their heart rate in standing versus sitting posture. Of those, 30.65% reported an increase in heart rate of at least 30 beats per minute on standing, suggesting the possibility of POTS.[23] Within the context of long COVID, reports suggest that between 2% and 14% of survivors may develop POTS, with an additional 9% to 61% experiencing POTS-like symptoms within 6 to 8 months after SARS-CoV-2 infection, and up to 25% of long COVID patients reporting dysautonomia.[37,39–41] Equally important, orthostatic hypotension has been reported in 14% of subjects with long COVID symptoms.[42]

Select Endocrine Disparities

Endocrinologic changes related to reproductive health can also be seen in women with long COVID. Menstruating persons have reported menstrual cycle irregularities (eg, changes to the length of the cycle, duration, and intensity of the menses).[43] More than a third of menstruating participants experienced non-reproductive long COVID symptom exacerbations during or before menstruation.[23,43] In a cross-sectional survey in Ecuador, the most common long COVID symptoms in pregnant women were fatigue (10.6%), hair loss (9.6%), and difficulty concentrating (6.2%).[44] Perimenopausal women with long COVID are more likely to demonstrate more frailty-related factors and experience a higher rate of disability.[45] Surprisingly, postmenopausal bleeding has been reported in 4.5% of 1123 cisgender women aged 49 years or older.[43] Future patient-centered research should focus on the impact of long COVID and associated conditions for menstruating persons at various stages of their reproductive life.

ASSESSMENT/EVALUATION

The comprehensive assessment and evaluation protocol for long COVID patients is designed to address the multifaceted nature of this condition, recognizing its wide-ranging impacts on physical health, cardiopulmonary health, neurologic function, cognitive abilities, and mental well-being. Beyond the initial evaluation, ongoing monitoring over time and management are essential components of care. Regular reassessment of activity performance and functional status allows for adjustments in treatment strategies to meet evolving patient needs. By incorporating standardized measures and patient-reported outcomes, health care providers can track progress, identify areas of improvement, and tailor interventions accordingly. Moreover, the psychosocial aspect of long COVID cannot be understated. The integration of mental health screening and consideration of social determinants of health ensures a holistic approach to patient-care. Collaborative efforts with specialists across disciplines facilitate a comprehensive understanding of the condition and enable a coordinated approach to management. Regular follow-up appointments serve not only to monitor physical and cognitive progress but also to provide ongoing support and guidance to patients as they navigate the challenges of long COVID.

Performing a thorough physical examination is crucial for both ruling out treatable causes of the presenting symptoms and for clinically diagnosing long COVID. This examination should be preceded by a detailed history that also characterizes the severity of symptoms experienced and their impact on quality-of-life. Key areas of focus during the physical examination include neurologic, cardiovascular, pulmonary, musculoskeletal, and psychiatric assessments. It is important to review vital signs and consider additional components such as 10-minute passive stand test for those with postural symptoms, dizziness, fatigue, cognitive impairment, or malaise. Ambulatory pulse oximetry may be warranted for those with respiratory symptoms, fatigue, or malaise. Given the high prevalence of autonomic dysfunction and orthostatic intolerance in women with long COVID, further autonomic testing could include a National Aeronautics and Space Administration (NASA) lean test, tilt table testing, and/or thermoregulatory sweat testing.[8]

In evaluating persons who menstruate and pregnant persons with long COVID, a comprehensive and sensitive approach is paramount. Health care providers should consider the unique physiologic and hormonal influences that may influence symptom presentation and severity. The history should include menstruation history and exogenous hormone use. Pregnant individuals may also require alternative diagnostic testing that prioritizes the safety of both the woman and the developing fetus while ensuring accurate diagnosis and appropriate management of the health condition. See **Table 1** for selected considerations and recommendations related to biologic sex and gender.

Finally, as our understanding of long COVID evolves, it becomes necessary to adopt a flexible and adaptive approach to both assessment and management. Ongoing research into the long-term effects of COVID-19 plays a pivotal role in informing clinical practice and will prompt refinements in treatment protocols and rehabilitation strategies. Continuous education and training for health care professionals are vital to keep pace with emerging evidence and best practices in the care of individuals with long COVID. By remaining receptive to evolving knowledge and patient needs, health care teams can uphold the delivery of high-quality, evidence-based care.

PATHOGENESIS

As research on long COVID starts to shed light on the pathophysiologic mechanisms involved, a growing number of publications highlight persistent inflammation and immune activation as a key feature of long COVID but without considering how females are more likely than males to experience these symptoms. A recent sex difference study in long COVID highlights the potentially crucial role of immune-endocrine dysregulation in sex-specific pathology. They found an overall higher symptom burden in females, an immune profile with exhausted T-cells, cytokine-secreting T cells, higher antibody reactivity to latent herpes viruses including epstein-barr virus (EBV), herpes simplex virus-2 (HSV-2), and cytomegalovirus (CMV), and lower testosterone levels than controls. Interestingly, higher testosterone levels were significantly associated with lower symptom burden in long COVID participants over sex designation.[46]

There is also evidence on how the menstrual cycle influences long COVID symptoms, with over one-third of pre-menopausal women with long COVID experiencing worsening of premenstrual symptoms and/or exacerbation of long COVID symptoms

Table 1
Selected health equity clinical recommendations and considerations related to sex included in the American Academy of Physical Medicine and Rehabilitation post-acute sequelae of severe acute respiratory syndrome coronavirus 2 consensus guidance statements

Health Equity Category	Autonomic Dysfunction[8]	Breathing Discomfort[12]	Cardiovascular Symptoms[11]	Cognitive Symptoms[10]	Fatigue[9]
Biologic sex	Clinicians should be aware of sex-related bias, which may add to diagnostic delays faced by female patients.	Pregnant people may have baseline respiratory discomfort exacerbated by COVID-19/PASC; Alternative diagnostic testing and treatment may be required.	Clinicians should be aware that females may be underdiagnosed and undertreated for cardiac conditions (including referrals to cardiac rehabilitation) and should work to ensure equitable care.	Pregnant/postpartum people may experience cognitive dysfunction difficult to differentiate from PASC; Alternative diagnostic testing and treatment may be needed.	Pregnant people may experience pregnancy-related fatigue and require alternative diagnostic testing and treatment to differentiate from PASC.
Gender				Women may report PASC cognitive dysfunction more than men.	Gender affirming care should be considered regarding impact on fatigue (eg, exogenous hormone use, sleep, mental health).

related to their menstrual cycle.[23] Women experiencing long COVID are often middle-aged and may also be experiencing symptoms and hormonal changes associated with peri-menopause and post-menopause syndromes. Another study reported changes in menstrual cycle duration, bleeding between periods, increased menstrual flow, and missed periods associated to long COVID.[47]

Regarding acute COVID-19, males are at higher risk than females for severe disease and carry a higher risk of mortality.[43,48] The plausible mechanisms behind this finding are the upregulation of ACE2 receptors in the lungs mediated by testosterone, imbalance of expression on genes, epigenetic modification, and direct effects of sex hormones on immunologic pathways.[43,48]

BURDEN OF DISEASE

Individuals with long COVID report protracted, multisystem derangement resulting in significant disability.[23] Women have an additional burden not only on the physiologic effects of long COVID, but also with the societal consequences of ongoing disability after COVID-19 infection. Loss of school and work participation is especially common in young women,[49] having psychological and economic consequences. By 7 months, many patients express significant ongoing symptoms and are unable to return to previous levels of work.[23] Due to persistent illness, nearly half of the unrecovered respondents were working reduced hours, and 23.3% were unable to work.[23] Individuals with long COVID have a myriad of concerns that plague (eg, applying for sick leave, qualifying for disability leave, being fired from their current position, quitting their employment, and being unable to find a job that will accommodate them).[23] Autonomic dysfunction in long COVID has been shown to have a substantial impact on an individual's functioning and quality-of-life in the short-term, medium-term, and long-term.[50] In a study involving 20 patients with long COVID (70% female), residual autonomic symptoms persisted in 85% of participants 6 to 8 months after COVID-19, with 60% unable to return to work.[51] Halloot and colleagues investigated a sample of 40 long COVID POTS patients and found that disabling symptoms persisted in 100% of previously high-functioning participants even after 6 months, indicating the enduring impact of long COVID POTS.[52] Studies show that women, people of color, sexual and gender minorities, and people without college degrees are more likely to have symptoms of long COVID and resultant activity limitations from long COVID.[25,28] Clinical care should take into account social determinants of health to overcome barriers including economic (medical expenses, lack of insurance, etc.), geographic (underserved areas, access to care, etc.), housing, and segregation, and occupational factors that negatively impact vulnerable and minoritized populations.[28,31]

MANAGEMENT IN WOMEN AND IN PREGNANCY

The current medical interventions for long COVID are based on symptomatic management, and there are no Food and Drug Administration-approved medications for the treatment of post-COVID Conditions. The Multidisciplinary PASC Collaborative of the American Academy of Physical Medicine and Rehabilitation (AAPM&R) has published guidance statements with recommendations on the pharmacologic management of common long COVID presentations.[8–15] Special consideration should be given regarding medication management for autonomic dysfunction in the female patient, particularly those of reproductive age. Most first-line medications are considered category C for pregnancy, meaning the increased risk during pregnancy cannot be ruled out. There are no pregnancy or lactation studies on fludrocortisone specifically; however, the data concerning glucocorticoid use in pregnancy suggest an increased risk for cleft palate and possible impaired fetal growth and an otherwise a relatively safe profile.[53] The American Academy of Pediatrics classifies glucocorticoids as compatible with breastfeeding.[54] As midodrine is an alpha-1 agonist, there is a theoretic concern that it might cause uterine arterial constriction and therefore be associated with intra-uterine growth retardation. There are no abundant human data on pregnancy or lactation concerning this agent. The pregnancy data for propranolol have not indicated an increased risk for teratogenicity; however, an association with neonatal apnea, respiratory distress, bradycardia, and hypoglycemia has been suggested.[55] The American Academy of Pediatrics classifies propranolol as compatible with breastfeeding.[54] Second-line agent use in the management of POTS, pyridostigmine, has no data indicating an increased risk for teratogenicity or adverse perinatal outcomes and is classified as category B for pregnancy.[56] The World Health Organization and the American Academy of Pediatrics classify pyridostigmine as compatible with breastfeeding.[54] Patients being started on ivabradine, a second-line medication used for heart rate control in POTS, must be advised to use contraception as this medication is considered category D for pregnancy. Animal studies have revealed evidence of embryo fetal toxicity, teratogenicity, increased post-implantation loss, and increased intrauterine and postnatal mortality.[57] There are no controlled data on human pregnancy for ivabradine.

From a clinical perspective, it is notable that during pregnancy, patients often notice that they have better control of their orthostatic symptoms, usually beginning at the end of the first trimester. This occurs in part because blood volume is increased by about 2 L during pregnancy. This often enables a reduction or elimination of helpful medications before the pregnancy.

DISCUSSION

Early in the pandemic, when intensive care units (ICUs) were full of gravely ill patients, physiatrists, and rehabilitation professionals provided rehabilitative care for persons who were impacted by more severe SARS-CoV-2 infections. Once deemed less/non-contagious, hospitalized patients with COVID-19 began to get therapy services based on prior protocols developed for ICU rehabilitation, including for ventilated patients. This was at times limited by access to personal protective equipment and fears of the spread of an airborne virus outside of the room. Despite the gravity of the situation and at times the need to close rehabilitation units, the field of rehabilitation medicine stepped up to provide rehabilitation across the continuum for persons with sequelae of COVID-19.[58,59] Inpatient rehabilitation units/hospitals prepared themselves and also began to take patients with effects of critical illness, transplants, strokes, and other devastating sequelae of COVID-19.[60,61] Much of the rehabilitations occurred in hospitals and inpatient units at the start of the pandemic and then there was a realization of a new group of persons who were not hospitalized were having ongoing or new symptoms requiring attention and rehabilitation services. Those persons who often developed long COVID had mild initial infections and did not get any medical attention early in the pandemic. Again, physiatrists stepped up to address this gap to address the many needs of patients with long COVID.[61]

A comprehensive rehabilitation plan should be created based on a patient's specific diagnosis and symptoms. Timing of initiation can occur concurrently with additional workup if there is low concern for an urgent or life-threatening additional disease process. Services considered should include physical therapy, occupational therapy, speech and language therapy, vocational therapy (along with guidance for return-to-work with or without accommodations), and neurologic rehabilitation for cognitive symptoms, including neuropsychologist evaluation and treatment. Some patients may also benefit from a multidisciplinary team inclusive of social work, psychology, and nutrition.

A physiatrist can help create a rehabilitation plan, inclusive of an individualized return to activity program. Specification of duration and intensity is recommended as some patients (those with PEM and fatigue) may benefit from much slower-paced rehabilitation strategies.[9,62] The strategy of the 4 P's can be used in determining a rehabilitation plan: pacing, prioritizing, positioning, and planning. Pacing avoids PEM and/or a crash following activity that is too intense for the patient's current functional level, which could result in prolonged periods of more intense fatigue and functional limitations. Prioritizing works on energy conservation strategies in identifying necessary tasks to prevent overexertion that may come from tackling additional tasks that can be postponed or avoided. Positioning involves modifying the placement of items to make activities easier, such as using a shower chair. Planning allows patients to plan ahead into the week by matching activities to times during the week and/or days when they may experience relatively higher energy levels.

Individuals with cognitive impairment can benefit from speech and language therapy for cognitive evaluation and treatment, as well as a neuropsychology evaluation and treatment. Those who experience mental fatigue may also benefit from pacing of cognitive activity with gradual increase as tolerated.[10] Other neurologic and neuromuscular symptoms may benefit from aqua therapy, vision therapy, vestibular therapy, olfactory training, and/or taste recall training programs.[13] Therapeutic modalities can be considered for musculoskeletal and pain-related symptoms (ice/heat, myofascial release, massage, transcutaneous electrical stimulation, kinesiotaping, and desensitization techniques).

Individuals with cardiac symptoms may benefit from cardiac rehabilitation with monitoring and pacing of their activity level with a gradual increase as tolerated. However, those with new cardiac diagnoses should receive cardiac clearance prior to participation.[11,63] Those with pulmonary symptoms may benefit from a formal pulmonary rehabilitation program, as well as breathing techniques and airway clearance exercises and/or devices.[12] Of note, insurance coverage for outpatient pulmonary rehabilitation was expanded to include those with suspected or confirmed COVID-19 who are experiencing persistent pulmonary symptoms for at least 4 weeks.[64]

Autonomic rehabilitation programs should be considered for those with orthostatic intolerance or dysautonomia. Recumbent, semi-recumbent, and mat-level exercises can be utilized in those who have trouble maintaining or excessive symptoms in a standing position. Breathwork exercise, careful titration of exercises, and restorative and adaptive therapies are important components for these patients.[8,65] There have also been case reports for enhanced external counterpulsation as a suitable treatment method for autonomic dysfunction, fatigue, and cognitive dysfunction.[65,66] It cannot be understated that rehabilitation strategies after COVID-19 are individualized. The rehabilitation team should help avoid acute events and symptom flare-ups, facilitate expectations, provide psychological and emotional support, and in some cases, improve/maintain general function.[67]

A challenge exists in rehabilitating individuals with long COVID who exhibit a phenotype similar to ME/CFS. The Institute of Medicine 2015 diagnostic criteria for ME/CFS include daily activity limiting profound fatigue for greater than 6 months, post-exertional malaise, and unrestful sleep, as well as the presence of cognitive dysfunction and/or orthostatic intolerance.[68] These symptoms do overlap with those of long COVID and require careful consideration when creating a rehabilitation plan tailored to the specific needs and limitations of the individual. Traditional approaches such as graded exercise therapy (GET) may not be suitable for the subgroup of long COVID patients that present with PEM and or meet diagnostic criteria for ME/CFS. GET can inadvertently exacerbate symptoms of PEM and fatigue in this population.[9,66] Similarly, excessive aerobic or cognitive activity may also prove detrimental, triggering symptom flare-ups and prolonging recovery. It is crucial for clinicians to adopt a cautious and individualized approach to return-to-activity, prioritizing symptom management and pacing strategies over aggressive exercise regimens. In developing rehabilitation plans for individuals with long COVID resembling ME/CFS, interdisciplinary collaboration among health care professionals—physicians, nurses, physical therapists, occupational therapists, speech and language pathologists, and mental health professionals—is essential. The goal of rehabilitation in this population is not to push individuals beyond their energy envelope but rather to support them in improving functional capacity, reducing the frequency and intensity of PEM episodes, managing symptoms, and enhancing overall well-being and quality-of-life. By recognizing the potential complications associated with traditional rehabilitation approaches (eg, GET) and adopting a holistic patient-centered approach, clinicians can better support individuals with long COVID on their journey toward recovery.

There are specific considerations for long COVID rehabilitation in those with biologic sex differences, including pregnant persons, persons who menstruate, and persons who may be lactating. Some of these are expanded on in **Table 1**, which comes from the AAPM&R consensus guidance statements.[8-15] As always, clinicians should be aware of sex-related bias, which may add to diagnostic delays faced by female patients. This has occurred in women with dysautonomia who have been told their palpitations are due to stress and therefore delaying a diagnosis of POTS. Even prior to the pandemic, women were underdiagnosed and undertreated for cardiac conditions, inclusive of cardiac rehabilitation programs.[11] Given this, clinicians must work to ensure equitable care and referrals. Given their changing physiology, pregnant people may experience pregnancy-related fatigue and require alternative diagnostic testing and treatment to differentiate the fatigue from long COVID. Gender-affirming care should be considered regarding its impact on fatigue (eg, exogenous hormone use, sleep, and mental health). Pregnant people may also have baseline respiratory discomfort that can be exacerbated by the effects of COVID-19. Furthermore, therapy may need to be adjusted for pregnant persons given limitations to positioning later in pregnancy. Clinicians should be aware of sex-related bias, which may add to diagnostic delays faced by female patients. Finally, when pharmaceutical treatments are being considered for pregnant or lactating persons, the pregnancy category of medications must be looked at to see if they are appropriate to be given during pregnancy or while lactating.

More research and clinical understanding of the impacts of acute COVID-19 and long COVID on historically marginalized and underrepresented populations, including females, are needed. The goal will be for clinicians to provide access to more effective rehabilitative care for all persons with long COVID.

CHALLENGES

The challenges surrounding long COVID and other infection-associated chronic conditions underscore a longstanding issue of underfunding and under-research related to these topics in health care systems worldwide. Historically, diseases that do not fit neatly into established categories or lack immediate, high-profile attention often struggle to secure the resources necessary for thorough investigation and treatment development. Long COVID, with its complex and varied persisting symptoms, exemplifies this disparity in research and funding allocation. As previously discussed, the individuals most affected by long COVID and similar conditions often find themselves marginalized within health care systems. Women, in particular, who have higher rates of long COVID, report their experiences are frequently dismissed or minimized. This further exacerbates the under-researched nature of these conditions, perpetuating a cycle of neglect and inadequate support.

Addressing these challenges requires a concerted interdisciplinary effort. Health care professionals, researchers, policymakers, patients, and advocacy groups must come together to advocate for increased funding and dedicated research into long COVID and related infection-associated chronic conditions. This interdisciplinary approach is crucial for understanding the multifaceted nature of these illnesses and developing comprehensive, patient-centered health care strategies. In addition to increased funding and research, there is a pressing need to reconstruct healthcare policy to prioritize the needs of those affected by long COVID and similar conditions.[69] This includes ensuring that marginalized groups have equitable access to health care services and are actively involved in decision-making processes that affect their care. Creating advocacy platforms for these groups to voice their concerns and experiences is essential for promoting inclusivity and improving outcomes.

The COVID-19 pandemic exposed pre-existing health care disparities and magnified the intricate intersectionality faced by women who are from racial/ethnic minoritized groups. Across the spectrum of COVID-19 impacts, persons from racial/ethnic minoritized groups have borne a disproportionate burden, experiencing higher rates of acute infection, hospitalization, hospital readmission, death, and are now grappling with the enduring challenges of long COVID.[70,71] Within this context, inequities persist for individuals with long COVID who require specialized rehabilitation care, with historic trends indicating they are less likely to access the comprehensive support they require.[72–74] Addressing these disparities demands a multifaceted approach that acknowledges the complex interplay of race, gender, and health care access, ensuring that marginalized communities are not further marginalized in their journey toward recovery.

SUMMARY

Dedicated research and further clinical guidance are needed to provide equitable, culturally competent, and individualized care to women with long COVID. Addressing the challenges associated with long COVID and other infection-associated chronic conditions requires a shift in health care systems toward a more holistic and patient-centered approach. By recognizing and actively working to overcome the disparities that exist, we can strive toward better outcomes and decreased disability for women and all individuals affected by these conditions.

CLINICS CARE POINTS

- Women are overrepresented and overburdened in long COVID and may face unique challenges in diagnosis and management.
- Common symptoms of long COVID in women may include fatigue, cognitive dysfunction, respiratory issues, cardiac symptoms, and autonomic dysfunction, but there are many more.
- Individualized and situation-dependent treatment is needed when caring for individuals with long COVID.

- Biologic sex differences must be considered regarding symptom presentation, response to treatment, and health care needs. Clinicians should be mindful of the impact of pregnancy, menstruation, and lactation on long COVID symptoms and treatment.
- Recognize and address the psychological impact of long COVID on women, but clinicians should not psychologize their symptoms.

DISCLOSURES

Dr M. Verduzco-Gutierrez is a Co-PI for AHRQ. Other authors have nothing to disclose.

REFERENCES

1. National Academies of Sciences, Engineering, and Medicine. A long COVID definition: a chronic, systemic disease state with profound consequences. Washington, DC: The National Academies Press; 2024. https://doi.org/10.17226/27768.
2. Sudre CH, Murray B, Varsavsky T, et al. Attributes and predictors of long COVID. Nat Med 2021;27(4):626–31.
3. Huang C, Huang L, Wang Y, et al. 6-month consequences of COVID-19 in patients discharged from hospital: a cohort study. Lancet 2023;401(10393):e21–33.
4. Kozak R, Armstrong SM, Salvant E, et al. Recognition of long-COVID-19 patients in a Canadian tertiary hospital setting: a retrospective analysis of their clinical and laboratory characteristics. Pathogens 2021;10(10):1246.
5. Fernández-de-Las-Peñas C, Martín-Guerrero JD, Pellicer-Valero ÓJ, et al. Female sex is a risk factor associated with long-term post-COVID related-symptoms but not with COVID-19 symptoms: the LONG-COVID-EXP-CM Multicenter Study. J Clin Med 2022;11(2):413.
6. The sex, gender and COVID-19 project. The COVID-19 sex-disaggregated data tracker. Cambridge: global health 50/50. Available at: https://globalhealth5050. org/the-sex-gender-and-covid-19-project/the-data-tracker. Accessed April 7, 2024.
7. Adjaye-Gbewonyo D, Vahratian A, Perrine CG, et al. Long COVID in adults: United States, 2022. NCHS Data Brief 2023;(480):1–8.
8. Blitshteyn S, Whiteson JH, Abramoff B, et al. Multi-disciplinary collaborative consensus guidance statement on the assessment and treatment of autonomic dysfunction in patients with post-acute sequelae of SARS-CoV-2 infection (PASC). Pharm Manag PM R 2022;14(10):1270–91.
9. Herrera JE, Niehaus WN, Whiteson J, et al. Multidisciplinary collaborative consensus guidance statement on the assessment and treatment of fatigue in postacute sequelae of SARS-CoV-2 infection (PASC) patients. Pharm Manag PM R 2021;13(9):1027–43 [published correction appears in PM R. 2022 Jan;14(1):164].
10. Fine JS, Ambrose AF, Didehbani N, et al. Multi-disciplinary collaborative consensus guidance statement on the assessment and treatment of cognitive symptoms in patients with post-acute sequelae of SARS-CoV-2 infection (PASC). Pharm Manag PM R 2022;14(1):96–111.
11. Whiteson JH, Azola A, Barry JT, et al. Multi-disciplinary collaborative consensus guidance statement on the assessment and treatment of cardiovascular complications in patients with post-acute sequelae of SARS-CoV-2 infection (PASC). Pharm Manag PM R 2022;14(7):855–78.

12. Maley JH, Alba GA, Barry JT, et al. Multi-disciplinary collaborative consensus guidance statement on the assessment and treatment of breathing discomfort and respiratory sequelae in patients with post-acute sequelae of SARS-CoV-2 infection (PASC). Pharm Manag PM R 2022;14(1):77–95.

13. Melamed E, Rydberg L, Ambrose AF, et al. Multidisciplinary collaborative consensus guidance statement on the assessment and treatment of neurologic sequelae in patients with post-acute sequelae of SARS-CoV-2 infection (PASC). Pharm Manag PM R 2023;15(5):640–62.

14. Cheng AL, Anderson J, Didehbani N, et al. Multi-disciplinary collaborative consensus guidance statement on the assessment and treatment of mental health symptoms in patients with post-acute sequelae of SARS-CoV-2 infection (PASC). Pharm Manag PM R 2023;15(12):1588–604.

15. Malone LA, Morrow A, Chen Y, et al. Multi-disciplinary collaborative consensus guidance statement on the assessment and treatment of postacute sequelae of SARS-CoV-2 infection (PASC) in children and adolescents. Pharm Manag PM R 2022;14(10):1241–69.

16. Chen C, Haupert SR, Zimmermann L, et al. Global prevalence of post-coronavirus disease 2019 (COVID-19) condition or long COVID: a meta-analysis and systematic review. J Infect Dis 2022;226(9):1593–607.

17. Wu Y, Sawano M, Wu Y, et al. Factors associated with long COVID: insights from two nationwide surveys. Am J Med 2024. https://doi.org/10.1016/j.amjmed.2024. 02.032.

18. Subramanian A, Nirantharakumar K, Hughes S, et al. Symptoms and risk factors for long COVID in non-hospitalized adults. Nat Med 2022;28(8):1706–14.

19. Bai F, Tomasoni D, Falcinella C, et al. Female gender is associated with long COVID syndrome: a prospective cohort study. Clin Microbiol Infect 2022;28(4): 611.e9.

20. McEvedy CP, Beard AW. Royal free epidemic of 1955: a reconsideration. Br Med J 1970;1(5687):7–11.

21. Thaweethai T, Jolley SE, Karlson EW, et al. Development of a definition of posta-cute sequelae of SARS-CoV-2 Infection. JAMA 2023;329(22):1934–46 [published correction appears in JAMA. 2024 Apr 10.

22. Sigfrid L, Drake TM, Pauley E, et al. Long Covid in adults discharged from UK hospitals after Covid-19: a prospective, multicentre cohort study using the ISA-RIC WHO Clinical Characterisation Protocol. Lancet Reg Health Eur 2021;8: 100186.

23. Davis HE, Assaf GS, McCorkell L, et al. Characterizing long COVID in an interna-tional cohort: 7 months of symptoms and their impact. EClinicalMedicine 2021; 38:101019.

24. Centers for Disease Control and Prevention. Long COVID in adults: United States. 2022. Available at: https://www.cdc.gov/nchs/products/databriefs/db480.htm# section_1. Accessed April 27, 2024.

25. Cohen J, van der Meulen Rodgers Y. An intersectional analysis of long COVID prevalence. Int J Equity Health 2023;22(1):261.

26. Matsumoto C. The necessity of investigations to clarify sex and racial disparities in pathophysiology of Long COVID. Hypertens Res 2024;47(4):984–6.

27. Ferretti VV, Klersy C, Bruno R, et al. Men with COVID-19 die. Women survive. Ma-turitas 2022;158:34–6.

28. National Academies of Sciences, Engineering, and Medicine. Long-term health ef-fects of COVID-19: disability and function following SARS-CoV-2 infection. Wash-ington, DC: The National Academies Press; 2024. https://doi.org/10.17226/27756.

29. Cho SM, Premraj L, Battaglini D, et al. Sex differences in post-acute neurological sequelae of SARS-CoV-2 and symptom resolution in adults after coronavirus disease 2019 hospitalization: an international multi-centre prospective observational study. Brain Commun 2024;6(2):fcae036. https://doi.org/10.1093/braincomms/fcae036.

30. Vásconez-González J, Izquierdo-Condoy JS, Fernandez-Naranjo R, et al. A systematic review and quality evaluation of studies on long-term sequelae of COVID-19. Healthcare (Basel) 2022;10(12):2364. Published 2022 Nov 24.

31. Jacobs MM, Evans E, Ellis C. Racial, ethnic, and sex disparities in the incidence and cognitive symptomology of long COVID-19. J Natl Med Assoc 2023;115(2):233–43.

32. Zakia H, Pradana K, Iskandar S. Risk factors for psychiatric symptoms in patients with long COVID: a systematic review. PLoS One 2023;18(4):e0284075. https://doi.org/10.1371/journal.pone.0284075.

33. Sylvester SV, Rusu R, Chan B, et al. Sex differences in sequelae from COVID-19 infection and in long COVID syndrome: a review. Curr Med Res Opin 2022;38(8):1391–9.

34. Zhao S, Tran VH. Postural orthostatic tachycardia syndrome. [Updated 2023 Aug 7]. In: StatPearls [Internet]. Treasure Island (FL): StatPearls Publishing; 2024. Available at: https://www.ncbi.nlm.nih.gov/books/NBK541074/.

35. Bhatia R, Kizilbash SJ, Ahrens SP, et al. Outcomes of adolescent-onset postural orthostatic tachycardia syndrome. J Pediatr 2016;173:149–53.

36. Arnold AC, Ng J, Raj SR. Postural tachycardia syndrome - diagnosis, physiology, and prognosis. Auton Neurosci 2018;215:3–11.

37. Narasimhan B, Calambur A, Moras E, et al. Postural orthostatic tachycardia syndrome in COVID-19: a contemporary review of mechanisms, clinical course and management. Vasc Health Risk Manag 2023;19:303–16.

38. Amekran Y, Damoun N, El Hangouche AJ. Postural orthostatic tachycardia syndrome and post-acute COVID-19. Glob Cardiol Sci Pract 2022;2022(1–2):e202213. https://doi.org/10.21542/gcsp.2022.13.

39. Kavi L. Postural tachycardia syndrome and long COVID: an update. Br J Gen Pract 2021;72(714):8–9. Published 2021 Dec 31.

40. Ladlow P, O'Sullivan O, Houston A, et al. Dysautonomia following COVID-19 is not associated with subjective limitations or symptoms but is associated with objective functional limitations. Heart Rhythm 2022;19(4):613–20.

41. Raj SR, Arnold AC, Barboi A, et al. Long-COVID postural tachycardia syndrome: an American Autonomic Society statement. Clin Auton Res 2021;31(3):365–8.

42. Buoite Stella A, Furlanis G, Frezza NA, et al. Autonomic dysfunction in post-COVID patients with and witfhout neurological symptoms: a prospective multidomain observational study. J Neurol 2022;269(2):587–96.

43. Pollack B, von Saltza E, McCorkell L, et al. Female reproductive health impacts of Long COVID and associated illnesses including ME/CFS, POTS, and connective tissue disorders: a literature review. Front Rehabil Sci 2023;4:1122673. https://doi.org/10.3389/fresc.2023.1122673.

44. Vásconez-González J, Fernandez-Naranjo R, Izquierdo-Condoy JS, et al. Comparative analysis of long-term self-reported COVID-19 symptoms among pregnant women. J Infect Public Health 2023;16(3):430–40.

45. Navas-Otero A, Calvache-Mateo A, Martín-Núñez J, et al. Characteristics of frailty in perimenopausal women with long COVID-19. Healthcare (Basel) 2023;11(10):1468.

46. Silva J, Takahashi T, Wood J, et al. Sex differences in symptomatology and immune profiles of Long COVID. Preprint. medRxiv 2024;24303568. https://doi.org/10.1101/2024.02.29.24303568.

47. Alvergne A, Kountourides G, Argentieri MA, et al. A retrospective case-control study on menstrual cycle changes following COVID-19 vaccination and disease. iScience 2023;26(4):106401.

48. Lott N, Gebhard CE, Bengs S, et al. Sex hormones in SARS-CoV-2 susceptibility: key players or confounders? Nat Rev Endocrinol 2023;19(4):217–31.

49. Bourne KM, Nerenberg KA, Stiles LE, et al. Symptoms of postural orthostatic tachycardia syndrome in pregnancy: a cross-sectional, community-based survey. BJOG 2023;130(9):1120–7.

50. Carmona-Torre F, Mínguez-Olaondo A, López-Bravo A, et al. Dysautonomia in COVID-19 patients: a narrative review on clinical course, diagnostic and therapeutic strategies. Front Neurol 2022;13:886609. https://doi.org/10.3389/fneur.2022.886609.

51. Blitshteyn S, Whitelaw S. Postural orthostatic tachycardia syndrome (POTS) and other autonomic disorders after COVID-19 infection: a case series of 20 patients [published correction appears in Immunol Res. 2021 Apr 13;:]. Immunol Res 2021;69(2):205–11.

52. Haloot J, Kabbani M, Verduzco-Gutierrez M, et al. Ce-541-02 post-covid and postural orthostatic tachycardia syndrome. Heart Rhythm 2022;19(5 Supplement):S54.

53. Park-Wyllie L, Mazzotta P, Pastuszak A, et al. Birth defects after maternal exposure to corticosteroids: prospective cohort study and meta-analysis of epidemiological studies. Teratology 2000;62(6):385–92.

54. American Academy of Pediatrics Committee on Drugs. Transfer of drugs and other chemicals into human milk. Pediatrics 2001;108(3):776–89. https://doi.org/10.1542/peds.108.3.776.

55. Campbell JW. A possible teratogenic effect of propranolol. N Engl J Med 1985;313(8):518.

56. Heinonen OP, Slone D, Shapiro S. In: Birth defects and drugs in pregnancy. Littleton, MA: Publishing Sciences Group; 1977. p. 345–56.

57. Hoeltzenbeln M, Lehmann ML, Beck E, et al. Ivabradine use in pregnant women—treatment indications and pregnancy outcome: an evaluation of the German Embryotox database. Eur J Clin Pharmacol 2021;77:1029–37.

58. Carda S, Invernizzi M, Bavikatte G, et al. COVID-19 pandemic. What should Physical and Rehabilitation Medicine specialists do? A clinician's perspective. Eur J Phys Rehabil Med 2020;56(4):515–24.

59. Carda S, Invernizzi M, Bavikatte G, et al. The role of physical and rehabilitation medicine in the COVID-19 pandemic: the clinician's view. Ann Phys Rehabil Med 2020;63(6):554–6.

60. McNeary L, Maltser S, Verduzco-Gutierrez M. Navigating coronavirus disease 2019 (Covid-19) in physiatry: a CAN report for inpatient rehabilitation facilities. Pharm Manag PM R 2020;12(5):512–5.

61. Whiteson JH, Escalón MX, Maltser S, et al. Demonstrating the vital role of physiatry throughout the health care continuum: lessons learned from the impacts of the COVID-19 pandemic on inpatient rehabilitation. Pharm Manag PM R 2021;13(6):554–62.

62. Centers for Disease Control and Prevention. Post-COVID Conditions: information for healthcare providers. 2023. Available at: https://www.cdc.gov/coronavirus/2019-ncov/hcp/clinical-care/post-covid-conditions.html. Accessed November 7, 2023.

63. Terzic CM, Medina-Inojosa BJ. Cardiovascular complications of coronavirus disease-2019. Phys Med Rehabil Clin 2023;34(3):551–61.
64. Whiteson JH. Pulmonary sequelae of coronavirus disease 2019. Phys Med Rehabil Clin 2023;34(3):573–84.
65. Haloot J, Bhavaraju-Sanka R, Pillarisetti J, et al. Autonomic dysfunction related to postacute SARS-CoV-2 syndrome. Phys Med Rehabil Clin 2023;34(3):563–72.
66. Sathyamoorthy M, Sevak RJ, Cabrera J, et al. Enhanced external counterpulsation improves cognitive function of persons with long COVID. Am J Phys Med Rehabil 2024. https://doi.org/10.1097/PHM.0000000000002433.
67. DeMars J, Brown DA, Angelidis I, et al. What is safe long COVID rehabilitation? J Occup Rehabil 2023;33(2):227–30.
68. Committee on the diagnostic criteria for myalgic encephalomyelitis/chronic fatigue syndrome; board on the health of select populations; Institute of medicine. *Beyond myalgic encephalomyelitis/chronic fatigue syndrome: Redefining an illness.* Washington (DC): National Academies Press (US); 2015.
69. Jesus TS, Kamalakannan S, Bhattacharjya S, et al. PREparedness, REsponse and SySTemic transformation (PRE-RE-SyST): a model for disability-inclusive pandemic responses and systemic disparities reduction derived from a scoping review and thematic analysis. Int J Equity Health 2021;20(1):204.
70. Muñoz-Price LS, Nattinger AB, Rivera F, et al. Racial disparities in incidence and outcomes among patients with COVID-19. JAMA Netw Open 2020;3(9): e2021892. https://doi.org/10.1001/jamanetworkopen.2020.21892.
71. Tanne JH. Covid-19: US studies show racial and ethnic disparities in long covid. BMJ 2023;380:535.
72. Odonkor CA, Esparza R, Flores LE, et al. Disparities in health care for black patients in physical medicine and rehabilitation in the United States: a narrative review. Pharm Manag PM R 2021;13(2):180–203.
73. Flores LE, Verduzco-Gutierrez M, Molinares D, et al. Disparities in health care for hispanic patients in physical medicine and rehabilitation in the United States: a narrative review. Am J Phys Med Rehabil 2020;99(4):338–47.
74. Harden JK, Blauwet CA, Silver JK, et al. Health and health care disparities related to rehabilitation and COVID-19. Pharm Manag PM R 2022;14(2):273–9.

Rehabilitation of Women with Neurodegenerative Diseases

Check for updates

Steven Markos, MD[a,b,c,*], Michael Galibov, DO[a]

KEYWORDS

- Neurodegenerative disorders • Parkinson's disease • Multiple sclerosis
- Alzheimer's disease • Motor neuron disease • Progressive supranuclear palsy
- Multiple system atrophy • Huntington's disease

KEY POINTS

- Important differences exist between women and men in the prevalence, natural course, symptomatic features, treatment response, health care utilization patterns, and outcomes in regards to Parkinson's disease.
- Sex-related differences in multiple sclerosis include incidence, progression, genetic and hormonal factors, and radiologic findings.
- Alzheimer's disease has a female predominance, both due to longevity as well as other factors.
- Other neurodegenerative disorders, such as typical and atypical presentations of motor neuron disease, may also have a slight gender predominance toward male individuals; however, these discrepancies remain somewhat poorly understood and not fully explored.

INTRODUCTION

Neurodegenerative diseases are a group of conditions that cause progressive injury of neurons.[1] The brain is the predominant site where injury and loss of neurons occur within the neurodegenerative diseases in general.[1,2] Parkinson's disease, multiple sclerosis (MS), Alzheimer's disease, motor neuron disease (MND) including amyotrophic lateral sclerosis (ALS), progressive supranuclear palsy (PSP), multiple system atrophy (MSA), and Huntington's disease (HD) are examples of neurodegenerative disease and will be discussed here. While these are a heterogenous group of conditions with their own sets of features, all are incurable and grow increasingly difficult

[a] Department of Physical Medicine and Rehabilitation, JFK Johnson Rehabilitation Institute, 65 James Street, Edison, NJ 08820, USA; [b] Rutgers Robert Wood Johnson Medical School; [c] Hackensack Meridian School of Medicine
* Corresponding author. Department of Physical Medicine and Rehabilitation, JFK Johnson Rehabilitation Institute, 65 James Street, Edison, NJ 08820.
E-mail address: Steven.Markos@hmhn.org

Phys Med Rehabil Clin N Am 36 (2025) 389–398
https://doi.org/10.1016/j.pmr.2024.11.006
1047-9651/25/© 2024 Elsevier Inc. All rights reserved, including those for text and data mining, AI training, and similar technologies.

to treat as the condition progresses. The human impact of neurodegenerative disease is significant; for instance, dementia alone is considered to be responsible for the greatest societal and economic burden of all diseases in developed countries.[2] With a growing interest in and evidence for the role that sex plays in neurodegenerative disease, we will review this topic to help seek a better understanding of these conditions.

PARKINSON'S DISEASE
Background

Parkinson's disease (PD) is the second-most prevalent neurodegenerative disease behind only Alzheimer's disease.[3] The multitude of potential motor and nonmotor symptoms of PD include resting tremor, bradykinesia, rigidity, multifactorial gait impairments, autonomic dysfunction, cognitive impairment, and sleep disorders, among others.[4] The sequelae of the motor and nonmotor symptoms of PD can negatively affect quality of life, increase fall risk, impair mobility and functional independence, and affect social, emotional, and medical well-being.[5,6] By 2037, the total US economic burden of the disease is estimated to reach US$79.1 billion.[7] The exact cause of PD is unknown, but it is believed to be influenced by genetics, age-related changes in neurons, and the presence of abnormal proteins called Lewy bodies, resulting in the main pathology of a deficiency of dopamine in the substantia nigra of the brainstem.[3]

Discussion

The role of biological sex has gained increasing attention as an important component in the development and impact of PD. Generally speaking, the prevalence of PD is twice as high in men compared to women.[8] Sex-related differences exist in some motor manifestations of the disease process. Women are more likely than men to present with tremor as their initial symptom.[8] Women have a slightly older age of onset and have a shorter time to and higher likelihood of developing levodopa-induced dyskinesias.[9,10] Women also tend to have a lower likelihood of rigidity but a higher likelihood to develop postural instability.[11]

Sex also appears to play a role in the prevalence of multiple nonmotor symptoms. Women more often present with depression, fatigue, lack of motivation, nervousness, constipation, pain, and restless legs and report worse disability and quality of life.[8,9] Compared to women, men appear to have more common and severe symptoms of daytime sleepiness, drooling, and sexual dysfunction, which includes altered interest in sex as well as increased frequency of compulsive sexual behavior.[8,12]

Health care disparities between men and women also appear to exist. A retrospective observational cohort study of Medicare beneficiaries with PD published in 2011 revealed that women were statistically significantly less likely than men to obtain care from a neurologist, even after the adjustment for comorbid disease and socioeconomic barriers to specialty care.[12] There is evidence that sex is a strong, independent predictor of receiving a deep brain stimulator (DBS), with women being disproportionately less likely than men to receive a DBS for reasons that remain unclear.[13] In a retrospective cohort study of over 133,000 Medicare beneficiaries diagnosed with PD and followed through 2008, compared to men, women had higher utilization of advanced nursing care (skilled nursing facility, home health, and hospice) and lower utilization of direct physician contact.[9] A 2018 study of 7209 patients at 21 centers in the United States, Canada, the Netherlands, and Israel, revealed that women were less likely than men to receive caregiver support from a spouse, family, or friends and utilized paid caregiver services less often than men.[14]

Response to treatment can vary between sexes. Multiple studies have demonstrated that compared to men and controlling for other factors, women have higher blood levels and bioavailability of levodopa following oral carbidopa–levodopa administration.[15–17] One review article presented interesting findings for patients with PD following DBS implantation; women tended to report more improvement in activities of daily living, while motor improvement appeared to be equal between both sexes.[18]

Estrogens also appear to play a potential protective role in both the risk of PD development and symptom reduction. A prospective cohort study concluded that women with a higher cumulative exposure to both endogenous and exogenous estrogens throughout life had a significantly reduced PD risk.[19] In a double-blind, placebo-controlled, crossover study[20] and a double-blind, parallel-group, prospective study,[21] both among postmenopausal women, estrogen replacement therapy reduced levodopa-induced dyskinesias. Furthermore, in this study by Tsang and colleagues,[21] estrogen replacement also improved "on/off" times and motor symptoms as measured by the Unified Parkinson's disease rating scale subscale III.

A 2020 cross-sectional case–control research study revealed important findings relating to osteoporosis in PD, 2 age-related diseases that can affect mobility and disability.[22] Women with PD were compared to age-similar women without PD. Women with PD had lower bone mineral density of the lumbar spine, femoral neck, distal radius, and total body compared to women without PD. The frequency of history of osteoporotic fractures in women with PD was higher compared to women without PD, at 51.7% versus 11.3%, respectively. Additionally, the future 10 year probability of major osteoporotic and hip fractures were higher in women with PD compared to women without PD, as projected by FRAX (Sheffield, UK), a well-known calculator for the assessment of fracture risk. The authors thus conclude that with lower bone mineral density indices, higher rates of osteoporosis and fractures, and higher risk of future low-energy fractures, this osteoporosis and fracture risk should be taken into consideration with the clinical management of women with PD.

MULTIPLE SCLEROSIS
Background

MS is an autoimmune disease that affects the central nervous system (CNS) and involves a pattern of demyelination, inflammation, and neuronal insult.[23] Colloquially characterized as disseminated in time and space, lesions that develop within the CNS often present in different areas and at different times.[23] Initial presentations have a wide range, including visual deficits, sensorimotor effects, cognitive implications, and bowel/bladder problems. Wherever a lesion is present, downstream symptoms can be seen. Progression of MS can be gradual or rapid based on MS subtypes, including relapsing-remitting, primary progressive, secondary progressive, and progressive relapsing.[23] Worldwide, 2.5 million individuals live with MS, with an overall prevalence of 1 in 1000 in populations of European ancestry.[24] Notably, MS has a predilection for women, with a woman:man prevalence ranging from 2:1 to 3:1, with numbers as high as 3.2:1 in patient populations below the age of 20 years.[25]

Discussion

The immune system and the CNS are closely linked, with implications of the immune system commonly seen in many CNS disorders.[26] MS specifically is thought to be an autoimmune disorder of TH1 cell-mediated immunity, similar to rheumatoid arthritis and psoriasis.[24,27] Autoreactive CD4[+] T cells go on to attack myelinated proteins found on neurons, which leads to the development of plaques and astrocytic scars.[28,29] Gender differences of the immune system have been observed in humans and also experimentally in mice, with one disease being studied at the forefront— experimental autoimmune encephalomyelitis (EAE).[24] Within the confines of this disease, which is akin to MS, special attention was paid to peroxisome proliferator-activated receptor-α, which is involved in gender differences of lipid metabolism. This receptor also exerted gender-specific effects in EAE, indicating a potential interaction between sex-related factors and diet in autoimmunity.[30] Further gender differences can be stratified as related to incidence and progression.

Between 65% and 70% of new MS diagnoses are in women, with this trend steadily increasing in recent years.[24] Many mechanisms may be behind this pattern, with the Y chromosome offering a level of protection by way of the *SrY* gene. If this *SrY* gene is transposed to the X chromosome, disease progression has been witnessed to worsen.[24] Additionally, physiologic testosterone is protective, where castration of mice worsens established EAE and places the mice at higher risk of disease onset and incidence.[24] Looking further into hormonal impacts, pregnancy has often shown a consistent and profound beneficial impact on nearly all aspects of MS.

From an overarching stance, pregnancy modifies disease most significantly in the third trimester; MS has the lowest relapse risk during this time, with an overall reduction of nearly 70%.[24] Important shifts at this time period include peak levels of estradiol, estriol, and progesterone, which are all thought to be protective modulating factors.[24] This is further drawn home by an increased presence of relapse at 6 months postpartum, where many of these hormones either normalize or downregulate considerably.[24] In fact, 2 recent pilot studies examined the use of oral estriol in women with MS with definitively positive impacts.[28] Current MS treatment regimens diminish relapse risk by an average of 30% to 60%, thereby indicating that pregnancy confers even higher protection than current pharmacologic modulations.[24] On a more macroscopic level, the previously noted increase in new diagnoses among women could be explained by a waning tendency of many young women in society today to be multiparous, therein evading the summative protection of multiple pregnancies in the context of MS.[24]

Beyond the above gender-specific differences on incidence and in the context of pregnancy, specific differences were also seen in MS effects on men and women, both clinically and radiologically. Despite women receiving MS diagnoses more often, men with the disease tend to progress differently than women, and often more rapidly especially in the context of gray matter volumes.[24] A recent examination conducted by Antulov and colleagues[31] looked at 763 total patients with MS, 171 of which were men (22%), and identified considerably less gray matter volumes within the men of this group. Interestingly, women had less white matter volumes in comparison, yet many of MS sequelae are related directly to gray matter changes that may explain why men develop more rampant symptoms at times and more often are implicated in the progressive variants of the disease.[31,32] Gray matter atrophy has also been shown to correlate stronger with permanent disability than does white matter atrophy.[32] Transdermal testosterone has been utilized in men that suffer from MS similarly to the regimen of oral estriol in women, with similarly positive outcomes. Hormonal fluctuations of testosterone may potentially play a role in pathogenesis of MS, with perhaps a diminished level of protection compared to estrogens. Estrogen and testosterone levels thus could affect clinical outcomes in men compared to women based on hormonal differences.[28]

ALZHEIMER'S DISEASE
Background

Alzheimer's disease (AD) has had a profound, multifaceted impact on the world. Examining just the United States, approximately 5.2 million Americans carry the diagnosis, with 5 million of these individuals being older than 65 years.[33] This number is expected to nearly triple by 2050, with a high burden on morbidity and mortality as well, with AD currently being the sixth leading cause of death in the United States.[33] Fiscal cost and opportunity cost revolving this disease are dramatic, with Medicare estimates in congruence with the 17.7 billion hours of care given to family members affected leading to a cost of nearly US$214 billion for the former and US$220 billion for the latter.[33] The aim of this review is to dive deeper into the discrepancies of men and women who are diagnosed with AD.

Discussion

On the surface, women appear to be further affected by this disease in particular, as women are more likely to develop the disease and also twice as prevalent in caregiver roles compared to men.[33] Several mechanisms may be at play but all boil down to a simple concept—longevity.

Two-thirds of novel cases of AD are women, with a common explanation being offered of dementia risk correlating with age.[34] Swedish twin studies from the 1960s and stratified studies from the 1980s both concluded that men overall are not expected to live as long as women, with a significant dichotomy observed in the incidence of AD above the age of 85 years in particular.[34,35] These studies, thus, did not identify sex-specific rationales for the differences in incidence and prevalence, rather attributing it all to age and life expectancy.[34,35]

More recent investigations have added some components to the argument beyond longevity, albeit supporting the notion that a difference in age remains the primary culprit of discrepancies. Sporadic AD is strongly linked to the APOE4 allele (apolipoprotein E4), with statistically stronger evidence of gene conversion in women compared to men.[36] For instance, one copy of this allele in a woman increases the risk of developing AD 4 fold, while only marginally increasing the risk in a man with only one copy of this allele.[37] Beyond simply the genetic background, some experts consider AD a subset of an autoimmune condition, which women are at greater risk for, because one of the first actual signs of damage seen pathologically in the brain was microglial infiltration of macrophages.[38,39] This inflammatory component has several downstream implications for those actually afflicted with the disease, as Irvine and colleagues[40] identified that women tend to demonstrate a more profound cognitive decline compared to men. A reduction in estrogen in postmenopausal women has been posited as a potential explanation for this phenomenon, as estrogen has been shown to serve a protective factor in numerous neurologic and autoimmune conditions.[40] However, more consistent with principles discussed initially, perhaps cognitive performance is swayed simply by a greater number of women diagnosed with AD who continue to live longer than their male counterparts. Yet another study saw an explanation revolving around brain anatomy, as men tended to have up to 10% larger brain volumes than women, which therefore may lend itself to a greater resilience of a gradual degeneration.[37] This concept was later reinforced by an autopsy study declaring women are much more likely to be clinically diagnosed with AD compared to men at similar levels of actual brain pathology.[37]

Another interesting parallel uniquely seen in women involves the relation of menopause and eventual Alzheimer's dementia risk. As a review, following menopause, certain sex hormones begin to rapidly decline—most notably 17 beta-estradiol and progesterone.[37] If a bilateral oophorectomy is indicated and performed for a female patient prior to menopause, similar rampant declines are witnessed in these patients, along with testosterone and the totality of the hypothalamic-pituitary-ovarian axis.[37] The Mayo Clinic Cohort Study of Oophorectomy and Aging examined patients longitudinally to try and understand how this significant change could impact the remaining lifespan of patients moving forward. An almost doubled risk of all-cause dementia was seen in this population; yet, if women began hormone replacement therapy after their oophorectomies until the age of expected natural menopause, the risk of AD was synonymous with the general female population.[37]

OTHER NEURODEGENERATIVE DISORDERS

Other neurodegenerative disorders exist, which are relatively rare and therefore less elucidated. MND, including the most common subtype ALS as well as others, demonstrates differences in male and female disease onset and prognosis. Men have a higher prevalence of the disease at a rate of 1.6:1 as well as an earlier age of onset.[41] Women tend to demonstrate symptoms of this disease more readily after menopause and are more likely to succumb to the sequela of MND.[41] Overall, for ALS, incidence rate is 1.7 per 100,000 person-years, and the prevalence is 4.5 per 100,000 people.[41] A large Belgian cohort study sought out to seek gender differences in an additional neurodegenerative disorder, PSP, which is characterized by gait disturbance, ocular disturbance, and often significant dysphagia.[42] This study acknowledged the limitations of such a venture but did ultimately recruit more men than women in their study, at a similar 1.6:1 ratio.[42] Men had a longer time of symptom onset prior to eventual diagnosis and tended to be older at time of diagnosis. Women were seen to be able to ambulate without a wheelchair for longer than men.[42] PSP has an estimated annual prevalence of 5 to 7 per 100,000 people.[42] MSA has an estimated prevalence of 1.9 to 4.9 per 100,000 people and equal between sexes.[43–45] Compared to men, women with MSA appear more likely to demonstrate motor symptoms prior to diagnosis.[43] Additionally, women were seen to live about 1 year longer in a study by Coon and colleagues.[43] Lastly, HD is an autosomal dominant neurodegenerative disorder with an equal prevalence (globally 2.71 per 100,000) but variable phenotypes between the sexes.[46,47] Women have shown a higher frequency of past and current depression as well as faster rates of progression in the Unified Huntington's Disease Rating Scale functional assessment, motor assessment, and independence scale.[47] Overall, neurodegenerative disorders may also have a concrete explanation for gender differences that are beginning to be elucidated, but fledgling research has not yet compiled all of the patterns.

SUMMARY

Regarding PD, important differences exist between women and men in the prevalence, natural course, symptomatic features, treatment response, health care utilization patterns, and outcomes in regards to PD. Ongoing prospective, long-term, high-quality studies will be important to further elucidate the extent and mechanisms of these differences so that maximal care can be provided to every individual.

With respect to MS, the aforementioned observations offer a clear pattern for many aspects of MS, especially in the context of gender differences. By definition, MS symptoms are highly variable based on the position of the plaques and neurologic insults.[23] Some common presentations are observed, but every patient must be viewed as unique in terms of progression, disability, and morbidity.[25] The variable character of

MS also extends into the gender of the patients afflicted, with some of the fundamentals necessitating a clear understanding in order to best approach these patients and their challenges.[25]

In regard to AD, there remains a considerable amount of rationales to explore in order to gain further knowledge regarding the differences of development of AD in men and women. Women appear to be more affected in many milieus—as currently diagnosed patients, family and caregivers, and women that seemingly are addressing other concerns, such as oophorectomies. Longevity remains at the heart of the argument, but is likely not the sole mechanism behind gender-related differences in AD.

Other neurodegenerative diseases such as MND, PSP, MSA, and HD to varying degrees appear to display some differences in prevalence and/or phenotype between men and women. Ongoing studies of these relatively rare diseases will be needed to further discover how sex may affect items such as natural course, symptomatic features, and treatment response.

CLINICS CARE POINTS

- Women with PD are more likely than men to present with tremor as their initial symptom.
- Women with PD have a shorter time to and higher likelihood of developing levodopa-induced dyskinesias.
- Women with PD tend to have a higher likelihood to develop postural instability.
- Women with PD more often present with depression, fatigue, lack of motivation, nervousness, constipation, pain, and restless legs and report worse disability and quality of life.
- Pregnancy modifies MS and most significantly in the third trimester, with an overall relapse reduction of nearly 70%.
- Despite women receiving MS diagnoses more often, men with the disease tend to progress differently than women, and often more rapidly, especially in the context of gray matter volumes.
- Regarding AD, women are more likely to develop the disease (two-thirds of novel cases of AD are women) and carry out caregiver roles compared to men.
- Other neurodegenerative conditions are rarer and less understood. Some have equal prevalence among sexes while MND has a male predominance. Some phenotypic differences between men and women may exist.

DISCLOSURE

The authors have nothing to disclose.

REFERENCES

1. Davenport F, Gallacher J, Kourtzi Z, et al. Neurodegenerative disease of the brain: a survey of interdisciplinary approaches. J R Soc Interface 2023; 20(198):20220406.
2. Gao HM, Hong JS. Why neurodegenerative diseases are progressive: uncontrolled inflammation drives disease progression. Trends Immunol 2008;29(8):357–65.
3. Prajjwal P, Flores Sanga HS, Acharya K, et al. Parkinson's disease updates: addressing the pathophysiology, risk factors, genetics, diagnosis, along with the medical and surgical treatment. Ann Med Surg 2023;85(10):4887–902.

4. Tolosa E, Garrido A, Scholz SW, et al. Challenges in the diagnosis of Parkinson's disease. Lancet Neurol 2021;20(5):385–97.

5. Hermanowicz N, Jones SA, Hauser RA. Impact of non-motor symptoms in Parkinson's disease: a PMDAlliance survey. Neuropsychiatr Dis Treat 2019;15:2205–12.

6. Bock MA, Brown EG, Zhang L, et al. Association of motor and nonmotor symptoms with health-related quality of life in a large online cohort of people with Parkinson disease. Neurology 2022;98(22):e2194–203.

7. Yang W, Hamilton JL, Kopil C, et al. Current and projected future economic burden of Parkinson's disease in the U.S. NPJ Park Dis 2020;6:15.

8. Solla P, Cannas A, Ibba FC, et al. Gender differences in motor and non-motor symptoms among Sardinian patients with Parkinson's disease. J Neurol Sci 2012;323(1–2):33–9.

9. Fullard ME, Thibault DP, Todaro V, et al. Sex disparities in health and health care utilization after Parkinson diagnosis: rethinking PD associated disability. Parkinsonism Relat Disord 2018;48:45–50.

10. Haaxma CA, Bloem BR, Borm GF, et al. Gender differences in Parkinson's disease. J Neurol Neurosurg Psychiatry 2007;78(8):819–24.

11. Cerri S, Mus L, Blandini F. Parkinson's disease in women and men: what's the difference? J Park Dis 2019;9(3):501–15.

12. Willis AW, Schootman M, Evanoff BA, et al. Neurologist care in Parkinson disease: a utilization, outcomes, and survival study. Neurology 2011;77(9):851–7.

13. Willis AW, Schootman M, Kung N, et al. Disparities in deep brain stimulation surgery among insured elders with Parkinson disease. Neurology 2014;82(2):163–71.

14. Dahodwala N, Shah K, He Y, et al. Sex disparities in access to caregiving in Parkinson disease. Neurology 2018;90(1):e48–54.

15. Martinelli P, Contin M, Scaglione C, et al. Levodopa pharmacokinetics and dyskinesias: are there sex-related differences? Neurol Sci 2003;24(3):192–3.

16. Kompoliti K, Adler CH, Raman R, et al. Gender and pramipexole effects on levodopa pharmacokinetics and pharmacodynamics. Neurology 2002;58(9):1418–22.

17. Kumagai T, Nagayama H, Ota T, et al. Sex differences in the pharmacokinetics of levodopa in elderly patients with Parkinson disease. Clin Neuropharmacol 2014;37(6):173–6.

18. Georgiev D, Hamberg K, Hariz M, et al. Gender differences in Parkinson's disease: a clinical perspective. Acta Neurol Scand 2017;136(6):570–84.

19. Lifetime exposure to estrogens and Parkinson's disease in California teachers. Parkinsonism Relat Disord 2014;20(11):1149–56.

20. Nicoletti A, Arabia G, Pugliese P, et al. Hormonal replacement therapy in women with Parkinson disease and levodopa-induced dyskinesia: a crossover trial. Clin Neuropharmacol 2007;30(5):276–80.

21. Tsang KL, Ho SL, Lo SK. Estrogen improves motor disability in parkinsonian postmenopausal women with motor fluctuations. Neurology 2000;54(12):2292–8.

22. Bystrytska M, Povoroznyuk V, Grygorieva N, et al. Bone mineral density and risk of osteoporotic fractures in women with Parkinson's disease. J Osteoporos 2020;2020:5027973.

23. Tafti D, Ehsan M, Xixis K. Multiple sclerosis. 2022. Available at: https://www.ncbi.nlm.nih.gov/books/NBK499849/.

24. Didonna A, Oksenberg JR. The genetics of multiple sclerosis. In: Zagon IS, McLaughlin PJ, editors. Multiple sclerosis: perspectives in treatment and

pathogenesis. Codon Publications; 2017. https://doi.org/10.15586/codon.multiplesclerosis.2017.ch1.

25. Voskuhl RR, Gold SM. Sex-related factors in multiple sclerosis susceptibility and progression. Nat Rev Neurol 2012;8(5):255–63.

26. Confavreux C, Vukusic S, Adeleine P. Early clinical predictors and progression of irreversible disability in multiple sclerosis: an amnesic process. Brain J Neurol 2003;126(Pt 4):770–82.

27. Hemmer B, Archelos JJ, Hartung HP. New concepts in the immunopathogenesis of multiple sclerosis. Nat Rev Neurosci 2002;3(4):291–301.

28. Gold SM, Voskuhl RR. Estrogen and testosterone therapies in multiple sclerosis. Prog Brain Res 2009;175:239–51.

29. McFarland HF, Martin R. Multiple sclerosis: a complicated picture of autoimmunity. Nat Immunol 2007;8(9):913–9.

30. Dunn SE, Ousman SS, Sobel RA, et al. Peroxisome proliferator-activated receptor (PPAR)alpha expression in T cells mediates gender differences in development of T cell-mediated autoimmunity. J Exp Med 2007;204(2):321–30.

31. Antulov R, Weinstock-Guttman B, Cox JL, et al. Gender-related differences in MS: a study of conventional and nonconventional MRI measures. Mult Scler Houndmills Basingstoke Engl 2009;15(3):345–54.

32. Ge Y, Grossman RI, Udupa JK, et al. Brain atrophy in relapsing-remitting multiple sclerosis and secondary progressive multiple sclerosis: longitudinal quantitative analysis. Radiology 2000;214(3):665–70.

33. Alzheimer's disease facts and figures. Alzheimers Dement J Alzheimers Assoc 2014;10(2):e47–92.

34. Beam CR, Kaneshiro C, Jang JY, et al. Differences between women and men in incidence rates of dementia and Alzheimer's disease. J Alzheimers Dis JAD 2018;64(4):1077–83.

35. Hebert LE, Scherr PA, McCann JJ, et al. Is the risk of developing Alzheimer's disease greater for women than for men? Am J Epidemiol 2001;153(2):132–6.

36. Altmann A, Tian L, Henderson VW, et al. Sex modifies the APOE-related risk of developing Alzheimer disease. Ann Neurol 2014;75(4):563–73.

37. Mielke MM, Vemuri P, Rocca WA. Clinical epidemiology of Alzheimer's disease: assessing sex and gender differences. Clin Epidemiol 2014;6:37–48.

38. Hanamsagar R, Bilbo SD. Sex differences in neurodevelopmental and neurodegenerative disorders: focus on microglial function and neuroinflammation during development. J Steroid Biochem Mol Biol 2016;160:127–33.

39. Rogers J, Mastroeni D, Leonard B, et al. Neuroinflammation in Alzheimer's disease and Parkinson's disease: are microglia pathogenic in either disorder? Int Rev Neurobiol 2007;82:235–46.

40. Irvine K, Laws KR, Gale TM, et al. Greater cognitive deterioration in women than men with Alzheimer's disease: a meta analysis. J Clin Exp Neuropsychol 2012;34(9):989–98.

41. Park J, Kim JE, Song TJ. The global burden of motor neuron disease: an analysis of the 2019 global burden of disease study. Front Neurol 2022;13:864339. PMID: 35528743; PMCID: PMC9068990.

42. Mahale RR, Krishnan S, Divya KP, et al. Gender differences in progressive supranuclear palsy. Acta Neurol Belg 2022;122(2):357–62. Epub 2021 Feb 17. PMID: 33595832.

43. Coon EA, Nelson RM, Sletten DM, et al. Sex and gender influence symptom manifestation and survival in multiple system atrophy. Auton Neurosci 2019;219:49–52. Epub 2019 Apr 24. PMID: 31122601; PMCID: PMC6684211.

44. Barer Y, Chodick G, Cohen R, et al. Epidemiology of progressive supranuclear palsy: real world data from the second largest health plan in Israel. Brain Sci 2022;12(9):1126. PMID: 36138862; PMCID: PMC9496895.
45. Goh YY, Saunders E, Pavey S, et al. Multiple system atrophy. Pract Neurol 2023; 23(3):208–21. Epub 2023 Mar 16. PMID: 36927875; PMCID: PMC10314081.
46. Medina A, Mahjoub Y, Shaver L, et al. Prevalence and incidence of Huntington's disease: an updated systematic review and meta-analysis. Mov Disord 2022; 37(12):2327–35. Epub 2022 Sep 26. PMID: 36161673; PMCID: PMC10086981.
47. Zielonka D, Marinus J, Roos RA, et al. The influence of gender on phenotype and disease progression in patients with Huntington's disease. Parkinsonism Relat Disord 2013;19(2):192–7. Epub 2012 Oct 25. PMID: 23102616.

Reproductive and Sexual Health Considerations for Adolescent Females with Disabilities

Amanda Appel, MD, MPH[a,b,c], Carly Rothman, DO[d,*]

KEYWORDS

- Disability • Sexual health • Sexuality • Puberty • Menstruation
- Menstrual suppression • Pregnancy • Sexual abuse

KEY POINTS

- Sexuality is an activity of daily living and a human right. Unfortunately patients with disabilities are not receiving adequate, disability specific sexual healthcare and education.
- As physicians with general medicine training and an expertise in caring for people with disabilities, physiatrists are uniquely qualified to address sexual health with patients.
- Disability-specific education and anticipatory guidance regarding puberty, menstruation, menstrual suppression, pregnancy, and general sexual health is vital for adolescents with disabilities.

INTRODUCTION

Sex and sexuality are integral parts of the everyday lives of most of the population. According to the World Health Organization's key conceptual elements of sexual health, sexuality is a human right and should be viewed as part of a rights-based approach to sexual health.[1] In other words, sex is an activity of daily living (ADL) and a right and should be treated as such in all aspects of a person's care. It has been well-documented in the literature that individuals with disabilities are often viewed as asexual, or "child-like" and not interested, or able, to participate in sexual activity, which is simply not true.[2] Individuals with physical disabilities are as sexually

[a] Department of Pediatric Rehabilitation Medicine, Children's Hospital Colorado, Aurora, USA; [b] Department of Pediatrics, Children's Hospital Colorado, Aurora, USA; [c] Department of Physical Medicine and Rehabilitation, University of Colorado Anschutz School of Medicine, 13123 East 16th Avenue, Aurora, CO 80045, USA; [d] Department of Pediatric Physical Medicine & Rehabilitation, Joseph M. Sanzari Children's Hospital, Hackensack Meridian Health, 30 Prospect Avenue, Hackensack, NJ 07601, USA
* Corresponding author.
E-mail address: carly.rothman@hmhn.org
Twitter: @carlyrothmanDO (C.R.)

Phys Med Rehabil Clin N Am 36 (2025) 399–414
https://doi.org/10.1016/j.pmr.2024.11.013
1047-9651/25/© 2024 Elsevier Inc. All rights are reserved, including those for text and data mining, AI training, and similar technologies.

pmr.theclinics.com

Abbreviations	
ADL	activity of daily living
IEP	Individualized Education Plan
IUD	intrauterine device
POTS	postural orthostatic tachycardia syndrome
STI	sexually transmitted disease
US MEC	United States Medical Eligibility Criteria for Contraceptive Use
VTE	venous thromboembolism

experienced as their nondisabled counterparts,[3] and people with disabilities often report wanting to learn more about sexual health.[4–6] Therefore, we should be providing adequate, appropriate, and disability specific sexual health education and health care.

DISPARITIES IN SEXUAL HEALTH EDUCATION

Sexual development spans the entire lifespan from infancy, childhood, adolescence, adulthood, and beyond. Arguably, one's exposure to sexual health education, or lack thereof, is the foundation upon which an individual's sexuality, identity, and relationships are built. It is impossible to make informed decisions about your body, health, relationships, and behaviors without access to comprehensive sexual health education. Unfortunately, individuals with disabilities or medical complexities do not have access to the same resources as their counterparts in the general population when it comes to sexual health education, despite the fact that many people with disabilities are sexually active.[3] The most common places adolescents are learning about sexual health include school-based sexual health education programs, medical providers, parents or guardians, friends, and media. However, it seems that many of these resources do not provide adequate, appropriate, or disability-specific information. Most importantly, people with disabilities are interested in learning more about sexual health and report the need for more disability-specific sexual health education.[4–6]

School-based sexual health education programs can be a great resource if they are comprehensive in nature. Unfortunately, the quality of the information taught in school-based programs varies significantly based on state laws and regulations.[7] In addition, most school-based programs provide sexual health education as it pertains to the majority of students and often does not address disability-specific topics, adjust the delivery of the topics for those with intellectual disability, or have representation of individuals with disabilities in the material. Individuals with disabilities are less likely to receive school-based sexual health education, and their teachers are less likely to deem it beneficial or appropriate.[8] Depending on the state, opt-in or opt-out policies may preclude individuals with disabilities from participating in sexual health classes if a guardian or teacher does not deem it pertinent or appropriate. They also may not be in the classroom during sexual health education classes depending on the specifications of their Individualized Education Plan (IEP). Finally, most people who are teaching sexual health education are not trained to do so and therefore, do not feel comfortable with the topic of sexual health, let alone adapting the curriculum for their students with disabilities.

Medical providers can also be a great source of sexual health information for their patients, but this is often not the case for individuals with disabilities. In a study published in the Journal of Pediatric Rehabilitation Medicine in 2019, primary care providers were less likely to adhere to sexual health guidelines for their patients with disabilities compared to the general population.[9] Specifically, they were less likely to document a sexual history, less likely to document a pregnancy history, less likely to document menstrual history, and less likely to screen for human immunodeficiency virus in patients with disabilities compared to their matched counterparts. Medical providers often state that they do not feel that they have adequate training, do not have time, and do not feel comfortable discussing sexual health with people with disabilities.[5] Patients also report issues with being perceived as asexual or infantilized, finding accurate and appropriate information, lack of accessibility of the examination room, and clinician discomfort with discussing sexual health.[5,10]

THE PHYSIATRIST'S ROLE IN SEXUAL HEALTH

Arguably, every medical professional should be discussing sexual health with their patients as it pertains to their specialty. Physiatrists are experts in maximizing patients' independence in ADLs and functional mobility, with the goal of improving overall quality-of-life. As an ADL, sexual health should be a part of any holistic approach to a patient's health and well-being. As noted earlier, many primary care providers and other subspecialists are not discussing sexual health with their patients with disabilities for a myriad of reasons, but often it is because they simply do not feel knowledgeable about or comfortable with their disability. As disability experts, physiatrists can provide a unique perspective when it comes to the sexual health of their patients and can advocate for their patients to receive the information and health care that they deserve. Therefore, physiatrists should be addressing sexual health as a routine part of each visit or inpatient rehabilitation course.

PUBERTY

Puberty, and the emotional and physical changes that accompany it, can be stressful for adolescents and their caregivers especially when they are not given proper anticipatory guidance.[11] Caregivers of people with disabilities report significant anxiety surrounding puberty and menarche.[6,12] Due to the inaccurate infantilization of people with disabilities, the initiation of a process that signals that one's body is ready to reproduce can be disconcerting for caregivers. This, along with concerns about hygiene, additional caregiver burden, and menstrual symptoms can add to the caregivers' distress.[6] On the other hand, adolescents with disabilities may be more concerned with sexuality, body image, and the social impact of menarche. A qualitative study performed by Gray and colleagues showed that there is marked variation in parental perception of the significance of puberty for their daughters with cerebral palsy.[6] Due to the wide variety of concerns held by adolescents with disabilities and their caregivers, it is essential that an open line of communication is started early between providers, adolescents, and their caregivers surrounding puberty and menstruation. This is especially important for adolescents with intellectual disability who would benefit from early and repeated education surrounding the changes that will happen to their body.

MENARCHE AND MENSES

The median age of menarche in the general population in the United States is around 12 to 13 years of age.[13,14] Some females with disabilities are at risk of precocious or delayed adrenarche, pubarche, or menarche. For example, individuals with Spina Bifida and hydrocephalus,[15] Down Syndrome,[16] and Fragile X,[17] acquired brain injury, and neurodevelopmental disabilities[18] tend to experience puberty precociously, whereas individuals with autism spectrum disorder,[19] Noonan syndrome,[20] cerebral palsy,[21] Rhett Syndrome,[22] or disabilities that may affect their ability to receive proper nutrition may experience delayed completion of puberty.[23] In addition to the disability specific physiology affecting the timing of puberty, menstrual cycle regularity can be affected by commonly used medications including antiepileptic drugs,[24] dopaminergic agents,[25] and antipsychotics.[24] Therefore, prior to the initiation of menarche, it is important for providers, patients, and caregivers to discuss the possible effects of their diagnoses and medications on the initiation and regularity of their menstrual cycles. It is also important to provide anticipatory guidance to patients and families regarding menstrual management and hygiene at home and in the community. Starting discussions early allows for the creation of a patient-centered management plan that promotes patient independence.

In addition to variations in timing of puberty, individuals with disabilities may have differences in symptoms associated with the timing of menses including worsening seizures, behavioral problems, increased tone, migraines or headaches, and iron-deficiency anemia. These symptoms can worsen around the time of menarche and some patients continue to have cyclical increases in symptoms around the time of their menses. Patients who experience these types of fluctuations in symptoms may benefit from menstrual manipulation or improved medical management of symptoms around menses.

IRON DEFICIENCY

As mentioned earlier, iron deficiency is a common complication of menses and is the most common micronutrient deficiency worldwide.[26] Iron deficiency is underdiagnosed in adolescents, causes a plethora of symptoms, increases the risk of pregnancy and peripartum complications, and may cause potentially irreversible neurologic changes to the developing fetus. Symptoms of iron deficiency, including fatigue, dizziness, and headache[27,28] can be present without anemia and are common in adolescents with disabilities. Patients with chronic migraine have significantly lower hemoglobin and serum ferritin levels compared to controls and their symptoms improve with iron repletion.[29,30] In addition, many symptoms of the post-concussion syndrome and postural orthostatic tachycardia syndrome (POTS) overlap with the symptoms of iron deficiency. One of the diagnostic criteria of POTS includes ruling out other causes of sinus tachycardia such as anemia, and low iron storage has been found to be more frequent in adolescents with POTS compared to the general population. However, it is unclear whether low iron storage is a consequence, cause, or exacerbating factor in POTS.[31] Treatment for POTS is focused on symptomatic treatment, which includes treating iron deficiency.[32]

Due to improvements in symptom burden with treatment, all menstruating people, including those with disabilities, should be screened for iron deficiency.[33] Unfortunately, the current threshold of ferritin concentration to assess iron status (<15 μg/L) is likely too low, with symptoms arising in many patients prior to ferritin values dropping to these levels.[34,35] Thus, higher thresholds have been proposed,[36–38] and it is reasonable to consider treatment of any symptomatic patient with ferritin less than 75 to 100 μg/L.[39] If identified, the underlying cause of iron deficiency should be investigated and treated. Initial treatment includes dietary and oral iron supplementation, though some patients may benefit from intravenous iron formulations due to poor oral supplementation tolerance or the need for rapid repletion.[33,40]

MENSTRUAL SUPPRESSION

Many individuals with disabilities and their caregivers opt to pursue menstrual suppression to help alleviate the symptoms associated with menses, improve hygiene, or increase independence. Menstrual suppression refers to the use of an intervention, often medications and devices, to decrease the frequency or intensity of menses. Menstrual suppression can be initiated after menarche, but is not recommended prior.[41] While complete amenorrhea is often desired by patients and caregivers, it is very difficult to achieve, and expectations should be managed appropriately.[42] The goal of menstrual suppression should always be to use the lowest-risk, reversible method while maximizing patient autonomy.[43] While there are many options for menstrual suppression, care must be taken to choose the appropriate method that aligns with the patient and caregiver's goals while minimizing risk factors and adverse events (**Table 1**).

The first thing a provider should do prior to discussing the available options for menstrual suppression with a patient and their caregivers is check the US Medical Eligibility Criteria for Contraceptive Use (US MEC). The US MEC provides evidence-based guidance on contraceptive selection taking different comorbidities and medical conditions into account.[44] In addition, the American Academy of Pediatrics released guidelines for the menstrual management for adolescents with disabilities in 2016, which serves as a great source of disability specific considerations for menstrual suppression and management.[45] If a provider is unsure of the most appropriate methods of menstrual suppression for their patient, it is recommended to confer with someone who specializes in Adolescent Medicine or Gynecology.

Additional considerations when choosing a menstrual suppression method for a patient with a physical disability includes venous thromboembolism (VTE) risk, dexterity, weight, and bone health. Prior to choosing a method for a patient with a physical disability, their functional mobility should be fully assessed. Patients with upper extremity weakness, tone, or contractures may have difficulty self-administering pills, placing a patch or vaginal ring, or checking the strings of an intrauterine device (IUD). Similarly, someone with lower extremity weakness, tone, or contractures may have difficulty with the positioning necessary to place a vaginal ring or check IUD strings. The use of estrogen-containing methods for patients with decreased mobility is controversial because estrogen-containing methods can increase the risk of VTE. However, the US MEC does not list physical disability or wheelchair use as a contraindication to estrogen-containing contraceptives. Estrogen-containing methods should be avoided in individuals with any additional risk factors for VTE including personal or family history of clot, smoking, obesity, age greater than 35, or being within 3 months of traumatic spinal cord injury. Additionally, patients with significant weakness often have decreased bone mineral density at baseline. Studies have shown that the Depo Medroxyprogesterone Acetate shot can decrease bone density when used long-term. This decrease in bone density resolves with discontinuation of the medication.[46] However, it is unknown whether or not this has a significant effect on bone density or fracture risk for patients with physical disabilities. Finally, the unwanted side effect of weight gain with the use of hormonal methods is controversial with inconclusive evidence.[43] However, the potential of even a small increase in weight should not be ignored as it can significantly affect a patient's ability to transfer, reposition, or perform ADLs, which can be detrimental to their independence.

Individuals with intellectual disability can also benefit from menstrual suppression but present a unique set of ethical and legal considerations when a caregiver is making medical decisions for them. It is important that the decisions be made in the best interest of the patient and not solely for caregiver convenience. It is vital to ensure that the patient is included in all discussions and is provided developmentally-appropriate education. This patient population may also benefit from placement of IUDs or implants under sedation. In a prospective cohort study done by Buyers and colleagues,

Table 1
Comparison of menstrual suppression methods

Method	Dosing Schedule	Hormones Utilized	Effect on Menstruation	Effect on Fertility (% of Females Who Experienced Unintended Pregnancy Within First y of Typical Use)[67]	Considerations for Individuals with Disability	Considerations for Patients with Seizure Disorders
Combined oral contraceptives	Daily	Estrogen and progestin	Can use continuously or for extended cycling	9%	• Can have break through bleeding if not taken continuously • Can use chewable pills or crush pills if patient is unable to swallow pills safely	Not recommended for use when taking cytochrome p450 inducing AEDs
Progestin only oral contraceptives	Daily	Progestin	Can cause irregular bleeding		• Can have break through bleeding if not taken continuously • Can use chewable pills or crush pills if patient is unable to swallow pills safely	Not recommended for use when taking cytochrome p450 inducing AEDs
GnRH agonists	Daily to every 3 mo (formulation dependent)	Gonadotropin releasing hormone agonists	Can cause increased bleeding initially but eventually result in suppression		• Can cause decreased bone density • Can cause menopausal symptoms	

Patch	Weekly	Estrogen and progestin	Can use continuously or for extended cycling	9%	• Can be difficult to place for people with poor dexterity • For patients with ID, should place the patch in an area that is difficult for the patient to reach • Can cause skin irritation	Not recommended for use when taking cytochrome p450 inducing AEDs
Vaginal ring	Monthly	Estrogen and progestin	Breakthrough bleeding	9%	• Can be difficult to place for people with poor dexterity or lower extremity tone • Very invasive to have placed by someone else	Not recommended for use when taking cytochrome p450 inducing AEDs
Implant	5 y	Progestin	Breakthrough bleeding	0.05%	Pain and discomfort of insertion	
Shot (DMPA)	3 mo	Progestin	Can have breakthrough bleeding but risk decreases the longer you use this method.	6%	• Can cause weight gain • Can cause decreased bone density	May need to increase frequency of dosing to every 10 w[51]
LNG-IUD	Up to 8 y depending on type	Progestin	Breakthrough bleeding	0.2%	• For patients with ID, may need to be placed under sedation	

(continued on next page)

Table 1
(continued)

Method	Dosing Schedule	Hormones Utilized	Effect on Menstruation	Effect on Fertility (% of Females Who Experienced Unintended Pregnancy Within First y of Typical Use)[67]	Considerations for Individuals with Disability	Considerations for Patients with Seizure Disorders
					• For patients with significant tone or contractures positioning for placement may be difficult • Patients with poor dexterity may have difficulty checking strings	
Copper IUD	Up to 12 y	Copper		0.8%	• For patients with ID, may need to be placed under sedation • For patients with significant tone or contractures positioning for placement may be difficult • Patients with poor dexterity may have difficulty checking strings	

NSAIDs	Every 6 h during menses	None	Does not have significant effect on bleeding	No known effect on fertility	• Does not cause amenorrhea • Need to consider renal health • Can help with pain associated with menstruation	Unethical
Surgical methods (Sterilization or endometrial ablation)	Permanent	None	Amenorrhea	0.5% with sterilization	Unethical	Unethical

the most common method of menstrual suppression chosen by patients and their caregivers with developmental disabilities was the levonorgestrel intrauterine device, and all of these were placed under anesthesia at their institution.[47] If the patch is being considered for a patient with intellectual disability, appropriate placement should be thought about if the patient is at high risk of picking at or removing the patch. In these cases, it should be placed in an area that is difficult to reach. Finally, due to the invasive and uncomfortable nature of having a caregiver place the vaginal ring, it should only be utilized in this population if the patient is able to consistently and successfully place it themselves.

Considering many people with disabilities are sexually active, it is important to address the role that the methods used for menstrual suppression also play in contraception. Providers should discuss the risk of pregnancy with each method, as well as the importance of the use of condoms and other barriers for prevention of sexually transmitted diseases (STIs).

SEXUALITY AND GENDER IDENTITY

Exploring sexuality and gender identity is a normal part of adolescence. In a study by Cheng and colleagues, people with disabilities were as sexually experienced as their peers, and those classified as having severe disability were more likely to report being unsure about their sexual preference and reported less romantic attraction to the opposite sex. Those with mild disabilities had a higher tendency for same-sex attraction than their nondisabled peers.[3] Additionally, gender-dysphoric or gender-incongruent individuals are nearly twice as likely to report having a disability than as their cisgender peers, and transgender people with disabilities have more general unmet health needs than their cisgender counterparts.[44,45] One additional unmet health need unique to this population is gender affirming care for which interested parties can be referred to an endocrinologist.[46]

PREVENTATIVE HEALTHCARE

Patients with disabilities should receive the same preventative health care as their peers as described by the US Preventive Services Task Force.[18] Despite this guideline, individuals with disabilities are less likely to receive pap smears,[49–51] breast examinations[52](although outdated), mammograms,[49] human papilloma virus (HPV) vaccination,[53] and routine STI testing.[9] Physiatrists should advocate for their patients to receive the recommended preventive care interventions.

SEXUAL ACTIVITY

Despite having the potential for a very satisfying sex life, many people with disabilities report dissatisfaction with their sexual function and encounters,[5,54,55] reporting limitations due to bowel/bladder incontinence, pain, libido, vaginal lubrication, bone health, fatigue, tone, and range-of-motion. The unique knowledge and skill set of physiatrists makes us particularly suited to guide patients with disabilities to achieve a satisfying sexual experience. A thorough musculoskeletal and neurologic examination can help identify insensate areas and regions at risk for injury (dislocation, fracture, skin breakdown, etc.). Many of the principles in the Consortium for Spinal Cord Medicine's Clinical Practice Guideline for Sexuality and Reproductive Health can be adapted for a range of other conditions seen by physiatrists.[56]

Recommendations for people with disabilities to optimize their sexual experience include but are not limited to:

- Encourage them to explore their body using mirrors to see parts of the body that are difficult to see, touching every part of their body to see what feels good including using different pressures, vibrations, or textured materials.
- Environmental modifications can help to enhance sexual experience by stimulating all the senses, such as music, temperature, mirrors, lighting, images in movies or books, or arousing smells or tastes.
- Trial different strategies for fatigue management.
- If having partnered sex, encourage open communication with their partner regarding all aspects of the sexual encounter.
- Explore different positions, including the use of props or furniture, to maximize comfort and mobility. Partners or caregivers may need to assist with safe and comfortable positioning, and if wheelchairs or other adaptive equipment is being used all should be aware of the safety and weight limitations.
- People with sensory deficits should be educated on the risk of injury with certain positions or with certain devices, lubricants, or oils. Insensate skin surfaces are at risk for injury and thus, should be carefully examined after sexual activity.
- Bladder and bowel care prior to sexual activity can decrease risk of incontinence, but it is recommended to also have a contingency plan in case it does occur.[56]
- Stimulation of erogenous zones other than genitals (ear, neck, wrist, nipple, thigh, lips, fingers, foot, etc.) can be helpful for people with mobility limitations, sensory deficits, or both. Some people can achieve orgasm with stimulation of these zones in the absence of penetration.[57] People with sensory deficits may report the transitional zone between where they are sensate and insensate as an erogenous zone.

PREGNANCY AND FERTILITY

The majority of females with physical disability have normal fertility and many desire pregnancy and parenthood.[54] People with disabilities who are thinking of becoming pregnant should meet early with an obstetrician for preconception counseling and often benefit from referral to a high-risk obstetrician. Some individuals may require prenatal interventions, evaluation of uterine or vaginal anatomy, or higher levels of prenatal supplementation. For example, females with Spina Bifida require a higher level of folic acid supplementation than the general population prior to conception and during pregnancy. Depending on diagnosis people may experience a myriad of complications during pregnancy and delivery including autonomic dysreflexia, worsening seizures, changes in tone, increased number of urinary tract infections, intensive care unit admissions, exacerbation of constipation, skin injury such as pressure injuries, worsening respiratory function, ventriculoperitoneal (VP) shunt malfunction, difficulties with prior surgical continence procedure sites, pelvic organ prolapse, higher rates of cesarean sections, and fetal complications.[58–61] People with mobility disabilities may be significantly impacted by the change in distribution of weight and may experience more falls or significant changes in function. People with Cerebral Palsy report not receiving appropriate referrals to physical and occupational therapy despite experiencing loss of mobility during pregnancy.[59] Despite the relative increased risk of pregnancy and delivery for individuals with disabilities, many individuals safely and effectively reproduce, and all people who desire pregnancy should be encouraged to meet with an obstetrician.

SEXUAL ABUSE

It is well-documented that people with disabilities are at much higher risk of sexual abuse than the general population,[62–66] and in reality the number of abused individuals is probably much larger than reported. To reduce the risk of sexual abuse, it is important that individuals receive appropriate sexual health education, consent, and are empowered to be in control of their own bodies. Without being able to name body parts appropriately, understand sexual acts, or differentiate between appropriate and inappropriate touch, it is difficult to communicate with others regarding inappropriate or uncomfortable situations. This is particularly crucial for people with intellectual disability, or those with childhood onset disability who are constantly being examined by physicians, having diapers changed by caregivers, and having their bodies manipulated by therapists throughout their lifespan. It is also important to discuss capacity and consent with patients and their caregivers, and to remind caregivers that having capacity does not mean someone will make good decisions. Finally, one of the easiest interventions a provider can implement is to allow each adolescent or young adult time to speak with the provider alone without a caregiver present. This not only empowers the individual to take a more active role in their health care, but it also provides the space for them to discuss topics they may not want to discuss with their caregiver present, including reporting mistreatment.

In conclusion, patients with disabilities are sexually active, fertile, less likely to receive preventative health care, at risk for sexual abuse, and want to learn more about sexual health. It is irresponsible to care for any patient of reproductive age without discussing general sexual health education including sexuality, gender, puberty, pregnancy, sexuality, STIs, HPV vaccination, papanicolaou (PAP) smears, sexual abuse, and so forth. As physicians with general medicine training and an expertise in caring for people with disabilities, physiatrists are uniquely qualified to address sexual health with their patients.

SUMMARY

As experts in the care of people with disability, physiatrists are well-equipped to address reproductive and sexual health needs for female adolescents with disability. We recommend that any physiatrist caring for this population discuss these topics with patients and their caregivers. Even if we do not have all the answers, having these discussions gives us a more comprehensive assessment of our patient's functioning in their everyday life and is greatly appreciated by patients and their caregivers.

CLINICS CARE POINTS

- Education and anticipatory guidance regarding puberty and menstruation is important for female adolescents with disability.
- Physiatrists should screen for iron deficiency in female adolescents presenting with fatigue, dizziness, sleep dysfunction, and headaches.
- There are many options for menstrual suppression, physiatrists should be aware of the risks and benefits of these options for females with disability.
- The majority of females with disability have normal fertility; however, certain conditions carry specific risks that may need special attention or monitoring.
- Sexual health and safety are important for females with disability. Conversations regarding safe sexual practices and sexual abuse should start before adolescence with both patient and caregivers.

DISCLOSURES

The authors have nothing to disclose.

REFERENCES

1. Organization WH. Defining sexual health. Report of a technical consultation on sexual health 2002;28:31.
2. Esmail S, Darry K, Walter A, et al. Attitudes and perceptions towards disability and sexuality. Disabil Rehabil 2010;32(14):1148–55.
3. Cheng MM, Udry JR. Sexual behaviors of physically disabled adolescents in the United States. J Adolesc Health 2002;31(1):48–58.
4. Cho S-R, Park ES, Park CI, et al. Characteristics of psychosexual functioning in adults with cerebral palsy. Clin Rehabil 2004;18(4):423–9.
5. Streur CS, Schafer CL, Garcia VP, et al. "If everyone else is having this talk with their doctor, why am I not having this talk with mine?": the experiences of sexuality and sexual health education of young women with spina bifida. J Sex Med 2019; 16(6):853–9.
6. Gray SH, Wylie M, Christensen S, et al. Puberty and menarche in young females with cerebral palsy and intellectual disability: a qualitative study of caregivers' experiences. Dev Med Child Neurol 2021;63(2):190–5.
7. SIECUS. State profiles. Available at: https://siecus.org/state-profiles/. Accessed June 3, 2024.
8. Barnard-Brak L, Schmidt M, Chesnut S, et al. Predictors of access to sex education for children with intellectual disabilities in public schools. Ment Retard 2014; 52(2):85–97.
9. Roden RC, Oholendt K, Lange H, et al. Primary care provider adherence to reproductive healthcare guidelines in adolescents and young adults with disabilities: a retrospective matched cohort study. J Pediatr Rehabil Med 2019;12:317–24.
10. Gray SH, Byrne R, Christensen S, et al. Women with cerebral palsy: a qualitative study about their experiences with sexual and reproductive health education and services. J Pediatr Rehabil Med 2021;14(2):285–93.
11. Streur CS, Kreschmer JM, Ernst SD, et al. "They had the lunch lady coming up to assist": the experiences of menarche and menstrual management for adolescents with physical disabilities. Disabil Health J 2023;16(4):101510.
12. Zacharin M, Savasi I, Grover S. The impact of menstruation in adolescents with disabilities related to cerebral palsy. Arch Dis Child 2010;95(7):526–30.
13. Diaz A, Laufer MR, Breech LL. Menstruation in girls and adolescents: using the menstrual cycle as a vital sign. Pediatrics 2006;118(5):2245–50.
14. Martinez GM. Trends and patterns in menarche in the United States: 1995 through 2013-2017. Natl Health Stat Report 2020;146:1–12.
15. Dahl M, Proos LA, Arnell K, et al. Swedish cohort study found that half of the girls with shunted hydrocephalus had precocious or early puberty. Acta Paediatr 2024;113(4):827–32.
16. Erdoğan F, Güven A. Is there a secular trend regarding puberty in children with down syndrome? Front Endocrinol 2022;13:1001985.
17. McLay L, Carnett A, Tyler-Merrick G, et al. A systematic review of interventions for inappropriate sexual behavior of children and adolescents with developmental disabilities. Review Journal of Autism and Developmental Disorders 2015/12/01 2015;2(4):357–73.
18. Siddiqi SU, Van Dyke DC, Donohoue P, et al. Premature sexual development in individuals with neurodevelopmental disabilities. Dev Med Child Neurol 1999; 41(6):392–5.
19. Knickmeyer RC, Wheelwright S, Hoekstra R, et al. Age of menarche in females with autism spectrum conditions. Dev Med Child Neurol 2006;48(12):1007–8.

20. Patti G, Scaglione M, Maiorano NG, et al. Abnormalities of pubertal development and gonadal function in Noonan syndrome. Front Endocrinol 2023;14:1213098.
21. Worley G, Houlihan CM, Herman-Giddens ME, et al. Secondary sexual characteristics in children with cerebral palsy and moderate to severe motor impairment: a cross-sectional survey. Pediatrics 2002;110(5):897–902.
22. Killian JT, Lane JB, Cutter GR, et al. Pubertal development in Rett syndrome deviates from typical females. Pediatr Neurol 2014;51(6):769–75.
23. Zacharin M. Endocrine problems in children and adolescents who have disabilities. Horm Res Paediatr 2013;80(4):221–8.
24. Joffe H, Hayes FJ. Menstrual cycle dysfunction associated with neurologic and psychiatric disorders: their treatment in adolescents. Ann N Y Acad Sci 2008; 1135:219–29.
25. Kinon BJ, Gilmore JA, Liu H, et al. Hyperprolactinemia in response to antipsychotic drugs: characterization across comparative clinical trials. Psychoneuroendocrinology 2003;28(Suppl 2):69–82.
26. World Health Organization. Haemoglobin concentrations for the diagnosis of anaemia and assessment of severity (No. WHO/NMH/NHD/MNM/11.1). 2011, World Health Organization.
27. Ghazzay H, Jasim A, Shukur A. Mahasinaltaha. Low ferritin with normal hemoglobin, a common neglected and hidden hematological disorder. Ann Trop Med Publ Health 2021;24:242–50.
28. National Collaborating Centre for Women's and Children's Health (UK). Heavy Menstrual Bleeding. London: RCOG Press; 2007.
29. Saleem MI, Haqnawaz K, Jadoon SB, et al. Association between iron deficiency anemia and chronic daily headache. Journal of Health and Rehabilitation Research 2023;3(2):676–81.
30. Casazza K, Swanson E. Nutrition as medicine to improve outcomes in adolescents sustaining a sports-related concussion. Exploratory Research and Hypothesis in Medicine 2017;2:1–9.
31. Jarjour IT, Jarjour LK. Low iron storage and mild anemia in postural tachycardia syndrome in adolescents. Clin Auton Res 2013;23(4):175–9.
32. Fedorowski A. Postural orthostatic tachycardia syndrome: clinical presentation, aetiology and management. J Intern Med 2019;285(4):352–66.
33. Munro MG. Heavy menstrual bleeding, iron deficiency, and iron deficiency anemia: framing the issue. Int J Gynaecol Obstet 2023;162(Suppl 2):7–13.
34. World Health Organization. WHO guideline on use of ferritin concentrations to assess iron status in populations. Geneva: World Health Organization; 2020.
35. Sezgin G, Loh T, Markus C. Functional reference limits: a case study of serum ferritin. J Lab Med 2021;45:69–77.
36. Mei Z, Addo OY, Jefferds ME, et al. Physiologically based serum ferritin thresholds for iron deficiency in children and non-pregnant women: a US National Health and Nutrition Examination Surveys (NHANES) serial cross-sectional study. Lancet Haematol 2021;8(8):e572–82.
37. Al-Jafar H. Treatment of serum ferritin deficiency regardless haemoglobin level. Blood 2012;120:5166.
38. Soppi ET. Iron deficiency without anemia - a clinical challenge. Clin Case Rep 2018;6(6):1082–6.
39. Al-Naseem A, Sallam A, Choudhury S, et al. Iron deficiency without anaemia: a diagnosis that matters. Clin Med 2021;21(2):107–13.
40. Stoffel NU, Cercamondi CI, Brittenham G, et al. Iron absorption from oral iron supplements given on consecutive versus alternate days and as single morning

doses versus twice-daily split dosing in iron-depleted women: two open-label, randomised controlled trials. Lancet Haematol 2017;4(11):e524–33.

41. Committee opinion No. 668: menstrual manipulation for adolescents with physical and developmental disabilities. Obstet Gynecol 2016;128(2):e20–5.

42. Dural Ö, Taş İS, Akhan SE. Management of menstrual and gynecologic concerns in girls with special needs. J Clin Res Pediatr Endocrinol 2020;12(Suppl 1):41–5.

43. Gallo MF, Lopez LM, Grimes DA, et al. Combination contraceptives: effects on weight. Cochrane Database Syst Rev 2014;2014(1):Cd003987.

44. Smith-Johnson M. Transgender adults have higher rates of disability than their cisgender counterparts: study examines rates of disability among transgender adults and cisgender adults. Health Aff 2022;41(10):1470–6.

45. Mulcahy A, Streed CG Jr, Wallisch AM, et al. Gender identity, disability, and unmet healthcare needs among disabled people living in the community in the United States. Int J Environ Res Publ Health 2022;19(5).

46. Hembree WC, Cohen-Kettenis PT, Gooren L, et al. Endocrine treatment of gender-dysphoric/gender-incongruent persons: an endocrine society clinical practice guideline. J Clin Endocrinol Metabol 2017;102(11):3869–903.

47. Buyers EM, Hutchens KJ, Kaizer A, et al. Caregiver goals and satisfaction for menstrual suppression in adolescent females with developmental disabilities: a prospective cohort study. Disability and Health Journal 2023;16(4):101484.

48. USPSTF. Published guidelines. Available at: https://www.uspreventiveservicestaskforce. org/uspstf/topic_search_results?topic_status=P. Accessed May 22, 2024.

49. Jackson AB, Mott PK. Reproductive health care for women with spina bifida. Sci World J 2007;7:1875–83.

50. Baruch L, Bilitzky-Kopit A, Rosen K, et al. Cervical cancer screening among patients with physical disability. J Wom Health 2022;31(8):1173–8.

51. Orji AF, Gimm G, Desai A, et al. The association of cervical cancer screening with disability type among US women (aged 25–64 Years). Am J Prev Med 2024;66(1): 83–93.

52. Nosek MA, Howland CA. Breast and cervical cancer screening among women with physical disabilities. Arch Phys Med Rehabil 1997;78(12 Suppl 5):S39–44.

53. O'Neill J, Newall F, Antolovich G, et al. Vaccination in people with disability: a review. Hum Vaccines Immunother 2020;16(1):7–15.

54. Lee NG, Andrews E, Rosoklija I, et al. The effect of spinal cord level on sexual function in the spina bifida population. J Pediatr Urol 2015;11(3):142. e1–e142. e6.

55. McCabe MP, Taleporos G. Sexual esteem, sexual satisfaction, and sexual behavior among people with physical disability. Arch Sex Behav 2003;32(4): 359–69.

56. Sexuality and reproductive health in adults with spinal cord injury: a clinical practice guideline for health-care professionals. J Spinal Cord Med 2010;33(3): 281–336.

57. Younis I, Fattah M, Maamoun M. Female hot spots: extragenital erogenous zones. Human Andrology 2016;6(1):20–6.

58. Auger N, Arbour L, Schnitzer ME, et al. Pregnancy outcomes of women with spina bifida. Disabil Rehabil 2019;41(12):1403–9.

59. Hayward K, Chen AY, Forbes E, et al. Reproductive healthcare experiences of women with cerebral palsy. Disability and Health Journal 2017;10(3):413–8.

60. Shah S, Taylor J, Bradbury-Jones C. Access to and utilisation of sexual and reproductive healthcare for women and girls with cerebral palsy: a scoping review. Disabil Soc 2024;39(1):105–25.

61. Abati E, Corti S. Pregnancy outcomes in women with spinal muscular atrophy: a review. J Neurol Sci 2018;388:50–60.
62. Jemtå L, Fugl-Meyer KS, Oberg K. On intimacy, sexual activities and exposure to sexual abuse among children and adolescents with mobility impairment. Acta Paediatr 2008;97(5):641–6.
63. Findley PA, Plummer SB, McMahon S. Exploring the experiences of abuse of college students with disabilities. J Interpers Violence 2016;31(17):2801–23.
64. Suris J-C, Resnick MD, Cassuto N, et al. Sexual behavior of adolescents with chronic disease and disability. J Adolesc Health 1996;19(2):124–31.
65. Mitra M, Mouradian VE, McKenna M. Dating violence and associated health risks among high school students with disabilities. Matern Child Health J 2013;17: 1088–94.
66. Wissink IB, Van Vugt E, Moonen X, et al. Sexual abuse involving children with an intellectual disability (ID): a narrative review. Res Dev Disabil 2015;36:20–35.
67. Trussell J. Contraceptive failure in the United States. Contraception 2011;83(5): 397–404.

www.ingramcontent.com/pod-product-compliance
Lightning Source LLC
Chambersburg PA
CBHW050458190326
41458CB00005B/1331